FIRST AID FOR THE®
USMLE STEP 2 CS

Fifth Edition

TAO LE, MD, MHS
Associate Clinical Professor of Medicine and Pediatrics
Chief, Section of Allergy and Immunology
Department of Medicine
University of Louisville

VIKAS BHUSHAN, MD
Diagnostic Radiologist

MAE SHEIKH-ALI, MD
Associate Professor of Medicine
Associate Program Director, Endocrinology Fellowship Program
Division of Endocrinology, Diabetes and Metabolism
University of Florida College of Medicine–Jacksonville

KACHIU CECILIA LEE, MD, MPH
Clinical and Research Fellow
Wellman Center for Photomedicine
Department of Dermatology
Massachusetts General Hospital, Harvard Medical School

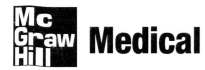

New York / Chicago / San Francisco / Lisbon / London / Madrid / Mexico City
Milan / New Delhi / San Juan / Seoul / Singapore / Sydney / Toronto

First Aid for the® USMLE Step 2 CS, Fifth Edition

Copyright © 2014, 2012, 2010, 2007, 2004 by Tao Le. All rights reserved. Printed in the United States of America. Except as permitted under the United States Copyright Act of 1976, no part of this publication may be reproduced or distributed in any form or by any means, or stored in a data base or retrieval system, without the prior written permission of the publisher.

First Aid for the® is a registered trademark of McGraw-Hill Education.

3 4 5 6 7 8 9 0   DOW/DOW   20 19 18 17 16 15

ISBN 978-0-07-180426-4
MHID 0-07-180426-9
ISSN 1930-5354

This book was set in Goudy Old Style by Rainbow Graphics.
The editors were Catherine A. Johnson and Peter J. Boyle.
Project management was provided by Rainbow Graphics.
The production supervisor was Jeffrey Herzich.
The designer was Mary McKeon.
RR Donnelley was printer and binder.

This book is printed on acid-free paper.

McGraw-Hill Education books are available at special quantity discounts to use as premiums and sales promotions, or for use in corporate training programs. To contact a representative please visit the Contact Us pages at www.mhprofessional.com.

DEDICATION

To the contributors of this and past editions, who took time to share their experience, advice, and humor for the benefit of future physicians.

and

To our families, friends, and loved ones, who supported us in the task of assembling this guide.

CONTENTS

SECTION 5   TOP-RATED REVIEW RESOURCES   541

CONTRIBUTING AUTHORS

Raeda Alshantti, MD
Hospitalist, Alshifa Hospital
University of Damascus School of Medicine

Melissa Marie Cranford, MD
Resident, Department of Psychiatry
Yale-New Haven Hospital

Kevin Day, MD
Resident, Department of Medical Imaging
University of Arizona Medical Center

Michael King, MD
Resident, Department of Anesthesiology
Massachusetts General Hospital

Jasmine Rassiwala, MD, MPH
Resident, Department of Internal Medicine
University of California, San Francisco

Ruba Sheikh-Ali, MD
Clinical Researcher
University of Florida College of Medicine–Jacksonville

Jody Tversky, MD
Assistant Professor
Clinical Director
Division of Allergy and Clinical Immunology
Johns Hopkins University School of Medicine

Jinyu (Jane) Zhang, MD
Resident, Department of Internal Medicine
Thomas Jefferson University

ASSOCIATE CONTRIBUTING AUTHOR

Mohammad Samer Agha, MD
Internal Medicine Consultant
Clinical Director, Internal Medicine
Al-Kalamoon University, Damascus

FACULTY REVIEWERS

Kelly A. Best, MD, FACOG
Associate Professor, Division of General Obstetrics and Gynecology
Department of Obstetrics and Gynecology
University of Florida College of Medicine–Jacksonville

Arkadiy Finn, MD
Clinical Instructor
Department of Medicine
Warren Alpert Medical School, Brown University

Nilmarie Guzman, MD
Assistant Professor, Division of Infectious Disease
Department of Medicine
University of Florida College of Medicine–Jacksonville

Jeffrey G. House, DO
Associate Professor, Division of General Medicine
Department of Medicine
University of Florida College of Medicine–Jacksonville

Nizar F. Maraqa, MD
Assistant Professor, Division of Pediatric Infectious Diseases and Immunology
Department of Pediatrics
University of Florida College of Medicine–Jacksonville

Carlos Palacio, MD, MPH
Associate Professor, Division of General Internal Medicine
Department of Medicine
University of Florida College of Medicine–Jacksonville

Jigme M. Sethi, MD, FCCP
Associate Professor
Department of Medicine
Warren Alpert Medical School, Brown University
Chief, Pulmonary, Critical Care, and Sleep Medicine
Memorial Hospital of Rhode Island

The USMLE Step 2 CS can be a source of stress and anxiety, especially among international medical graduates (IMGs), who often find themselves at a disadvantage because of their non-U.S. training background. *First Aid for the USMLE Step 2 CS* is our "cure" for this exam. This book represents a virtual medicine bag of high-yield tools for students and IMGs, including:

- An updated exam preparation guide for the new USMLE Step 2 CS, including proven study and exam strategies for clinical encounters based on the patient-centered interview.

- Expanded guidelines on how to deal with challenging situations, including a range of situations that pose ethical and confidentiality issues.

- Detailed descriptions of high-yield physical exam maneuvers that will win you points without costing time.

- Forty-four full-length practice cases that allow you to simulate the actual Step 2 CS exam, updated to reflect recent exam changes that test your ability to document the patient's most likely diagnoses and how they are supported by the history and physical exam findings.

- A revised and expanded set of minicases representing common complaints designed to help you rapidly develop a working set of differential diagnoses.

This book would not have been possible without the suggestions and feedback of medical students, IMGs, and faculty members. We invite you to share your thoughts and ideas to help us improve *First Aid for the USMLE Step 2 CS*. See How to Contribute, p. xvii.

Louisville	Tao Le
Los Angeles	Vikas Bhushan
Jacksonville	Mae Sheikh-Ali
Boston	Kachiu Cecilia Lee

ACKNOWLEDGMENTS

This has been a collaborative effort from the start. We gratefully acknowledge the thoughtful comments, corrections, and advice of the many medical students, residents, international medical graduates, and faculty who have supported the authors in the continuing development of *First Aid for the USMLE Step 2 CS*.

For support and encouragement throughout the process, we are grateful to Thao Pham, Isabel Nogueira, Louise Petersen, and Jonathan Kirsch.

Thanks to our publisher, McGraw-Hill, for the valuable assistance of its staff. For enthusiasm, support, and commitment to the *First Aid* series, thanks to our editor, Catherine Johnson. For outstanding editorial work, we thank Andrea Fellows, our developmental editor. Finally, a special thanks to Rainbow Graphics, especially David Hommel, Tina Castle, and Susan Cooper, for remarkable editorial and production support.

Louisville	Tao Le
Los Angeles	Vikas Bhushan
Jacksonville	Mae Sheikh-Ali
Boston	Kachiu Cecilia Lee

HOW TO CONTRIBUTE

First Aid for the USMLE Step 2 CS incorporates many contributions from students and faculty. We invite you to participate in this process. Please send us:

- Study and test-taking strategies for the Step 2 CS exam
- High-yield case topics that may appear on future Step 2 CS exams
- Personal comments on review books that you have examined

For each entry incorporated into the next edition, you will receive up to a $20 Amazon.com gift certificate and a personal acknowledgment in the next edition. Significant contributions will be compensated at the discretion of the authors. The preferred way to submit entries, suggestions, or corrections is via our blog:

www.firstaidteam.com

Otherwise, you can e-mail us directly at:

firstaidteam@yahoo.com

Contributions sent earlier will receive priority consideration for the next edition of *First Aid for the USMLE Step 2 CS*.

NOTE TO CONTRIBUTORS

All entries are subject to editing and reviewing. Please verify all data and spellings carefully. In the event that similar or duplicate entries are received, only the first entry received will be used. Please follow the style, punctuation, and format of this edition as much as possible. All contributions become property of the authors.

INTERNSHIP OPPORTUNITIES

The author team of Le and Bhushan is pleased to offer part-time and full-time paid internships in medical education and publishing to motivated medical students and physicians. Internships may range from two to three months (eg, a summer) up to a full year. Participants will have an opportunity to author, edit, and earn academic credit on a wide variety of projects, including the popular *First Aid* series. Writing/editing experience, familiarity with Microsoft Word, and Internet access are required. For more information, e-mail a résumé or a short description of your experience along with a cover letter and writing sample to **firstaidteam@yahoo.com.**

Guide to the USMLE Step 2 CS

INTRODUCTION

As a prerequisite to entering residency training in the United States, all U.S. and Canadian medical students as well as international medical graduates (IMGs) are required to pass a clinical skills exam known as the United States Medical Licensing Examination (USMLE) Step 2 Clinical Skills (CS)—a test involving clinical encounters with "standardized patients."

Even if you are a pro at taking standardized exams such as the USMLE Step 1 and Step 2 Clinical Knowledge (CK), you may find it challenging to prepare for the USMLE Step 2 CS, which distinguishes itself from other USMLE exams by using live patient actors to simulate clinical encounters. Common mistakes medical students and IMGs make in preparing for the Step 2 CS include the following:

- Panicking because of the unfamiliar format of the test
- Not practicing enough with mock patient scenarios before taking the actual exam
- Not developing a logical plan of attack based on patient "doorway information"
- Failing to understand the required objectives for each patient encounter
- Managing time poorly during patient encounters
- Becoming flustered by challenging questions or situations
- Taking unfocused histories and physical exams
- Failing to understand how to interact with a patient appropriately
- Neglecting to carry out easy but required patient interactions

This book will guide you through the process of efficiently preparing for and taking the Step 2 CS with five organized sections:

- **Section 1** introduces you to the Step 2 CS.
- **Section 2** reviews critical high-yield steps to take during the patient encounter.
- **Section 3** provides high-yield minicases for common doorway chief complaints to help you rapidly develop focused differentials during the exam.
- **Section 4** offers full-length practice cases to help you simulate the real thing.
- **Section 5** rates other resources that help you prepare for the Step 2 CS.

USMLE STEP 2 CS—THE BASICS

Introduction

Like other USMLE exams, the USMLE Step 2 CS is sponsored by the National Board of Medical Examiners (NBME) and the Federation of State Medical Boards (FSMB). According to the USMLE Web site (www.usmle.org), "Step 2 of the USMLE assesses the ability of examinees to apply medical knowledge, skills, and understanding of clinical science essential for the provision of patient care under supervision, and includes emphasis on health promotion and disease prevention. Step 2 ensures that due attention is devoted to the principles of clinical sciences and basic patient-centered skills that provide the foundation for the safe and effective practice of medicine."

An impressive statement, but what does it mean? Let's dissect the statement so that you can better understand the philosophy underlying the Step 2 CS and anticipate the types of questions and scenarios you may encounter on test day.

- **"Assesses the ability of examinees to apply medical knowledge, skills, and understanding of clinical science"**: This refers to anything and everything you have learned in medical school so far.
- **"Essential for the provision of patient care"**: This alludes to the minimum level of knowledge and skills needed to provide patient care.
- **"Under supervision"**: This signifies that as an intern, you'll typically have a resident and an attending watching over you.
- **"Includes emphasis on health promotion and disease prevention"**: Roughly stated, this means that it's not all about acute MIs, trauma, or sepsis, but also about enabling patients to take control of their own health.
- **"Attention is devoted to the principles of clinical sciences and basic patient-centered skills that provide the foundation for the safe and effective practice of medicine"**: Here again, emphasis is placed on the bare-bones clinical science knowledge and communication skills needed to help reduce morbidity and mortality.

In summary, the test designers want to evaluate your application of clinical knowledge and your ability to communicate well enough to work with other house staff on a joint mission to help keep patients alive and healthy.

Test designers aim to evaluate your application of clinical knowledge and ability to communicate on a solid level while maintaining a comfortable and professional rapport.

But precisely how does one demonstrate the ability to manage disease and promote good health by communicating? The answer is simple: practice. Do this by examining as many patients and colleagues as you can. Then logically synthesize what you uncovered by communicating your findings. For IMGs, we must emphasize that this practice should be done in English, ideally with native English speakers.

The underlying philosophy of the Step 2 CS, therefore, is not to cover the same factual knowledge tested on the Step 1 or Step 2 CK. Rather, its primary objective is to test your ability to apply a fundamental knowledge base by communicating with mock patients toward the goal of extracting enough information to generate a basic differential diagnosis and workup plan. So the best one can do to prepare for the exam is become familiar with its format, practice focused history taking and patient interactions, and present cases in a logical and well-rehearsed fashion.

What Is the USMLE Step 2 CS?

The USMLE Step 2 CS is a one-day exam whose objective is to ensure that all U.S. and Canadian medical students seeking to obtain their medical licenses—as well as all IMGs seeking to start their residencies in the United States—have the communication, interpersonal, and clinical skills necessary to achieve these goals. To pass the test, all examinees must show that they can speak, understand, and communicate in English as well as take a history and perform a brief physical exam. Examinees are also required to exhibit competence in written English and to demonstrate critical clinical skills by writing a brief patient note (PN), follow-up orders, and a differential diagnosis.

The Step 2 CS simulates clinical encounters that are commonly found in clinics, physicians' offices, and emergency departments. The test makes use of "standardized patients" (SPs), all of whom are laypersons who have been extensively trained to simulate various clinical problems. The SPs give the same responses to all candidates participating in the assessment. When you take the Step 2 CS, you will see 12 SPs over the course of about an eight-hour day, including a 30-minute break for lunch. Half of the cases are performed before the lunch break and half afterward. SPs will be mixed in terms of age, gender, ethnicity, organ system, and discipline.

For quality assurance purposes, a video camera will record all clinical encounters, but the resulting videotapes will not be used for scoring. The cases used in the Step 2 CS represent the types of patients who are typically encountered during core clerkships in the curricula of accredited U.S. medical schools. These clerkships are as follows:

- Internal medicine
- Surgery
- Obstetrics and gynecology
- Pediatrics
- Psychiatry
- Family medicine
- Emergency medicine

> *There is no physical exam in pediatric or phone encounters. Instead, you should focus on obtaining a thorough history and delivering effective closure.*

Examinees do **not** interact with children during pediatric encounters. Instead, SPs assuming the role of pediatric patients' parents recount patients' histories, and no physical exam is required under such circumstances.

How Is the Step 2 CS Structured?

Before entering a room to interact with an SP, you will be given an opportunity to review some preliminary information. This information, which is posted on the door of each room (and hence is often referred to as "doorway information"), includes the following:

- Patient characteristics (name, age, gender)
- Chief complaint and vitals (temperature, respiratory rate, pulse, blood pressure)

> *Many students choose to use a bullet-style format when typing the PN.*

You will be given 15 minutes (with a warning bell sounded after 10 minutes) to perform the clinical encounter, which includes reading the doorway information, entering the room, introducing yourself, obtaining an appropriate history, conducting a focused physical exam, formulating a differential diagnosis, and planning a diagnostic workup. You will also be expected to answer any questions the SP might ask, discuss the diagnoses being considered, and advise the SP about any follow-up plans you might have. After leaving the room, you will have 10 minutes to type a PN. Examinees will not be permitted to handwrite the PN unless technical difficulties on test day make the typing program unavailable.

If you happen to finish a clinical encounter early, there is no need for you to rush out the door. Once you leave the examination room, you may not reenter it. So if you find yourself running ahead of schedule, you might consider telling the patient that you are organizing your notes, as one or two last-minute questions might pop into mind.

How Is the Step 2 CS Scored?

Of your 12 patient encounters, 10 will be scored. Two people will score each encounter: the SP and a physician. The SP will evaluate you at the end of each encounter by filling out three checklists: one for the history, a second for the physical exam, and a third for communication skills. The physician will evaluate the PN you write after each encounter. Your overall score, which will be based on the clinical encounter as a whole and on your overall communication skills, will be determined by the following three components:

1. **Integrated Clinical Encounter (ICE) score.** The skills you demonstrate in the clinical encounter are reflected in your ICE score. This score will reflect your **data-gathering and data interpretation skills**.

    ▪ **Data gathering.** SPs will evaluate your data-gathering skills by documenting your ability to collect data pertinent to the clinical encounter. Specifically, they will note whether you asked the questions listed on their checklists, successfully obtained relevant information, and correctly conducted the physical exam (as indicated by your performance of the procedures on their checklists). If you asked questions or performed procedures that are not on an SP's checklist, you will not receive credit—but at the same time will not lose credit—for having done so.

    ▪ **Data interpretation.** To demonstrate your data interpretation skills, you will be asked to document, as part of the PN, your analysis of a patient's possible diagnoses and your assessment of how such diagnoses are supported or refuted by the evidence obtained from the history and physical exam. Although in actual practice physicians must develop the ability to recognize and rule out a range of disorders, you will be asked to record only the most likely diagnoses along with the positive and negative findings that support each. Physicians who score the PN make a global assessment based on documentation and organization of the history and physical exam; the relevance, justification, and order of the differential diagnosis; and the initial testing modalities proposed. Your final score will represent the average of your individual PN scores over all 10 scored clinical encounters.

    > *Do not list unlikely disorders in your differential, however important this may be in actual practice. Instead, focus on the differential diagnoses that are most likely.*

2. **Communication and Interpersonal Skills (CIS) score.** In addition to assessing your data-gathering abilities, SPs will evaluate your communication and interpersonal skills. According to the USMLE, these include fostering a relationship with the patient, gathering and providing information, helping the patient make decisions, and supporting the patient's emotions. You will be evaluated on your ability to tailor your questions and responses to the specific needs of the case presented and on your capacity to react to the patient's concerns. Overall, the CIS subcomponent focuses on your ability to conduct a *patient-centered interview* (discussed at length in Section 2) in which you identify and respond to the broader scope of the

patient's concerns beyond just the diagnosis. The CIS performance is documented by SPs with checklists.

3. **Spoken English Proficiency (SEP) score.** This component scores you on pronunciation, word choice, and the degree of effort the SP must make to understand your spoken English. The SEP score is based on SP evaluations that make use of rating scales.

The grade you receive on the Step 2 CS will be either a "pass" or a "fail." Your report will include a graphic representation of your strengths and weaknesses on all three components of the exam. Unlike Step 1 or Step 2 CK, you will not receive a numerical score. To pass the Step 2 CS overall, candidates must pass all three individual components. The good news is that most U.S. and Canadian medical students pass (see Table 1-1). However, the failure rate is higher among IMGs, with approximately one in four examinees failing.

> You must pass all three components of the Step 2 CS to pass the exam.

Relatively few U.S. students fail the CIS, and even fewer fail the SEP component. If U.S. students fail the exam as a whole, it is most likely due to poor ICE scores. For IMGs, the CIS is the most likely component to cause failure. The SEP is more of a challenge for IMGs compared to U.S. students but is still the least likely component to cause failure. Few IMGs fail all three subcomponents.

> Among students who fail the Step 2 CS, U.S. students are most likely to fail because of ICE scores, and IMGs are most likely to fail because of the CIS.

How Do I Register to Take the USMLE Step 2 CS?

Applicants can register directly for the Step 2 CS without having passed any other USMLE Step. However, registration information and procedures are constantly evolving. For the most current information on registering for the Step 2 CS, go to www.usmle.org or check with your dean's office. IMGs should also refer to the Web site of the Educational Commission for Foreign Medical Graduates (ECFMG) at www.ecfmg.org.

U.S. students must register using the NBME's interactive Web site for applicants and examinees (click the appropriate link at www.nbme.org). IMGs can either apply online using the ECFMG's Interactive Web Application (IWA) at https://iwa2.ecfmg.org/gradoverview.asp or download the paper application from the ECFMG Web site and mail it to the ECFMG with the registration fee. Although there is no specific application deadline, you should apply early to ensure that you get your preferred test date and center.

> Register as early as possible, as some test centers fill up months in advance.

After your application has been processed, you will receive a scheduling permit by e-mail. Orientation manuals and videos of sample encounters are available at www.usmle.org or can be obtained on CD when you register. The video is an excel-

TABLE 1-1. Step 2 CS Pass Rates				
	2010–2011		2011–2012	
	No. Tested	Passing	No. Tested	Passing
U.S./Canadian	18,361	98%	17,164	97%
IMGs	15,042	77%	13,780	77%

lent preparation resource that shows exactly how the Step 2 CS is administered as well as how you should conduct yourself during the exam. Once you have received your scheduling permit, you are eligible to take the Step 2 CS for one year, starting from the date your application was processed. Your scheduling permit will list your eligibility period, scheduling instructions, and identification requirements for admission to the exam. You can schedule the test through the NBME or ECFMG Web site or by telephone. Access information will be included with your registration materials. Note that test centers offer both morning and afternoon sessions. You may be offered an afternoon session if you select a date and center for which morning sessions are already filled. Try to select a date and center that offer you a morning session, when you are likely to be fresher and more relaxed (unless you are an inveterate night owl).

Although you cannot extend your eligibility period for the Step 2 CS, you can cancel or reschedule your examination date. You will not be charged a fee if you cancel or reschedule 14 calendar days before your scheduled test date, not including the day of the test. However, a fee of $150 will be levied if you cancel or reschedule at any time during the 14-day period before (but not including) your scheduled test date. You will need to pay $400 if you miss an appointment without canceling or rescheduling. These fees are subject to change, so please check the USMLE Web site (www.usmle.org) for the current fee schedule.

Finally, a word of caution regarding the exchange of scheduled test dates. Some applicants have been known to post requests on online forums to swap their appointment with another applicant. The Step 2 CS scheduling system does not allow anyone to schedule or reschedule an appointment on behalf of another applicant. In addition, the system works on a first-come, first-served basis—so if you cancel your appointment in anticipation of such an exchange, your test date might be claimed by someone else who happens to be logged onto the system at the same time. Applicants are therefore advised to avoid such exchanges and instead to reschedule test dates only within the formal protocols. If you have registered late and your only options are later than you would like, be sure to check back frequently for openings closer to your desired date.

Where Can I Take the Exam?

The Step 2 CS will be administered at five regional sites called Clinical Skills Evaluation Collaboration centers (see Figure 1-1). Additional centers are currently under consideration.

For detailed information about cities, hotels, and transportation, please refer to the USMLE Web site (www.usmle.org), the ECFMG Web site (www.ecfmg.org), and the Section 1 Supplement to this text.

How Long Will I Wait to Get My Scores?

Step 2 CS results are posted to your On-line Applicant Status and Information System (OASIS) account on the ECFMG/NBME Web site. An e-mail is sent to you once your score report has been uploaded onto your account page. A fixed schedule of

FIGURE 1-1. **Step 2 CS Test Centers**

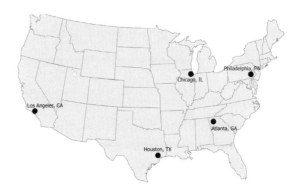

score-reporting periods is published on the USMLE Web site well in advance of your test date. Most examinees who take the Step 2 CS receive their scores on the first day of the corresponding reporting period, which is usually 1–3 months from the date of the test. If you do not receive your results within that time, you must send a written request for a duplicate report to the NBME or the ECFMG. Again, the score report you receive indicates only whether you passed or failed the exam. Your numerical score is not disclosed to you or to any of the programs to which you apply. Once you pass the Step 2 CS, your passing score remains valid for the purpose of applying for residency training.

What If I Fail?

If you fail the Step 2 CS, you can retake it, but not more than three times within any 12-month period. In addition, each time you take the exam you must submit a new application and an appropriate fee.

If for some reason you think that you received a failing score unfairly, you may be able to appeal and request a rescoring of your exam. However, doing so is unlikely to change your overall exam results, and little information is provided to explain exactly how or why you may have failed. Even if you feel your results are unjustified, it may be best to begin preparation to retest. Use the knowledge and experience you gained from your first attempt to optimize your preparation and improve your performance. It is worth recognizing that even though the NBME tries hard to design a test that is fair and accurate, the exam will always have a subjective component. Costly fees acknowledged, the most effective response to what you perceive may be an inaccurate assessment of your true clinical skills is to practice more and give it another shot. Check your orientation manual or the USMLE and/or ECFMG Web sites for the latest reexamination and appeal policies.

PREPARING FOR THE STEP 2 CS

In preparing for the Step 2 CS, keep in mind that you will need to demonstrate certain fundamental but critical clinical skills in order to pass. These skills include the following:

- Interacting with patients in a professional and empathetic manner
- Taking a good medical history
- Performing an appropriate and focused physical exam
- Counseling and delivering information
- Typing a logical and organized PN that includes a reasoned differential diagnosis

In this section, we will briefly explore a few of these skills. Section 2 reviews these skills in greater detail in addition to the mechanics of the clinical encounter and PN.

Ability to Interact with Patients in a Professional Way

There are several elements of the CIS component that you must incorporate into each encounter. These are simple and easy to learn but require practice.

- **Introduce yourself to the patient.** When you first meet a patient, be sure to smile, address the patient by his or her last name (eg, "Mr. Jones"), introduce yourself clearly, shake hands firmly, and establish good eye contact.
- **Actively listen to the patient.** Allow the patient to express his or her concerns without interrupting or interjecting your own thoughts. Your demeanor should be curious, nonjudgmental, and compassionate.
- **Wash your hands.** It is probably best to wash your hands just before the physical exam. Hand washing also gives you an opportunity to briefly reflect and perhaps ask a confirmatory question or two. It is acceptable to use gloves as an alternative.
- **Use "draping manners."** Always keep the patient well draped. You can cover the patient at any time before the physical exam, but it is better to do so at the beginning of the encounter. Do not expose large portions of the patient's body at the same time; instead, uncover only the parts that need to be examined, and only one at a time. Be sure to ask permission before you uncover any part of the body and explain why you are doing so. You should also ask permission to untie the patient's gown and should tie the gown again when you are done.
- **Be mindful of appearance.** In your encounters, you should appear confident, calm, and friendly as well as serious and professional. Wear a clean white lab coat over professional-looking but comfortable clothes. Do not wear shorts or jeans. Men should wear slacks, a shirt, and a tie. Women should consider slacks and low-heeled shoes and should avoid wearing skirts above the knee.
- **Maintain appropriate body language.** During the clinical encounter, look the patient in the eye, smile when appropriate, and show compassion. When trying to console a patient, you may place your hand on his or her shoulder or arm but not on the leg or hand. Do not exaggerate your facial expressions in an effort to convince the patient that you empathize with him or her. Never talk to a patient

while standing somewhere he or she cannot see you, especially during the history and closure.

- **Focus your concentration on the patient.** Ask permission before you examine any part of the patient's body, and explain what you intend to do. Pay attention to everything the patient says and does, because the behavior is most likely purposeful. It is more important to maintain good rapport than to perfect the nuances of your physical exam technique. You can show concern by doing the following:
  - **Keep the patient comfortable.** Help the patient sit up, lie down, and get onto and off the examination table. Do not repeat painful procedures.
  - **Show compassion for the patient's pain.** If the patient does not allow you to touch his or her abdomen because of severe pain, say, "I know that you are in pain, and I want to help you, but I need to examine you to locate the source of your pain and give you the right treatment."
  - **Show compassion for a patient's sadness.** To demonstrate empathy, you may take a brief moment of silence and place your hand lightly on the patient's shoulder or arm. You may then say something like "You must feel sad. Would you like to tell me about it?"
  - **Respect the patient's beliefs.** Do not reject a patient's beliefs even if they sound incorrect to you. A patient may tell you, "I am sure that the pain I have is due to colon cancer." You may respond to this with something like "That may be one possibility, but there are others that we need to consider as well."

> IMGs should focus on communication and interpersonal skills. U.S. medical students should be careful not to use complex language or medical jargon.

Ability to Take a Good Medical History

The interviewing techniques you use should allow you to collect a thorough medical history. It is true that you can prepare a list of questions to use for every system or complaint. However, be aware that you will not be able to cover everything. Therefore, you should ask only those questions that are relevant to the specific case; your goal is to direct each interview toward exploring the chief complaint and uncovering any hidden complaints. Remember that a good survey of the chief complaint with a goal of uncovering and acknowledging salient positives and negatives is more important than covering every single detail.

If you feel that a patient is not following your line of questioning, be careful, as this may indicate that you are drifting away from the correct diagnosis. You should also bear in mind that physical findings may be simulated and may not look the same as real ones (eg, simulation of wheezes during chest auscultation). In such circumstances, you should pretend that the findings are real.

Do not be intimidated by angry patients. Remember that SPs are only actors, so stay calm, firm, and friendly. Ask about the reason for a patient's anger or complaint, and address it appropriately. Do not be defensive or hostile.

If you do not understand what a patient has said or recognize a drug that has been prescribed, do not hesitate to ask, "Can you please repeat what you said?" or "What is the name of that drug again?"

Finally, remember to use the **summary technique** at least once during the interview. This technique, which involves briefly summarizing what the patient has just told you, often using the patient's own words, may be used either after you finish taking the history or after the physical exam. Summarizing will help ensure that you remember the details of the history before you leave the room to write the PN.

The summary technique is an excellent patient communication strategy.

Ability to Counsel and Deliver Information

At the end of each encounter, you will be expected to tell the patient about your findings, offer your medical opinion (including a concise differential diagnosis), describe the next step in diagnosis, and outline possible treatments. In doing so, you should always be clear and honest. Tell the patient only the things you know, and do not try to render a final diagnosis.

Before you leave, ask the patient if he or she still has any questions. After you respond, follow up by asking, "Did that answer your question?" Make sure the patient understands what you are saying, and avoid the use of complex medical jargon. It is much simpler to ask patients to gently lie back than to tell them to assume a reverse Trendelenburg position.

When counseling a patient, always be open. Tell the patient what you really think is wrong, and explain that the final diagnosis can be made only after some tests have been ordered. You should also explain some of the tests you are planning to conduct. Address any concerns the patient may have in a realistic manner, and never offer false reassurances.

TEST-DAY TIPS

The Step 2 CS is a one-day exam. Bring a stethoscope and a white coat. A limited number of stethoscopes will be provided if you happen to forget yours. Tendon hammers, tongue depressors, tuning forks, and pen lights are provided in the rooms. You will be scheduled for either the morning or the afternoon session. The duration of the Step 2 CS, including orientation, testing, and breaks, is approximately eight hours. Once you have entered the secured area of the assessment center for orientation, you may not leave that area until the exam has been completed. During this time, the following conventions should be observed:

- You may not use watches (analog or digital), cell phones, or beepers at any time during the exam. A locker will be provided to secure your items.
- The morning session starts at 8 A.M. and the afternoon session at 3 P.M. Test proctors will generally wait up to 30 minutes for latecomers, so the actual exam usually does not begin until 8:30 A.M. or 3:30 P.M. Nonetheless, you should plan to arrive 30 minutes before your session is scheduled to begin.
- Do not come to an afternoon session early in an attempt to meet candidates from the morning session, as they are not allowed to leave until you are safely secured in the exam room.
- Bring a government-issued photo ID (eg, a U.S. driver's license or a passport) that carries your signature.

No watches of any kind, either analog or digital, are allowed in the test area. Neither are pens/pencils or scratch paper.

■ Be sure to bring your admission permit! You will not be admitted to the test center without it.

After the 30-minute waiting period has ended, the staff will give you a name tag, a numbered badge to be worn around your arm, a pen, and a clipboard. There is no need to bring a pen of your own; in fact, you are not allowed to use anything other than the pen provided at the exam site.

If you are traveling with luggage, do not bring it to the test site, as the staff cannot store it for you. You will be provided only with a coat rack and a small storage locker for belongings that you are not allowed to carry during the encounter, such as watches, cell phones, purses, and handbags. If you are planning to travel immediately after the exam, you can keep your luggage at the front desk of your hotel.

At the beginning of your session, you will be asked to sign a confidentiality agreement. An orientation session will then be held to introduce you to the equipment that you will find in the examination rooms. Examine and become familiar with this equipment, especially the bed, foot extension, and head elevation. Do not hesitate to try each piece of equipment made available to you during this session.

You will be given two breaks during the exam. The first break lasts 30 minutes and takes place after the fourth encounter. During this break, the staff will serve you a meal. The second break lasts 15 minutes and takes place after the eighth encounter. Use the bathroom during these breaks, as you will not have time to do so during the encounters. Finally, remember that smoking is strictly prohibited not only during the exam but also during breaks. You cannot leave the center during break periods.

In the break room, you will be assigned a seat and a desk. You can keep your food or drink on this desk so that it will be accessible during break time. Although the testing staff will provide you with one meal, you may want to bring some high-energy snacks for your breaks. Also remember that your personal belongings will not be accessible to you until the end of the exam—so if you do plan to bring food with you, keep it on your assigned desk, not in the storage area.

The Step 2 CS is not a social event, so when you meet with other candidates during breaks, do not talk about the cases you encountered. During breaks (and, of course, during the encounters), speak only in English; doing otherwise will be considered irregular and may be questioned.

Finally, remember that even though all your encounters are videotaped, these tapes are not used for scoring purposes. To the contrary, they are used only to ensure the safety of the SPs and candidates and to ensure quality. So don't worry about the camera, and don't try to look for it during the encounters. Act as you would on a regular clinic day.

Some Final Words

The following general principles will help you excel on the Step 2 CS:

■ **Remember to rest before the exam.** Try to give yourself a few days to overcome jet lag, eat well, and get exercise. A sluggish affect and a cloudy mind can lead to

> *Don't bring your luggage to the test center. Check it with the hotel front desk.*

> *Bring water or energy snacks to keep at your desk if you need them.*

inefficiency and poor rapport. This is especially important if you are scheduled for an afternoon session, which can run as late as 11 P.M.

- **Think about the present, not the past.** Clear your head before proceeding to your next encounter. Thinking about what you should have done or should have asked will only distract you from your current encounter.

- **Passing does not require perfection.** You need not be perfect. In fact, given the time constraints involved, the Step 2 CS rewards efficiency and relative completeness over perfection.

- **There is a reason for everything you see.** If a patient is wearing a sombrero, inquire why this is the case. He might have been in Mexico, and the diarrhea he presents with may be a simple traveler's diarrhea. Similarly, a prominently placed tattoo might suggest certain risk behaviors, not just a keen appreciation of body art.

> *Go for efficiency, not perfection.*

FIRST AID FOR THE IMG

If you are an IMG candidate seeking to pass the Step 2 CS, you must take a number of variables into account, from plotting a timetable to mastering logistical details to formulating a solid test preparation strategy.

Determining Eligibility

Before contacting the ECFMG for a Step 2 CS application, you must first take several preliminary steps. Begin by ascertaining whether you are eligible (see Table 1-2). Check the ECFMG Web site for the latest eligibility criteria.

Once you have established your eligibility to take the exam, you will need to factor in the residency matching process (the "Match"). If you are planning to apply for a residency in the United States, your timetable should reflect that and should be carefully planned at least one year in advance.

You are allowed to **register** (pay the fee) for the Match regardless of your ECFMG status. To **participate** in the Match, however, the National Residency Matching Program (NRMP) requires that you be ECFMG certified (or that you meet ECFMG requirements for certification even if you have not received your certificate) by the rank-order-list deadline (typically in February of each year). Applicants who do not

TABLE 1-2. IMG Eligibility for the USMLE Step 2 CS[a]	
Medical Students	**Medical School Graduates**
You must be enrolled in a foreign medical school listed in the International Medical Education Directory (IMED, http://imed.ecfmg.org) both at the time you apply and at the time you take the assessment. You must also be within 12 months of graduation when you take the exam.	You must be a graduate of a medical school that was listed in the IMED at the time of your graduation.
[a] You are not required to have passed the English-language proficiency test or the Test of English as a Foreign Language to be eligible for the Step 2 CS.	

meet these requirements will automatically be withdrawn from the Match. Therefore, you should take the Step 2 CS no later than October in the year before your target Match Day (see Figure 1-2).

There is a significant advantage to obtaining ECFMG certification by the time you submit your application for residency in the fall. Should you do so, residency programs are likely to consider you a ready applicant and may favor you over other candidates who have yet to take the Step 2 CS—even if such candidates have more impressive applications. In addition, if you are certified early, you can take Step 3 and get your results back before the rank-order-list deadline. A good score on Step 3 can provide a perfect last-minute boost to your application and may also make you eligible for the H-1B visa. In summary, take the Step 2 CS as soon as you are eligible (see Table 1-2), but not before you are confident that you are fully prepared. Remember that to get ECFMG certification, you need to pass the Step 1, Step 2 CK, and Step 2 CS within a seven-year period. In deciding when to apply for the Step 2 CS, when to take it, and whether you are ready for it, keep the following points in mind:

> All the USMLE exams need to be passed within a seven-year period for ECFMG certification.

- Scheduling your test date can be difficult during busy seasons. Apply at least three months before your desired examination date. Ideally, you should aim to take the Step 2 CS in June or July in order to be certified when you apply for residency.
- Schedule your exam on the date that you expect to be fully prepared for it. For IMGs, preparation for the exam typically requires anywhere between 1 and 12 weeks, factoring in your level of English proficiency as well as your medical knowledge and skills.

FIGURE 1-2. Typical Step 2 CS Timeline for IMGs

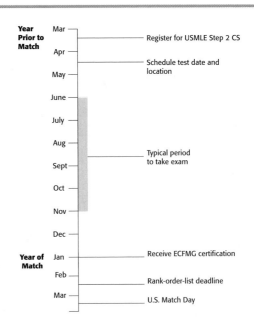

- If you choose to apply for the Step 2 CS using a paper application, it will take up to four weeks to receive your notification of registration, but it may take as few as 10 days to receive this information if you use the ECFMG's IWA.

> *Use the ECFMG's IWA to minimize delays and errors.*

Some residency programs use the Step 2 CS as a screening tool to select IMG applicants for interviews, so it is ideal to meet the deadline for the Match.

If you are an IMG living outside the United States, you must also factor in the time it may take to obtain a visa. You do not need a visa to come to the United States if you are a U.S. or Canadian citizen or a permanent resident. Citizens of countries participating in the Visa Waiver Program (such as European Union countries) may not need to obtain a visa either. You are responsible for determining whether you need a visa and, having done so, for obtaining that visa (regardless of how time-consuming and difficult this process may be). Before you apply to take the Step 2 CS, you should therefore complete the following tasks:

- Check with the U.S. embassy in your country to determine whether you need a visa.
- Determine how long it will take to get an appointment at the embassy.
- Find out how long it will take to get the visa and whether a clearance period is required.
- Check travel availability to the cities in which the exam centers are located.

As proof of the reason for your visit to the United States, the ECFMG will send you a letter to present to the U.S. consulate in your country. This letter will be sent to you only after you apply to take the Step 2 CS (ie, after you have paid the fee) and will not guarantee that you will be granted a visa. For this reason, it is wise not to schedule your actual exam day until you have arrived in the United States or have at least obtained your visa.

Application Tips

When you receive your application to take the Step 2 CS, be sure to read it carefully before filling it out. You do not want your application returned to you—thus wasting valuable time—simply because you forgot to answer a question or made a careless mistake. Applications that contain the following common errors will be returned:

- An application that is not written in ink or is illegible
- An incomplete application
- An application that is not the original document (ie, faxed or photocopied)
- An application that contains a nonoriginal signature or photograph
- An application that contains a photograph of the applicant that was taken more than six months before the date the application was submitted
- An application in which the signature of the medical school official or the notary public is more than four months old
- An application in which the medical school or notary public seal or stamp does not cover a portion of your photograph

- An application that does not explain why it was signed by a notary public but not by your medical school official
- An application that does not include full payment

Commonly encountered errors specific to IMGs include the following:

- Failure to send the ECFMG a copy of your medical school diploma with two full-face photographs
- Failure to send the ECFMG an English translation of your medical school diploma if the original is not in English
- Failure to staple together your medical school diploma and its English translation or to ensure that the translator's stamp covers both the original and the translation

Once you have completed your application and have double-checked it for errors, make every effort to send it by express mail or courier service. To check the status of your application online, you can use OASIS (https://oasis2.ecfmg.org).

Improving Your English Proficiency

For many IMGs taking the Step 2 CS, a critical concern lies in the demonstration of proficiency in spoken English. In Step 2 CS terms, this refers to the ability to speak English clearly and comprehensibly and to understand English when the SP speaks to you.

You may not have a problem with English proficiency if you are a native English speaker, have studied in a U.S. or other English-speaking school, have learned medicine in English in your medical school, or have spent at least a few months or years of your life in an English-speaking country. English proficiency may, however, be the main obstacle facing IMGs at the other end of the spectrum. The good news is that most IMGs who have already passed the USMLE Step 1 have the basic English language skills needed to pass the Step 2 CS. For such candidates, the key to passing the Step 2 CS lies in organizing these skills and practicing. Your spoken English proficiency is based on the following components:

- **The ability to speak in a manner that is easy for the SP to follow and understand.** Toward this goal, choose phrases that are simple, direct, and easy both for you to remember and for the SP to understand. Speaking slowly will also make it easier for SPs to understand you and will minimize the effect your accent has on your comprehensibility.
- **The correct use of grammar.** The key to mastering this element is to be familiar with commonly used statements, transitions, and questions and to practice them as much as possible. This will minimize the chance that you will make significant grammatical errors.
- **Comprehensible pronunciation.** Again, the key to good pronunciation lies in practicing common statements and questions, repeating them to yourself aloud, and asking someone (preferably a native English speaker) to listen to you and correct your mistakes. The more you practice, the better your chances will be of reaching an acceptable and even a superior level of clear, comprehensible English.

- **The ability to correct and clarify your English if necessary.** You may find it difficult to prepare for a situation in which an SP does not understand you and asks you for the meaning of something you have just said. Here again, you can avoid this situation by practicing common statements, questions, and transitions; speaking as slowly and clearly as possible; and using nontechnical words instead of complicated medical terms. If an SP still cannot understand something you have said, simply repeat the phrase or question, or restate it in simple lay terms.

> *The key to better spoken English is practicing commonly used statements, transitions, and questions.*

Make every effort to remain calm throughout your clinical encounters. Nervousness can cause you to mumble, making it difficult for the SP to understand you. Likewise, if you become nervous and start looking at the clock and rushing, you will further increase the likelihood of making mistakes. So remain calm, concentrate, and take your time.

Fifteen minutes may seem like a short time to do and say all the things you think are necessary, but it will be more than enough if you follow an organized plan. Most of the things you have to say in the exam are the same in each encounter, so by thoroughly studying common cases and medical conditions (see Sections 3 and 4), you can minimize this obstacle.

If you are still unsure about your English proficiency, the ECFMG suggests that you take the Test of Spoken English (TSE) to get a measure of your abilities. If you score higher than 35 on this exam, you have likely attained the level of English proficiency necessary for the Step 2 CS. You may also consider taking the Test of English as a Foreign Language (TOEFL) before you take the Step 2 CS. However, doing so is no longer a prerequisite to taking the Step 2 CS or to ECFMG certification. For more information about the TSE and the TOEFL, contact:

TOEFL/TSE Services
P.O. Box 6151
Princeton, NJ 08541-6151
609-771-7100
www.toefl.org

Getting Clinical Rotations and Observerships

Many IMGs may lack basic familiarity with the workings of U.S. medical schools. A clinical rotation or observership in the United States can prepare IMGs for the Step 2 CS by introducing them to the U.S. system and, in the process, immersing them in the "American" way of taking a history, performing a physical exam, and writing PNs. Clinical rotations are also good to have on your curriculum vitae when you apply for residency programs. Moreover, performing well on your rotation can earn you strong letters of recommendation, which are the most important part of your application after your USMLE scores. The more time you spend in such a rotation, the better.

Even if your Step 1 and Step 2 CK scores are impressive and you come highly regarded from a top international medical school, lack of proficiency in English will make it more challenging for you to pass the Step 2 CS. Participating in a formal clinical rotation in the United States is one of the best ways to polish your English skills. This will make the Step 2 CS experience more tolerable and may ultimately boost your communication skills if you are invited for residency interviews.

If you are still a **medical student,** it should not be difficult for you to find a clinical rotation. Check the Web sites of the universities in which you are interested and e-mail or write the program director and chairman of each. If you are already in the United States, call the relevant departments and make appointments to meet with the personnel responsible for the rotations. Most of the time, such personnel will send you an application by mail. For the purposes of your residency application, however, it is highly recommended that you also do a rotation in the specialty in which you are interested.

If you are a **medical graduate,** your mission is more difficult but not impossible. You are no longer eligible for clinical elective rotations (clerkships), but you can still apply for observerships and externships.

The observership is perhaps the least active function you can fill in a hospital, but it can still be highly useful. Getting an observership is not an easy task because most hospitals do not have any such formal rotation or training program. Nonetheless, here is some advice that may help you:

- Prepare a list of hospitals in your area or any area that interests you. Include all types of teaching hospitals: university, community, and Veterans Affairs medical centers.
- Contact people (attendings, senior residents, secretaries, administrators) whom you may know. Connections are an important way to uncover these unofficial rotations.
- Send e-mails and/or letters to the chairman and program director of each hospital. IMGs for whom English is not a first language should send targeted communication in the form of grammatically correct letters or e-mails. It is always better to address a physician by name and specifically mention your interest in the program and why. A generic e-mail blast composed of poorly written English is the best way to ensure that your message will end up in a spam folder.
- Call the office of the chairman or program director and try to set an appointment to meet him or her.
- Talk to other physicians who are doing or have done observerships and ask them where they did so and how to apply.

During your rotation, you will "officially" be an observer, which means that you cannot touch a patient or write on charts. The only things you will officially be allowed to do are observe, do rounds with your team, answer an occasional question, present some topics, and attend conferences. On rare occasions, you may be able to examine some patients and write some notes. Here is some advice for making the most of your observership:

- Show a high level of enthusiasm.
- Come early and stay late (not very late, though).
- Follow up on patients your team is taking care of and learn everything you can about them.

> *Internal medicine and emergency medicine are the best rotations for Step 2 CS preparation.*

> *Sending a generic e-mail blast composed of poorly written English is the best way to guarantee that your message will land in a spam folder.*

- Read about the cases your team is managing.
- Chat and spend time with the patients, but always let them know that you are an observer. This is the best way to practice taking histories and to improve your language skills.
- Write your own PNs and orders, ask your residents to correct them, and compare them to the official notes.
- Talk to the nurses, secretaries, and support staff. This will improve your communication skills.
- If you do not get a chance to examine patients, carefully observe the residents and medical students during the physical exam.
- Do as many presentations as you can.

Here is a partial list of hospitals that have been known to offer formal observerships or externships:

- Banner Good Samaritan Medical Center, Phoenix, AZ
- Emory University, Atlanta, GA
- Hahnemann Hospital, Philadelphia, PA
- Harbor Hospital, Baltimore, MD
- Harvard Medical School, Boston, MA (application and fees apply)
- Hospital of St. Raphael, New Haven, CT
- Maricopa Medical Center, Phoenix, AZ
- Mayo Clinic, Rochester, MN (visiting physicians program)
- Memorial Hospital, Pawtucket, RI
- Mount Sinai Medical Center, Miami, FL
- Providence Hospital, Washington, DC
- University of Miami, Miami, FL
- Veterans Administration Medical Center, Washington, DC

Some Final Tips

There are a few final practical measures you can take to help ensure your success on the Step 2 CS:

- Check and recheck the ECFMG and USMLE Web sites for the latest information about the Step 2 CS. This will help you get a clear idea about regulations, requirements, registration, examination dates, and all other details concerning the Step 2 CS.
- Carefully prepare for the exam using the preparation materials included in this book.
- Check other Web sites and discussion forums. They can be a good source of information.
- Review the steps of history taking (see Section 2). Choose and prepare common questions and cases (see Sections 3 and 4).
- Review the steps of the physical exam (see Section 2). Practice the physical exam as if you were performing the real exam.
- Practice writing PNs (see Section 4).

► **NOTES**

The USMLE Step 2 CS Travel Guide

Introduction
Traveling to the United States
Atlanta ("The Big Peach")
Chicago ("The Windy City")
Houston ("Space City")
Los Angeles ("The City of Angels")
Philadelphia ("The City of Brotherly Love")
Useful Web Sites

INTRODUCTION

After you've worked hard to prepare for the Step 2 CS, the last thing you need is extra travel stress—or, worse still, problems on the day of the exam. The best way to ensure that everything goes as smoothly as possible on test day is to plan ahead. Getting all the details in place well in advance of your trip will help you focus on what's really important: doing a great job on the exam!

The following quick guide can be used as a planning tool both before and during your travels. For each of the five cities with a Step 2 CS testing center (called Clinical Skills Evaluation Collaboration, or CSEC, centers), we have provided details on the best ways to get to your destination and some things to do once you have arrived. Since most of you will be flying, we have placed special emphasis on distances to the CSEC test sites and routes from the airports. Also listed are a number of nearby hotels, most of which are reasonably priced and within walking distance of the CSEC centers. As a cheaper option, we have included one youth hostel for each city. Finally, we have recommended a few well-known restaurants and tourist attractions for each destination.

All five CSEC destinations are amazing cities, and we do not want you to miss out on what they have to offer. Although you should not let sightseeing get in the way of your test, you might want to schedule at least a few hours to see the sights. Even better, think about giving yourself an extra day or two after the exam to relax and really enjoy yourself in a new and exciting city.

With that said, make sure to confirm the details of the destinations we've presented before you start your trip. We have compiled a broad range of suggestions for you, but by the time you get to your destination, some of the details may well have changed. Another great source of information is the travel section on the USMLE Web site. Also note that the Association of American Medical Colleges (AAMC) has negotiated reduced hotel rates with many nearby hotels for the Step 2 CS. We have included many of these hotels here, but be sure to check the updated list online. Links to these sites are provided at the end of this section.

TRAVELING TO THE UNITED STATES

We know that many of you who are planning to take the Step 2 CS may be coming to the United States for the first time—so here are a few things to keep in mind to help minimize travel hassles.

Arrange your documents. Generally, the most important document you will need for the Step 2 CS is your **scheduling permit.** However, other documents may be required as well, especially if you're coming from another country. These may include the following:

- Your **passport.**
- A U.S. **tourist visa** (usually a B-1/B-2 visa; apply at the nearest U.S. embassy in your country).

- An **international driver's license** (consider getting one if you're planning to drive to your testing center) and potentially an international driving permit. Check the U.S. government Web site (www.usa.gov/Topics/Foreign-Visitors-Driving.shtml) for links to the driving rules in your testing location.

Make sure your travel plans are in place. Be sure to make your reservations well in advance, and think about how you're going to get around in the test city. Once you've arrived at your destination, make sure you know how to get to the CSEC center on the day of your test, especially if you're planning to stay a bit farther away.

Consider travel safety. When traveling abroad, particularly in major U.S. population centers, it's important to follow a few general guidelines to ensure your safety:

- As a whole, Americans are friendly and willing to be of assistance, but not everyone has the best of intentions. Be particularly alert to individuals who seem a bit too eager to help or who go out of their way for you.
- Keep an eye on your baggage while traveling by taxi, train, or any form of public transportation. Pickpockets and petty thieves tend to target visitors.
- Never carry anything in your baggage that doesn't belong to you. You are responsible for the contents of your baggage, including anything illegal that might have been placed there by someone else.
- Avoid walking alone on deserted streets at night.

Pack appropriately. Packing before air travel requires a lot of preparation. Here are a few useful tips:

- There are many restrictions for carry-on luggage these days, particularly with regard to liquids. Check the U.S. Transportation Security Administration's Web site (www.tsa.gov) for the most up-to-date information.
- Prepare for lost or delayed baggage. Do not keep your scheduling permit, lab coat, or stethoscope in your checked baggage. Also remember to put a copy of your itinerary in your baggage so that authorities can locate you in the event that your baggage is lost.
- Using a mobile phone or a camera, take a photograph of your baggage to give to the authorities in the event that your baggage is delayed or lost.
- Tag your baggage with brightly colored tape or a distinguishing mark so that you can easily identify it at baggage carousels.

Plan, plan, plan. Here are some guidelines for planning your visit and booking your hotel:

- Try to schedule your exam well in advance. Doing so will make it easier for you to get a good price on your tickets and accommodations.
- Before you book a hotel or a flight, compare prices at multiple Web sites and at each organization's Web site (see "Useful Web Sites" at the end of this supplement). Vacation packages that include a combination of flight, lodging, and car rental are usually cheaper than purchasing individually.
- Before you choose a hotel, be sure to factor in the distance to the testing center as well as the services each hotel offers—for example, whether it has a free airport shuttle, free breakfast, and access to Wi-Fi. Bear in mind that staying in a

youth hostel may save you money on hotel accommodations but may increase travel time to the CSEC center on test day. Also, hotels that are closer to the test site may have services geared specifically toward examinees.

Choosing to drive. Rental cars are also an option for traveling to the site location. Don't forget your international driver's license! Also bear in mind that most companies require you to be 25 years old to rent a vehicle. The most popular companies in all the CSEC destinations are as follows:

- Alamo (www.alamo.com): 877-222-9075
- Avis (www.avis.com): 800-633-3469
- Budget (www.budget.com): 800-218-7992
- Dollar (www.dollar.com): 800-800-4000
- Enterprise (www.enterprise.com): 800-261-7331
- Hertz (www.hertz.com): 800-654-3131
- National (www.nationalcar.com): 877-222-9058
- Payless (www.paylesscarrental.com): 800-729-5377
- Thrifty (www.thrifty.com): 800-847-4389

ATLANTA ("THE BIG PEACH")

Clinical Skills Evaluation Collaboration Center
Two Crown Center
1745 Phoenix Boulevard, Suite 500 (5th Floor)
Atlanta, GA 30349-5585

The Atlanta metro area has a population of more than five million and is the capital city of the great state of Georgia. Throughout history, Atlanta has served as a main north-south and east-west railway hub; in fact, its name was derived from the Atlanta-Pacifica railway that ran through the town in the 1840s. Today, Atlanta is home to the Centers for Disease Control and Prevention as well as the headquarters of Coca-Cola. We know you'll enjoy your time in this diverse and thriving city!

Getting There

- **Air:** Atlanta's major airport is the Hartsfield-Jackson Atlanta International Airport (ATL) (www.atlanta-airport.com), located about 9 miles/14.5 km south of downtown and only a few blocks from the CSEC center.
- **Ground:**
  - Greyhound, 232 Forsyth Street Southwest (www.greyhound.com): The main bus terminal is located downtown, about 12 miles/19.3 km from the CSEC center, which is approximately 20 minutes by taxi for a flat rate of $25.
  - Amtrak, 1688 Peachtree Street Northwest (www.amtrak.com): The main train station is also located downtown, about 16 miles/25.7 km from the testing center. Atlanta is on the Crescent Line, which runs between New Orleans and New York.

Getting Around When You Arrive

- **Shuttles:** Most hotels offer free shuttle service to and from the airport. The airport Web site has a list of the hotels that offer complimentary service. There are also airport shuttle services available from the airport to downtown or other major attractions and surrounding cities. The airport Web site lists shuttle services by destination. Airport Metro Shuttle serves most of the metro area, and Atlanta Airport Shuttle serves the area within the corporate city limits of Atlanta (downtown, midtown, and Buckhead).
  - Atlanta Airport Shuttle (www.taass.net)
  - Airport Metro Shuttle (www.airportmetro.com)
- **Taxis:** Taxis are available at the airport and at the bus/train terminals and cost $30–$35 from the airport to downtown. The ride from the airport to the CSEC center is about 10 minutes. Local taxi companies include the following:
  - Atlanta Checker Cab: 404-351-1111
  - National: 404-752-6834
  - Day and Night Cab Co.: 404-767-7464
  - Yellow Cab: 404-521-0200
- **Rental cars:** All rental car companies are located at the Hartsfield-Jackson Rental Car Center (RCC). Once you pick up your luggage, follow the signs to the ATL SkyTrain for transport to the RCC. Visit the airport Web site for specific details.
- **Public transportation:** Atlanta has a regional metro system called MARTA (Metropolitan Atlanta Rapid Transit Authority, www.itsmarta.com), and it is by far the cheapest form of transit to and from the airport. To ride the train or bus, you will need to purchase a stored-value Breeze Card, which can be purchased for $1 at the MARTA Ride Store inside the Airport Station (located near the baggage claim area in the domestic terminal), from machines in MARTA stations, or from many retail outlets. You simply use cash to add value to the card and tap it at the MARTA station entry points for service. A trip downtown will take approximately 15–20 minutes and will cost $2.50. Hours of operation can be found on the MARTA Web site. Trip planning can be easily accomplished using the MARTA iPhone or Android app or the Web site. There is no access to the CSEC site via MARTA. For more information, check out this user-friendly guide: www.itsmarta.com/uploadedFiles/Using_Marta/How_to_ride_MARTA/RookiesGuide2013.pdf.

CSEC Center Location

The Atlanta CSEC center is located a few minutes to the south of the Hartsfield-Jackson airport, about 0.25 mile/0.4 km east of the intersection of West Fayetteville Road and Phoenix Boulevard. The V-shaped brown brick building that houses the CSEC center should be visible from the I-285 highway. The center is on the fifth floor, and plenty of free parking is available.

Where to Stay

The following list includes a few hotels located close to the test site as well as a youth hostel in the area. Most are located just outside the airport, but there are some highways around, so plan your walk carefully. Remember to ask hotels about their USMLE deals, listed on the AAMC Web site (marked with an asterisk below).

- ***Country Inn & Suites Atlanta Airport South ($$):** 5100 West Fayetteville Road (0.7 mile/1.1 km away); 770-991-1099. Just around the corner from the CSEC center, making it very convenient.
- ***Best Western Hotel & Suites Airport South ($$):** 1556 Phoenix Boulevard (about 0.7 mile/1.1 km away); 770-996-5800.
- ***Comfort Inn & Suites Airport South ($):** 2450 Old National Parkway (about 1.5 miles/2.4 km away); 404-684-9898.
- ***Sheraton Gateway Atlanta Airport ($$):** 1900 Sullivan Road (2.0 miles/3.2 km away); 770-997-1100.
- ***Hilton Garden Inn Atlanta Airport/Millenium Center ($$):** 2301 Sullivan Road (3.3 miles/5.3 km away); 404-766-0303.
- **Atlanta International Hostel ($):** 223 Ponce de Leon Avenue Northeast (14 miles/22.5 km away); 404-875-9449. A cheaper option with plenty of nightlife. A bit farther away from the CSEC center, but only a few blocks away from the MARTA North Avenue station.

Where to Eat and Play

Atlanta has amazing Southern food. Take advantage of this and enjoy some of our favorites:

- **The Varsity ($):** 61 North Avenue Northwest, Downtown; 404-881-1706. The world's largest drive-in restaurant, the Varsity is an Atlanta icon that has been serving burgers and hot dogs since 1928.
- **Sweet Auburn Curb Market ($):** 209 Edgewood Avenue Southeast, Downtown; 404-659-1665. A historic market with stalls that feature fresh produce and hot meals. Includes many small ethnic restaurants as well.
- **Fat Matt's Rib Shack ($):** 1811 Piedmont Avenue Northeast, Midtown; 404-607-1622. An Atlanta hot spot serving up Southern-style barbecue and playing live blues music every night.

What to See

Atlanta has much to see and do. Here are just a few places to consider seeing while you're in town:

- **Georgia Aquarium:** The world's largest aquarium, with more than 8.5 million gallons of water and 100,000 species of sea life.
- **World of Coca-Cola:** Come and celebrate the original home of this sugary drink in historic Piedmont Park.
- **Underground Atlanta:** A mall located under the streets in the Five Points neighborhood.

- **Sweet Auburn District:** Home to the Martin Luther King, Jr., National Historic Site.

For more information, check out:

- www.lonelyplanet.com/worldguide/usa/atlanta/
- www.atlanta.net

CHICAGO ("THE WINDY CITY")

Clinical Skills Evaluation Collaboration Center
8501 West Higgins Road, Suite 600
Chicago, IL 60631

Located on the shores of Lake Michigan, Chicago is the principal financial and cultural center of the Midwest and is currently the third-largest city in the United States. Chicago is known for its gangster lore, blues clubs, and biting cold winters. With plenty of history, shopping, and culture, today's Windy City is bursting with life, so be sure to enjoy your stay!

Getting There

- **Air:** Chicago has two major airports. The larger is O'Hare International Airport (ORD), which is about 20 miles/32.2 km northwest of downtown but only 5 miles/8 km from the CSEC center. The other is Chicago Midway Airport (MDW), located about 12 miles/19.3 km southwest of downtown and roughly 20 miles/32.2 km from the testing center. Both have easy public transportation within the city, but O'Hare may be more convenient given its closer proximity to the testing site.
- **Ground:**
  - Greyhound, 5800 North Cumberland Avenue (www.greyhound.com): The Chicago Cumberland Avenue Greyhound bus terminal is just a few blocks away from the CSEC center and is the closest of the six bus terminals in Chicago.
  - Amtrak, Canal Street between Adams and Jackson Boulevards (www.amtrak.com): The main train hub in Chicago is at downtown Union Station. This is a good choice, but you'll have to take public transportation or a taxi to get to the test site. The Chicago Transport Authority Blue Line runs to Cumberland Station from Union Station, taking you very close to the CSEC center.

Getting Around When You Arrive

- **Shuttles:** Most nearby hotels offer free shuttle service to and from the airport. You can also use either of the airport shuttle services. Schedules and up-to-date fares and booking are available online:
  - Continental Airport Express (www.airportexpress.com): 888-284-3826
  - Omega Airport Shuttle (www.omegashuttle.com): 773-734-6688

- **Taxis:** As in any big city, taxis are usually the most direct way to get around Chicago. They cost roughly $30–$40 from O'Hare to downtown and about $10 from O'Hare to the CSEC center:
  - American United: 773-248-7600
  - Des Plaines Cab Service: 847-826-8424
  - Flash Cab: 773-561-4444
  - Yellow Cab: 312-829-4222
- **Rental cars:** Rental car companies at O'Hare offer free shuttle service from the arrival terminal to the rental car site.
- **Public transportation:** Ride the famous Chicago "L," an easy-to-use and cheap light-rail system, or take a Chicago Transit Authority bus. Both the CSEC center and O'Hare are on the "L" Blue Line, and both connect to downtown. For the CSEC center, you'll want Cumberland Station (5800 North Cumberland Avenue). Single-ride fares are $2.25; multiple-day passes are also available. Fares are available at all stations. Check out fares and schedules online at www.transitchicago.com.

CSEC Center Location

The exam center is located on the northwest side of Chicago, about 15 miles/24.1 km from downtown and just 5 miles/8 km east of O'Hare along I-90 (Kennedy Expressway). From Cumberland Station, the CSEC center is a quick 0.8-mile/1.3-km walk or cab ride to the north over the highway. The CSEC center is located within the First Midwest Bank Building. There should be plenty of free parking at the site. **Note for drivers:** The signs in the visitor lot indicate one-hour-only parking. This does **not** apply to Step 2 CS examinees, so you are still free to park there. You may park in the visitor lot for the duration of the exam, but do not park in spaces reserved for other tenants, such as First Midwest Bank, Chicago Title, or Westwood College.

Where to Stay

The following hotels are good options near the testing center. Remember to ask hotels about their USMLE deals, listed on the AAMC Web site (marked with an asterisk below). If you have a car, you can also check out some of the hotels a bit farther west along I-90. You'll probably get a cheaper rate if you're willing to make a commute on the morning of the test.

- *Marriott Chicago O'Hare ($$$):** 8535 West Higgins Road (0.02 mile/0.03 km away); 773-693-4444. Right next door to the testing center!
- *SpringHill Suites Chicago O'Hare ($$):** 8101 West Higgins Road (0.04 mile/0.6 km away); 773-867-0000.
- *Renaissance Chicago O'Hare Suites ($$$):** 8500 West Bryn Mawr Avenue (0.7 mile/1.2 km away); 773-380-9600.
- *Holiday Inn Chicago O'Hare ($$):** 5615 North Cumberland Avenue (0.8 mile/1.3 km away); 773-693-5800. Very close to the Cumberland Blue Line stop.
- *Crown Plaza Chicago O'Hare ($$):** 5440 North River Road (2.1 miles/4.5 km away); 847-671-6350.

- ■ ***Sheraton Chicago O'Hare:** 6501 North Manheim Road (2.8 miles/3.3 km away); 847-699-6300.
- ■ **Hostelling International Chicago ($):** 24 East Congress Parkway (15 miles/24.1 km away); 312-360-0300. This large hostel is located downtown, about 15 miles/24.1 km from the testing center, so plan at least an hour to make the trip on the Blue Line.

Where to Eat and Play

Chicago has hundreds of amazing restaurants of all varieties; here are just a few.

- ■ **Giordano's Famous Chicago Pizza ($$):** 135 East Lake Street; 312-616-1200. Chicago is the town for pizza, and Giordano's delivers some of the best. There are branches all over the city, so find the one that works for you. This is likely to be the best and most filling meal you've had in a while.
- ■ **Café Spiaggia ($$):** 980 North Michigan Avenue; 312-280-2750. Try lunch at the café. This relaxed restaurant is just next door to the world-famous Italian restaurant Spiaggia, which is known to be a favorite of the Obamas.
- ■ **Blue Chicago ($$):** 736 North Clark Street; 312-642-6261. Check out one of Chicago's world-famous blues clubs, perhaps after you're done with the test.

What to See

Don't miss the sights of this amazing city just because you're staying near the airport and the testing center. After you're done taking the exam, think about booking a late flight and jumping on the "L" for an afternoon downtown.

- ■ **Willis Tower:** Visit the Skydeck for amazing views from the second-tallest building in North America.
- ■ **Navy Pier:** Features museums, shops, restaurants, and even a Ferris wheel on the shore of Lake Michigan.
- ■ **Magnificent Mile:** The heart of the city, with upscale shopping and fantastic restaurants running along Michigan Avenue.

For more information, check out:

- ■ www.lonelyplanet.com/worldguide/usa/chicago/
- ■ www.choosechicago.com
- ■ www.cityofchicago.org/tourism

HOUSTON ("SPACE CITY")

Clinical Skills Evaluation Collaboration Center
400 North Sam Houston Parkway, Suite 700
Houston, TX 77060

Houston was founded in 1836 on land near the Buffalo Bayou and was named after Sam Houston, then the president of the Republic of Texas. Today, Houston is one of the largest cities in the United States and is home to many major energy companies in addition to a substantial portion of the biomedical and aeronautical industries. It also boasts one of the best art festivals in the country, the Bayou City Art Festival, held here every spring and fall. Enjoy the show!

Getting There

- **Air:** Houston has two major airports: George Bush Intercontinental (IAH) and Hobby Airport (HOU). IAH is the larger of the two and is much closer to the CSEC center (8 miles/12.9 km); HOU is smaller and farther away (27 miles/43.5 km).
- **Ground:**
  - Greyhound, 2121 Main Street (www.greyhound.com): Houston has a terminal downtown. Outside the station, there are plenty of taxis available. A ride to your hotel should take about 30 minutes.
  - Amtrak, 902 Washington Avenue (www.amtrak.com): Houston is on the Sunset Limited line, which runs all the way from Louisiana to California.

Getting Around When You Arrive

- **Shuttles:** Most hotels around the CSEC center offer free shuttle service. If your hotel doesn't provide service, check out SuperShuttle (www.supershuttle.com): 713-523-8888.
- **Taxis:** A number of taxi companies operate in Houston; below are just a few ($20–$40 to the CSEC center from the airport):
  - Liberty Cab: 713-695-6700
  - Square Deal Cab: 713-659-5105
  - United Cab: 713-699-0000
  - Yellow Cab: 713-236-1111
- **Rental cars:** Multiple rental car companies are available at the Consolidated Rental Car Facility (CRCF) at the Bush Intercontinental Airport. Check the list on the airport Web site. Follow the signs in the arrival terminal and you will see white and maroon buses that will take you to the CRCF. Check the USMLE Web site for driving directions.
- **Public transportation:** If you're really adventurous, try Houston's Metro, which includes bus routes and light rail (www.ridemetro.org). Lines 102, 56, and 86 serve the area around the airport, the CSEC center, and hotels. Buses run every 10–45 minutes, depending on the route and time of day. Visit the Web site for a trip planner, which will help you figure out the details.

CSEC Center Location

The CSEC center is located on the north side of Houston in a large office building at the intersection of Imperial Valley Drive and Beltway East Access Road. There is a parking garage with a large "400" on the side that is visible from the street. You'll see McDonald's and Arby's restaurants across the street. Free parking is available in the attached garage.

Where to Stay

The following hotels are located around the test site. You can walk from most, although the sidewalks aren't great. Remember to ask hotels about their USMLE deals, listed on the AAMC Web site (marked with an asterisk below).

- ***Baymont Inn & Suites ($):** 502 North Sam Houston Parkway East (0.2 mile/0.3 km away); 281-820-2101. The Baymont gets high marks for cleanliness and service and is a great value.
- ***Park Inn Houston North ($):** 500 North Sam Houston Parkway East (0.2 mile/0.3 km away); 281-931-0101.
- **Venetian Inn & Suites ($):** 6 North Sam Houston Parkway East (0.5 mile/0.8 km away); 281-447-6888. Cheap with good service, but there is no shuttle from the airport.
- ***Hyatt Place Houston/Greenspoint ($$):** 300 Ronan Park Place (0.7 mile/1.1 km away); 281-820-6060. The Hyatt is a good deal, is close to the CSEC center, and is well recommended.
- ***Super 8 IAH West/Greenspoint ($):** 1230 North Sam Houston Parkway East (1.8 miles/2.9 km away); 281-987-7100.
- ***Comfort Inn Greenspoint ($$):** 12701 North Freeway (1.9 miles/3.1 km away); 281-875-2000.
- ***Holiday Inn Houston Intercontinental Airport ($$):** 15222 JFK Boulevard (4.3 miles/6.9 km away); 281-449-2311.
- ***Sheraton North Houston at George Bush Intercontinental ($$):** 15700 JFK Boulevard (4.5 miles/7.2 km away); 281-442-5100.
- **Houston International Hostel ($):** 5302 Crawford Street (18 miles/28.9 km away); 713-523-1009. The hostel is very cheap ($15/night in a dormitory) and is located about 30 minutes away from the CSEC center.

Where to Eat and Play

Houston has cuisine from all around the world but is especially well known for its Latin American fare. The restaurants we've listed aren't necessarily close to the test center, but we thought it might be fun for you to get out!

- **Américas ($$$):** 2040 West Gray Street, 832-200-1492. Américas serves Central and South American cuisine with flair.
- **Spanish Village Restaurant ($$):** 4720 Almeda Road; 713-523-2861. A restaurant that has been serving "Tex-Mex" food since 1953. Try their delicious margaritas.
- **Dry Creek Café ($):** 544 Yale Street; 713-426-2313. Relaxing and fun. Go for one of their "Bad Ass" burgers.

What to See

If your exam is over by early afternoon, you might have some extra time to enjoy the sights and sounds of Houston.

- **Theater district:** Located downtown with five great venues. Check out Bayou Place, with its many theaters, bars, and restaurants.

- **Museum district:** Located downtown near Rice University, with many museums and parks. It would be a shame to pass up the John C. Freeman Weather Museum.
- **Sports:** Check out an Astros (www.astros.com) or Rockets (www.rockets.com) game while you're there.

For more information, check out:

- www.visithoustontexas.com
- www.lonelyplanet.com/destinations/north_america/houston

LOS ANGELES ("THE CITY OF ANGELS")

Clinical Skills Evaluation Collaboration Center
100 North Sepulveda Boulevard, 13th Floor
El Segundo, CA 90245

Los Angeles is one of the best-known cities in the United States and is rich in cultural and ethnic diversity. One of its most notable attractions, of course, is Hollywood, the hub of the U.S. motion picture industry. L.A. is also home to some amazing cultural sites, such as the Kodak Theatre, the Walt Disney Concert Hall, and all your favorite actors. Take in some stargazing while you're in town!

Getting There

- **Air:** Los Angeles is served by one major airport, Los Angeles International (LAX). It is one of the busiest airports in the world and is located only about 3 miles/4.8 km from the CSEC center.
- **Ground:**
  - Greyhound, 1716 East 7th Street (www.greyhound.com): L.A. has a terminal near downtown. Plenty of taxis are available outside the station. A ride to your hotel should take about 30 minutes.
  - Amtrak, 800 North Alameda Street (www.amtrak.com): L.A. is on multiple rail routes that connect it to cities like New Orleans, Chicago, and Seattle.

Getting Around When You Arrive

- **Shuttles:** Many hotels around the CSEC center offer free shuttle service from LAX. If your hotel doesn't provide such service, check out the following:
  - SuperShuttle (www.supershuttle.com): 800-258-3826
  - Prime Time Shuttle (www.primetimeshuttle.com): 800-733-8267
- **Taxis:** A number of taxi companies operate in L.A.; below are just a few ($10–$15 from the airport to the CSEC center):
  - Beverly Hills Cab: 310-273-6611
  - Independent Taxi Owners Association: 800-521-9294
  - L.A. Taxi/United Checker Cab: 213-627-7000
- **Rental cars:** Multiple rental car companies (nearly 40!) are available in the area. These include Advantage, Alamo, Avis, Dollar, Enterprise, Hertz, and National.

For a full list of rental companies, visit www.lawa.org/lax and see "Ground Transportation."

- **Public transportation:** Despite its reputation, L.A. does have public transportation, and the CSEC center is not far from rail and bus stops. There is also a free shuttle from LAX to the Aviation station on the Green Line, a rail line that is just two stops away from the El Segundo/Nash station. The Green Line runs every 7–15 minutes during rush hour. Get off at the El Segundo/Nash station, walk west on El Segundo Boulevard (0.5 mile/0.8 km) toward the park on the south side of El Segundo, and make a right on North Sepulveda Boulevard. The hotels listed are also generally within walking distance of the stop. You can find more information and a Metro trip planner on the public transportation Web site, www.metro.net.

CSEC Center Location

The CSEC center is located on the west side of L.A., only a few miles from LAX and about 20 miles/32.2 km from downtown. It is situated at the corner of North Sepulveda and El Segundo Boulevards. You'll see a series of large office towers; turn in the first driveway marked "Pacific Corporate Towers." Follow the signs to get to visitors' parking ($9/day).

Where to Stay

The following hotels are situated around the test site. You can walk from most, although not all have great walking routes. Remember to ask hotels about their USMLE deals, listed on the AAMC Web site (marked with an asterisk below).

- ***Residence Inn El Segundo ($$):** 2135 East El Segundo Boulevard (0.4 mile/0.6 km away); 310-333-0888. Great, quiet rooms and a good complimentary breakfast.
- ***Hacienda Hotel ($$):** 525 North Sepulveda Boulevard (0.4 mile/0.6 km away); 310-615-0015. A convenient 10-minute walk to the CSEC center. An older but decent choice—just be prepared for small elevators.
- ***Doubletree Hotel Los Angeles International Airport ($$):** 1985 East Grand Avenue (0.6 mile/1 km away); 310-322-0999. The Doubletree is routinely recommended by guests for its comfortable beds, clean rooms, and complimentary warm chocolate chip cookies.
- **Travelodge LAX South ($$):** 1804 East Sycamore Avenue (0.9 mile/1.4 km away); 310-615-1073. An acceptable budget option, but service can be spotty.
- ***Hilton Garden Inn El Segundo ($$):** 2100 East Mariposa Avenue (0.9 mile/1.4 km away); 310-726-0100.
- ***Sheraton Gateway Los Angeles ($$):** 6101 West Century Boulevard (2.3 miles/3.7 km away); 310-642-1111.
- **USA Hostels Hollywood ($):** 1624 Schrader Boulevard (24 miles/38.6 km away); 323-462-3777. This hostel is very cheap ($30–$80/night) and is about 30 minutes away from the center by car if traffic is normal. It's fun but loud, so if you plan on staying here, be sure to bring earplugs.

Where to Eat and Play

L.A. is one of the most ethnically diverse cities in the world, so you can find food for almost every taste. Here are just a few of our favorites:

- **Paradise Cove Beach Café ($$):** 28128 Pacific Coast Highway, Malibu; 310-457-2503. Situated off Pacific Coast Highway, this seaside restaurant offers a variety of fare, including great hamburgers and steaks. Hang out with the locals and enjoy a great meal on the beach.
- **WoodSpoon ($):** 107 West Ninth Street; 213-629-1765. Located in downtown L.A., this unassuming restaurant serves up Brazilian fare. Grilled plates come with rice, beans, plantains, and collard greens. Simple and delicious.
- **Medusa Lounge ($$$):** 3211 Beverly Boulevard; 213-382-5723. An exciting place to get dinner and enjoy the nightly DJs. Offers great beers, sushi, duck, and bratwurst. You'll have to see it to believe it.

What to See

If your exam is over by early afternoon, you might have some extra time to see a bit of L.A. As the locals say, L.A. is very "spread out," so the sights aren't always easy to reach without a car, but it's worth a try.

- **Hollywood:** Enjoy a stroll down Hollywood Boulevard and the Walk of Fame. If you don't have a car, you can ride the Metro Rail, but remember that this will take some time. From the test center, take the Green Line to the Blue Line and transfer to the Red Line. Exit at the Hollywood/Highland station.
- **Venice Beach:** Only 15 minutes away. Take in some of the uniqueness of L.A. with attractions like Muscle Beach and the area's renowned street performers!

For more information, check out:

- www.latourist.com
- www.laweekly.com

PHILADELPHIA ("THE CITY OF BROTHERLY LOVE")

Clinical Skills Evaluation Collaboration Center
3624 Market Street, 3rd Floor
Philadelphia, PA 19104

Philadelphia is a great city that is steeped in U.S. history. It was a nexus of political activity during the American Revolution, serving as the site of the First and Second Continental Congresses, and there is a wealth of places you can visit to soak it all up. Today, Philadelphia is thriving, boasting the fifth-largest metro area in the country. While you're in town, check out Independence Hall, where the Declaration of Independence was first signed on July 4, 1776. And be sure to eat a Philly cheesesteak!

Getting There

- **Air:** Philadelphia is served by one major airport, Philadelphia International Airport (PHL). It serves flights from all around the country and the world. PHL is located about 10 miles/16.1 km from the CSEC center.
- **Ground:**
  - Greyhound, 1001 Filbert Street (www.greyhound.com): The Greyhound terminal is located near the downtown area. Plenty of taxis are available outside the station. A ride to your hotel should take about five minutes.
  - Peter Pan Bus Lines, 1001 Filbert Street (www.peterpanbus.com): This bus line is located at the same address as Greyhound.
  - Amtrak, 30th and 2955 Market Street (www.amtrak.com): Philadelphia is on multiple Amtrak lines, including the high-speed Acela line, which connects Boston, New York, Philadelphia, and Washington, DC. Other lines connect Philadelphia to the South and the Midwest.

Getting Around When You Arrive

- **Shuttles:** There is limited shuttle service from the airport, but one does cover the area: Lady Liberty Company (www.ladylibertyshuttle.com): 215-724-8888.
- **Taxis:** A number of taxi companies operate in the city; below are just a few ($28.50 flat rate from the airport to downtown):
  - Liberty Cab: 215-389-8000
  - Olde City Taxi Coach Association: 215-338-0838
  - PHL Taxi: 800-936-5111
  - Yellow Cab: 215-333-3333
  - Quaker City Cab: 215-728-8000
- **Rental cars:** Multiple rental car companies are available. Follow directions at the airport to Zone 2 outside the baggage claim area for car pickup.
- **Public transportation:** Philadelphia has an extensive public transportation network, called SEPTA (www.septa.org). Buses and a high-speed rail line connect to the airport. Although the rail line is more expensive, it is easier to use. The Airport rail line (R1) costs an $8 (cash-only) one-way fare and connects all the terminals to the 30th Street station, which is six blocks from the testing center—or you can transfer to the Market-Frankford line and take it to 34th and Market Street, which is just two blocks from the testing center. Multiple-use passes are available. Fares within the city vary depending on the destination and payment method (cash vs. tokens). See the Web site for more information.

CSEC Center Location

The CSEC center is located downtown, near the University of Pennsylvania campus. It can be found near the intersection of Market and 36th Streets. There is a parking lot right across the street ($14/day).

Where to Stay

The following hotels are within walking distance of the test site. Since the CSEC center is downtown, these hotels are fairly expensive. Remember to ask hotels about their USMLE deals, listed on the AAMC Web site (marked below by an asterisk).

- ***Sheraton Philadelphia University City ($$):** 3549 Chestnut Street (two blocks away); 215-387-8000. Well recommended and one of the only moderately priced hotels close by.
- **Hilton Inn at Penn ($$$):** 3600 Sansom Street (0.2 mile/0.3 km away); 215-222-0200. Located on the University of Pennsylvania's campus, this hotel is close but expensive.
- ***Cornerstone Bed and Breakfast ($$):** 3300 Baring Street (0.6 mile/1 km away); 215-387-6065. This B&B is a wonderful place to stay. The breakfasts are delicious.
- ***Best Western Center City Hotel ($$):** 501 North 22nd Street (1.7 miles/2.7 km away); 215-568-8300.
- **Rodeway Inn Philadelphia ($$):** 1208 Walnut Street (2.1 miles/3.8 km away); 215-546-7000. An acceptable budget option but not walkable. You can, however, ride the Market-Frankford line from City Hall to the 34th Street station.
- **Apple Hostels of Philadelphia ($):** 32 South Bank Street (2.8 miles/4.5 km away); 877-275-1971. This hostel offers both dorm-style and private rooms and is very well recommended. It is located just a block from the Market-Frankford line, so you can take the rail line to the 34th Street station and walk to the CSEC center.

Where to Eat and Play

Philadelphia is a great city with a variety of great restaurants. Here are a few of the best:

- **Geno's Steaks/Pat's King of Steaks ($):** 1219 South 9th Street; 215-389-0659/215-468-1547. The Philly cheesesteak (or "hoagie"), perhaps one of the best-known foods in the country, was born here. Just remember to drop the "Philly" while you're in town. Keys to a proper order: Cheese Whiz or provolone with or without fried onion rings.
- **Audrey Claire ($$):** 276 South 20th Street; 215-731-1222. One of the best restaurants in town, located in the heart of Rittenhouse Square.
- **Tangerine ($$$):** 232 Market Street; 215-627-5116. This is one of the tastiest experiences you'll ever have. There are too many great dishes to single out just one, but try the lobster risotto or the chicken tagine.

What to See

If your exam is over by early afternoon, you are likely to have some extra time to see the sights of Philadelphia. And since the CSEC center is downtown, you're already in the heart of it.

- **Independence Hall/Liberty Bell:** Located in the block between 5th and 6th Streets and Market and Chestnut Streets, Independence Hall and the Liberty

Bell are two of the most iconic images in all of U.S. history. You may want to make a reservation beforehand (www.nps.gov/inde).

■ **Museum District:** Close by and home of the Philadelphia Museum of Art, the Franklin Institute of Science, the Philadelphia Zoo, Fairmont Park, and Eastern State Penitentiary.

For more information, check out:

■ www.philly.com
■ www.lonelyplanet.com/destinations/north_america/philadelphia

USEFUL WEB SITES

Here are a few other Web sites that you might find useful while you are planning your trip:

■ **USMLE travel site:**
http://www.usmle.org/step-2-cs/#testcenters
■ **AAMC accommodations site:**
www.aamc.org/meetings/153904/clinicalskills_mtgs_homepage_teaser.html
■ **Travel and hotel sites:**
  ▪ www.expedia.com
  ▪ www.travelocity.com
  ▪ www.orbitz.com
  ▪ www.hotwire.com
  ▪ www.hotels.com
  ▪ www.priceline.com

► **NOTES**

The Patient Encounter

INTRODUCTION

As described in Section 1, the Step 2 Clinical Skills (CS) exam consists of 12 clinical encounters with trained "standardized patients" (SPs). These encounters are designed to replicate situations commonly seen in clinics, doctors' offices, and emergency departments.

Each encounter in the Step 2 CS lasts 15 minutes. You will be given a warning when five minutes remain in the session. The 15-minute period allotted for each of your interviews includes meeting the patient, taking the history, performing the physical exam, discussing your findings and plans, and answering any questions the patient might have. After that, you will have 10 minutes to summarize the patient history and physical exam and to formulate your differential diagnosis and workup plan. All this may seem overwhelming, but it need not be. This chapter will guide you through the process step by step.

Fifteen minutes should be adequate for each patient encounter as long as you budget your time wisely. The most common reasons for running out of time are as follows:

- Taking an overly detailed history
- Conducting an unnecessarily detailed physical exam
- Carrying out the encounter in a slow or disorganized fashion
- Allowing the patient to stray away from relevant topics
- Failing to adapt to or redirect challenging (eg, unresponsive, angry, crying) patients

To best manage your encounter, it is recommended that you distribute your time judiciously. A recommended timetable is as follows:

- **Doorway information** (assessing preliminary information posted on the door of each room): 10–20 seconds
- **History:** 7–8 minutes
- **Physical exam:** 3–5 minutes
- **Closure:** 2–3 minutes

Of course, this is only an approximation. In reality, each encounter is different, so some encounters will require more time for taking the history or doing the physical exam, while others will necessitate that more time be spent on closure and patient counseling. You should thus tailor your time to the demands of each case. Here are some additional time management tips:

- Do not waste valuable time looking at the clock on the wall. Use the official announcement that five minutes remain in the encounter as your only time indicator. If you have not begun to perform the physical exam by that point, you should do so.
- An organized and well-planned history is key. Stay focused on asking questions that are pertinent to the chief complaint.

- A brief and focused physical exam is also critical. There is no need to conduct a comprehensive physical exam during encounters. Remember that points may be deducted for omitting critical exam findings, but no bonus points will be given for performing low-yield maneuvers.
- One of the principal objectives of the Step CS is to evaluate your ability to communicate with patients. Make sure you leave time to discuss your management plan, and never try to save time by ignoring the patient's questions, requests, or emotional status.
- Practice is the best way to improve your performance, efficiency, and sense of timing.

Figure 2-1 illustrates the key components and desired outcomes of the clinical encounter. The following sections will guide you through each.

> *Any time saved from the patient encounter can be used to write the patient note.*

FIGURE 2-1. Overview of the Clinical Encounter

Doorway Information
Must get: Chief complaint, age, sex, and abnormal vital signs.
Leads to: Forming a hypothesis (broad differential, relevant points that should be elicited in the history, systems to examine).

History
Must get: Details of the chief complaint, associated symptoms, and any other relevant information that will help rule in or rule out each item in the differential.
Leads to: A more well-defined differential diagnosis, which will help narrow down the procedures that should be performed and the systems that should be examined in the physical exam.

Physical Exam
Must get: Evaluation of the appropriate systems to help rule in or rule out each item in the differential; any additional information on the patient's history if required.
Leads to: A final differential and an appropriate workup plan.

Closure
Explaining the findings, differential, and workup plan to the patient.
Answering the patient's questions and addressing his concerns.

DOORWAY INFORMATION

As described, you will be given a chance to review preliminary patient information, known as "doorway information," at the outset of each encounter. This information, which is posted on the door of the examination room, includes the patient's name, age, and gender; the reason for the visit; the patient's vital signs (pulse, blood pressure, temperature in both Celsius and Fahrenheit, and respiratory rate); and the task you will be called on to perform.

You should begin by reading the doorway information carefully, checking the chief complaint, and trying to organize in your mind the questions you will need to ask and the systems you will have to examine. Toward this goal, you should look for abnormalities in vital signs without trying to memorize actual numbers. Assume that these vital signs are accurate.

Remain calm and confident by reminding yourself that what you are about to encounter is a common scenario found in routine medical practice. You should also bear in mind that SPs are easier to deal with than real patients in that they are more predictable and already know what you are expected to do. Remember that a second copy of the doorway information sheet will be available on the other side of the door, so you can review that information at the end of each encounter. Note, however, that the time you spend reading the doorway information is included in the 15-minute time limitation.

Your entrance into the examination room is a critical part of the encounter. So before you enter the room, be sure to **read and commit to memory the patient's last name,** and then knock on the door. Once you have entered the examination room, ask the patient if he or she is the person identified on the door (eg, "Mr. Smith?"). You will receive credit for having done so and will not have to worry about remembering the patient's name for the remainder of the encounter. If the patient does not respond to your query, consider the possibility that there may be a change in mental status and that the SP might have been instructed not to respond to his or her name.

> *Address the patient by his or her name when you enter the room. Always make eye contact with the patient.*

After your initial entrance, you should shake hands with the patient and introduce yourself in a confident yet friendly manner (eg, "Hi, I am Dr. Morton. Nice to meet you."). You may also add something like "I would like to ask you some questions and do a physical exam." Again, make an effort to establish eye contact with the patient during this initial period.

The Patient-Centered Interview

Conducting a patient-centered interview (PCI) is an essential component of successfully completing the encounter in the Step 2 CS. The main goals of the PCI are to establish a trusting doctor-patient relationship and to ensure that the encounter centers on the patient's concerns and needs, not on the disease or the doctor.

Building a trusting relationship with the patient starts from the moment you enter the examination room. It includes the simple but essential components described previously: calling the patient by his or her name, introducing yourself, and shaking hands. Remember that these steps are not just courtesies; they set a respectful and attentive tone to the entire encounter.

The next step in conducting a PCI involves **reflective listening.** Building trust with your patient requires that you be a good listener. Therefore, start the encounter by telling the patient what your role is and then asking about his or her concerns (eg, "I was asked to see you for your chest pain; what are your concerns?"). Once you have asked the patient to state his or her concerns, listen without interrupting or interjecting your own thoughts. Encourage the patient to express these issues by using phrases such as "Is there anything else?" or "Tell me more about that." When the patient has stated all of his or her concerns, summarize them using the patient's own words as much as possible. Doing so builds trust by showing the patient that you are actively listening. In some instances it is also appropriate to express empathy, particularly if the patient is distraught, by saying something like "This must be a difficult time for you," or "I can only imagine what you are going through."

The next step in the PCI involves setting a **joint agenda with the patient.** Once you have summarized the patient's concerns, you need to prioritize them and establish a joint agenda with the patient to address them. For example, you might say to the patient, "You are concerned about chest pain, cough, and smoking. I am concerned about all these things as well. Let's start by addressing whichever of these things concerns you the most." By doing this, you will make the patient feel that he or she is an active part of the interview and that you are indeed conducting a *patient-centered* interview and not a *doctor-centered* interview.

> The interview is patient centered, not disease centered or doctor centered.

Once this is established, you can begin gathering information and developing a diagnosis (discussed in the history-taking section below).

Throughout the encounter, you should aim to **connect with the patient.** The patient is likely to express emotions such as anger, fear, sadness, and anxiety. Be alert to these emotions, and be ready to respond with **"PEARLS"** (Partnership, Empathy, Apology, Respect, Legitimization, and Support). Look for opportunities to use PEARLS in every patient encounter. Of course, you will not need to use all six PEARLS elements in each of your encounters; instead, you will likely use only one or two, depending on the nature of the case. A brief description of each PEARLS component is given below:

- **Partnership** means that you and the patient are working together to identify his or her main concerns and to come up with solutions. Phrases that help facilitate partnership include "Let's deal with this together" and "We can do this."
- **Empathy** is shown by acknowledging and showing understanding of the patient's feelings. For example, you might respond to a patient who expresses fear or anger with "That sounds hard" or "You look upset."
- **Apology** refers to taking personal responsibility when it is appropriate to do so (eg, "I'm sorry I was late" or "I'm sorry this happened to you").
- **Respect** means valuing the patient's choices, behaviors, and decisions (eg, "You have obviously worked hard on this.").

- **Legitimization** validates the patient and shows understanding of his or her feelings and choices. An example of a legitimizing statement would be something like "Many of us would be confused or upset by this situation."
- **Support** should be continually offered to the patient. You can offer support by saying something as simple as "I'll be here when you need me."

Again, the PCI is patient centered, not disease centered or doctor centered. Following these principles in the CS exam will help you establish a trusting doctor-patient relationship. From there, you can move on to making appropriate medical decisions and developing the differential diagnosis.

TAKING THE HISTORY

Your ability to take a detailed yet focused history is essential to the formulation of a differential diagnosis and workup plan. The discussion that follows will help guide you through this process in a manner that will maximize your chances of success.

Guidelines

You may take the history while standing in front of the patient or while sitting on the stool that is provided, which is usually located near the bed. You will find a sheet placed on this stool. Begin by removing the sheet and draping the patient. Do this before taking the history to make sure you get credit for doing so early on.

Don't cross your arms in front of your chest when talking to the patient, especially with the clipboard in your hands. Instead, it is best to sit down on the stool, relax, and keep the clipboard on your lap. If you decide to stand, maintain a distance of approximately two feet between yourself and the patient.

As noted, the interview as a whole should take no more than 7–8 minutes. You can start your interview by asking the patient an open-ended question such as "So what brought you to the hospital/clinic today?" or "How can I help you today?" See Figure 2-2 for an overview of the process.

Additional Tips

Once the interview has begun, be sure to maintain a professional yet friendly demeanor. You should speak clearly and slowly, and your questions should be short, well phrased, and simple. Toward that end, avoid the use of medical terms; instead, use simple words that a layperson can understand (eg, don't use the term *renal calculus*; use *kidney stone* instead). If you find yourself obliged to use a medical term that the patient may not understand, offer a quick explanation. Don't wait for the patient to ask you for the meaning of a term, or you may lose credit.

Use simple, nontechnical terminology when speaking to the patient.

If you don't understand something the patient has said, you may ask him or her to explain or repeat it (eg, "Can you please explain what you mean by that?" or "Can you please repeat what you just said?"). At the same time, do not rush the patient. Instead, give him or her ample time to respond. In interacting with the patient, you should always remember to ask questions in a neutral and nonjudgmental way.

FIGURE 2-2. History-Taking Overview

Introductions

Knock on the door.
Verify the patient's name.
Introduce yourself and shake hands.
Make eye contact.
Drape the patient and cover the legs.

What History to Get

Start with an open-ended question.
Then focus on key organ systems and:
  Frequency
  Onset
  Relieving factors
  Duration
  Precipitating factors
  Associated symptoms
  Previous episodes
  Progression

How to Get It

Avoid technical medical terms.
Show **empathy** and address any patient concerns.
Maintain good **eye contact.**
Do not interrupt or rush the patient.

Before the Physical Exam

Summarize the history.
Ask if there is anything that was not covered.
Ask if patient has any **concerns** or questions.

You should also remember not to interrupt the patient unless it is absolutely necessary. If the patient starts telling lengthy stories that are irrelevant to the chief complaint, you can interrupt politely but firmly by saying something like "Excuse me, Mr. Johnson. I understand how important those issues are for you, but I'd like to ask you some additional questions about your current problem." You can also redirect the conversation by summarizing what the patient has told you thus far and then move to the next step (eg, "So as I understand it, your abdominal pains are infrequent, last a short time, and are always in the middle of your belly. Now tell me about . . .").

It is critical to summarize what the patient has told you, not only to verify that you have understood him but also to ensure that you receive credit. You need to use this summary technique no more than once during the encounter in order to get credit, but you may use it more often if you consider it necessary. It is recommended, however, that you give a summary (1) after you have finished taking the history and before you start examining the patient, or (2) just after you have finished examining the

Summarizing key facts for the patient will earn you credit.

Look for nonverbal clues.

patient and before you give him your medical opinion. In either case, your summary should include only the points that are relevant to the patient's chief complaint.

Minor transitions may also be used during the history. For example, when you want to move from the history of present illness (HPI) to the patient's past medical history or social and sexual history, you can say something like "I need to ask you some questions about your health in the past," or "I'd like to ask you a few questions about your lifestyle and personal habits."

To ensure that you stay on track in gathering information, you will also need to watch the patient carefully, paying attention to his or her every word, move, or sign. Remember that clinical encounters are staged, so it is uncommon for something to occur for no reason. Although accidents do happen (for example, an SP once started to hiccup inadvertently), an SP will most likely cough in an encounter because he or she is intending to depict bronchitis, not because of an involuntary reflex.

By the same logic, you should address every sign you see in the patient (eg, "You look sad; do you know the reason?" or "You look concerned; is there anything that is making you worry?"). If your patient is coughing, ask about the cough even if it isn't cited as the reason for the visit. If the patient is using a tissue, ask to see it so that you can check the color of the sputum. A spot of blood on the tissue may take you by surprise!

Finally, take brief notes throughout the interview, mainly to record relevant yet easy-to-forget pieces of information such as the duration of the chief complaint or the number of years the patient smoked. To facilitate this note taking, you will be given a clipboard with 12 blank blue sheets, one for each encounter. The extent of your note taking inside the encounter will depend on how much you trust your memory. Before you finish your interview and move to the physical exam, you may ask the patient something like "Is there anything else you would like to tell me about?" or "Is there anything else you forgot to tell me about?"

Common Questions to Ask the Patient

In this section, we will cover a wide spectrum of questions that you may need to pose in the course of each of your patient interviews. This is not intended to be a complete list, nor do you have to use all the questions outlined below. Instead, be selective in choosing the questions you ask in your efforts to obtain a concise, relevant history. You should also be sure to ask only one question at a time. If you ask complex questions (eg, "Is there any redness or swelling?"), the SP will likely answer only the last question you posed. Instead, you should slow down and ask about one symptom at a time.

Opening of the encounter:
- "Mr. Jones, hello; I am Dr. Singh. It's nice to meet you. I'd like to ask you some questions and examine you today."
- "How can I help you today?"
- "What brought you to the hospital/clinic today?"
- "What made you come in today?"
- "What are your concerns?"

Pain:

- "Do you have pain?"
- "When did it start?"
- "How long have you had this pain?"
- "How long does it last?"
- "How often does it come on?"
- "Where do you feel the pain?"
- "Can you show me exactly where it is?"
- "Does the pain travel anywhere?"
- "What is the pain like?"
- "Can you describe it for me?"
- "What is the character of the pain? For example, is it sharp, burning, cramping, or pressure-like?"
- "Is it constant, or does it come and go?"
- "On a scale of 1 to 10, with 10 being the worst pain you have ever felt, how would you rate your pain?"
- "What brings the pain on?"
- "Do you know what causes the pain to start?"
- "Does anything make the pain better?"
- "Does anything make it worse?"
- "Have you had similar pain before?"

Nausea:

- "Do you feel nauseated?"
- "Do you feel sick to your stomach?"

Vomiting:

- "Did you vomit?"
- "Did you throw up?"
- "What color was the vomit?"
- "Did you see any blood in it?"

Cough:

- "Do you have a cough?"
- "When did it start?"
- "How often do you cough?"
- "During what time of day does your cough occur?"
- "Do you bring up any phlegm with your cough, or is it dry?"
- "Does anything come up when you cough?"
- "What color is it?"
- "Is there any blood in it?"
- "Can you estimate the amount of the phlegm? A teaspoon? A tablespoon? A cupful?"
- "Does anything make it better?"
- "Does anything make it worse?"

Headache:

- "Do you get headaches?"
- "Tell me about your headaches."
- "Tell me what happens before/during/after your headaches."
- "When do your headaches start?"
- "How often do you get them?"
- "When your headache starts, how long does it last?"
- "Can you show me exactly where you feel the headache?"
- "What causes the headache to start?"
- "Do you have headaches at certain times of the day?"
- "Do your headaches wake you up at night?"
- "What makes the headache worse?"
- "What makes it better?"
- "Can you describe the headache for me, please? For example, is it sharp, dull, pulsating, pounding, or pressure-like?"
- "Do you notice any change in your vision before/during/after the headaches?"
- "Do you notice any numbness or weakness before/during/after the headaches?"
- "Do you feel nauseated? Do you vomit?"
- "Do you notice any fever or stiff neck with your headaches?"

Fever:

- "Do you have a fever?"
- "Do you have chills?"
- "Do you have night sweats?"
- "How high is your fever?"

Shortness of breath:

- "Do you get short of breath?"
- "Do you get short of breath when you're climbing stairs?"
- "How many steps can you climb before you get short of breath?"
- "When did it first start?"
- "When do you feel short of breath?"
- "What makes it worse?"
- "What makes it better?"
- "Do you wake up at night short of breath?"
- "Do you have to prop yourself up on pillows to sleep at night? How many pillows do you use?"
- "Have you been wheezing?"
- "How far do you walk on level ground before you have shortness of breath?"
- "Have you noticed any swelling of your legs or ankles?"

Urinary symptoms:

- "Has there been any change in your urinary habits?"
- "Do you have any pain or burning during urination?"
- "Have you noticed any change in the color of your urine?"
- "How often do you have to urinate?"
- "Do you have to wake up at night to urinate?"

- "Do you have any difficulty urinating?"
- "Do you feel that you haven't completely emptied your bladder after urination?"
- "Do you need to strain/push during urination?"
- "Have you noticed any weakness in your stream?"
- "Have you noticed any blood in your urine?"
- "Do you feel as though you need to urinate but then very little urine comes out?"
- "Do you feel as though you have to urinate all the time?"
- "Do you feel as though you have very little time to make it to the bathroom once you feel the urge to urinate?"

Bowel symptoms:
- "Has there been any change in your bowel movements?"
- "Do you have diarrhea?"
- "Are you constipated?"
- "How long have you had diarrhea/constipation?"
- "How many bowel movements do you have per day/week?"
- "What does your stool look like?"
- "What color is your stool?"
- "Is there any mucus or blood in it?"
- "Do you feel any pain when you have a bowel movement?"
- "Did you travel recently?"
- "Do you feel as though you strain to go to the bathroom or a very small amount of feces comes out?"
- "Have you lost control of your bowels?"
- "Do you feel as though you have very little time to make it to the bathroom once you have the urge to have a bowel movement?"

Weight:
- "Have you noticed any change in your weight?"
- "How many pounds did you gain/lose?"
- "Over what period of time did it happen?"
- "Was the weight gain/loss intentional?"

Appetite:
- "How is your appetite?"
- "Has there been any change in your appetite?"
- "Are you getting full too quickly during a meal?"

Diet:
- "Has there been any change in your eating habits?"
- "What do you usually eat?"
- "Did you eat anything unusual lately?"
- "Are there any specific foods that cause these symptoms?"
- "Is there any kind of special diet that you are following?"

Sleep:
- "Do you have any problems falling asleep?"
- "Do you have any problems staying asleep?"

- "Do you have any problems waking up?"
- "Do you feel refreshed when you wake up?"
- "Do you snore?"
- "Do you feel sleepy during the day?"
- "How many hours do you sleep?"
- "Do you take any pills to help you go to sleep?"

Dizziness:

- "Do you ever feel dizzy?"
- "Tell me exactly what you mean by dizziness."
- "Did you feel the room spinning around you, or did you feel lightheaded as if you were going to pass out?"
- "Did you black out or lose consciousness?"
- "Did you notice any change in your hearing?"
- "Do your ears ring?"
- "Do you feel nauseated? Do you vomit?"
- "What causes this dizziness to happen?"
- "What makes you feel better?"

Joint pain:

- "Do you have pain in any of your joints?"
- "Have you noticed any rash with your joint pain?"
- "Is there any redness or swelling of the joint?"
- "Are you having difficulty moving the joint?"

Travel history:

- "Have you traveled recently?"
- "Did anyone else on your trip become sick?"

Past medical history:

- "Have you had this problem or anything similar before?"
- "Have you had any other major illnesses before?"
- "Do you have any other medical problems?"
- "Have you ever been hospitalized?"
- "Have you ever had a blood transfusion?"
- "Have you had any surgeries before?"
- "Have you ever had any accidents or injuries?"
- "Are you taking any medications?"
- "Are you taking any over-the-counter drugs, vitamins, or herbs?"
- "Do you have any allergies?"

Family history:

- "Does anyone in your family have a similar problem?"
- "Are your parents alive?"
- "Are they in good health?"
- "What did your mother/father die of?"
- "Are your brothers or sisters alive?"

Social history:

- "Do you smoke?"
- "How many packs a day?"
- "How long have you smoked?"
- "Do you drink alcohol?"
- "What do you drink?"
- "How much do you drink per week?"
- "Do you use any recreational drugs such as marijuana or cocaine?"
- "Which ones do you use?"
- "How often do you use them?"
- "Do you smoke or inject them?"
- "What type of work do you do?"
- "Where do you live? With whom?"
- "Tell me about your life at home."
- "Are you married?"
- "Do you have children?"
- "Do you have a lot of stressful situations on your job?"
- "Are you exposed to environmental hazards on your job?"

Alcohol history:

- "How much alcohol do you drink?"
- "Tell me about your use of alcohol."
- "Have you ever had a drinking problem?"
- "When was your last drink?"
- Administer the CAGE questionnaire:
  - "Have you ever felt a need to **cut down** on drinking?"
  - "Have you ever felt **annoyed** by criticism of your drinking?"
  - "Have you ever had **guilty** feelings about drinking?"
  - "Have you ever had a drink first thing in the morning (**'eye opener'**) to steady your nerves or get rid of a hangover?"

Sexual history:

- "I would like to ask you some questions about your sexual health and practice."
- "Are you sexually active?"
- "Do you use condoms? Always? Other contraceptives?"
- "Are you sexually active? With men, women, or both?"
- "Tell me about your sexual partner or partners."
- "How many sexual partners have you had in the past year?"
- "Do you currently have one partner or more than one?"
- "Have you ever had a sexually transmitted disease?"
- "Do you have any problems with sexual function?"
- "Do you have any problems with erections?"
- "Do you use any contraception?"
- "Have you ever been tested for HIV?"

Gynecologic/obstetric history:

- "At what age did you have your first menstrual period?"
- "How often do you get your menstrual period?"
- "How long does it last?"
- "When was the first day of your last menstrual period?"
- "Have you noticed any change in your periods?"
- "Do you have cramps?"
- "How many pads or tampons do you use per day?"
- "Have you noticed any spotting between periods?"
- "Have you ever been pregnant?"
- "How many times?"
- "How many children do you have?"
- "Have you ever had a miscarriage or an abortion?"
- "Do you have pain during intercourse?"
- "Do you have any vaginal discharge?"
- "Do you have any problems controlling your bladder?"
- "Have you had a Pap smear before?"

Pediatric history:

- "Was your pregnancy full term (40 weeks or 9 months)?"
- "Did you have routine checkups during your pregnancy? How often?"
- "Did you have any complications during your pregnancy/during your delivery/after delivery?"
- "Was an ultrasound performed during your pregnancy?"
- "Did you smoke, drink, or use drugs during your pregnancy?"
- "Was it a vaginal delivery or a C-section?"
- "Did your child have any medical problems after birth?"
- "When did your child have his first bowel movement?"

Growth and development:

- "When did your child first smile?"
- "When did your child first sit up?"
- "When did your child start crawling?"
- "When did your child start talking?"
- "When did your child start walking?"
- "When did your child learn to dress himself?"
- "When did your child start using short sentences?"

Feeding history:

- "Did you breast-feed your child?"
- "When did your child start eating solid food?"
- "How is your child's appetite?"
- "Does your child have any allergies?"
- "Is your child's formula fortified with iron?"
- "Are you giving your child pediatric multivitamins?"

Routine pediatric care:

- "Are your child's immunizations up to date?"
- "When was the date of your child's last routine checkup?"

- "Has your child had any serious illnesses?"
- "Is your child taking any medications?"
- "Has your child ever been hospitalized?"

Psychiatric history:
- "Tell me about yourself and your future goals."
- "How long have you been feeling unhappy/sad/anxious/confused?"
- "Do you have any idea what might be causing this?"
- "Would you like to share with me what made you feel this way?"
- "Do you have any friends or family members you can talk to for support?"
- "Has your appetite changed lately?"
- "Has your weight changed recently?"
- "Tell me how you spend your time/day."
- "Do you have any problems falling asleep/staying asleep/waking up?"
- "Has there been any change in your sleeping habits lately?"
- "Do you enjoy any hobbies?"
- "Do you take interest or pleasure in your daily activities?"
- "Do you have any memory problems?"
- "Do you have difficulty concentrating?"
- "Do you have hope for the future?"
- "Have you ever thought about hurting yourself or others?"
- "Do you think of killing yourself or ending your own life?"
- "Do you have a plan to end your life?"
- "Would you mind telling me about it?"
- "Do you ever see or hear things that others can't see or hear?"
- "Do you hold beliefs about yourself or the world that other people would find odd?"
- "Do you feel as if other people are trying to harm or control you?"
- "Has anyone in your family ever experienced depression?"
- "Has anyone in your family ever been diagnosed with a mental illness?"
- "Would you like to meet with a counselor to help you with your problem?"
- "Would you like to join a support group?"
- "What do you think makes you feel this way?"
- "Have you lost any interest in your social activities or relationships?"
- "Do you feel hopeless?"
- "Do you feel guilty about anything?"
- "How is your energy level?"
- "Can you still perform your daily functions or activities?"
- "Whom do you live with?"
- "How do they react to your behavior?"
- "Do you have any problems in your job?"
- "How is your performance on your job?"
- "Have you had any recent emotional or financial problems?"
- "Have you had any recent traumatic event in your family?"

Daily activities (for dementia patients):
- "Tell me about your day yesterday."
- "Do you need any help bathing/getting dressed/feeding yourself?"

- "Do you need any help going to the toilet?"
- "Do you need any help transferring from your bed to the chair?"
- "Do you ever have accidents with your urine or bowel movements?"
- "Do you ever not make it to the toilet on time?"
- "What do you need help with when you eat?"
- "Do you need any help taking your medications/using the telephone/shopping/ preparing food/cleaning your house/doing laundry/getting from place to place/ managing money?"

Abuse:

- "Are you safe at home?"
- "Is there any threat to your personal safety at home or anywhere else?"
- "Does anyone (your husband/wife/parents/boyfriend) treat you in a way that hurts you or threatens to hurt you?"
- "Can you tell me about the bruises on your arm?"

THE PHYSICAL EXAM

Guidelines

The key is a focused physical exam.

In this section, we will recommend a systematic way to perform the physical exam. You can use this method or any other system with which you feel comfortable. Regardless of the method you choose, however, it is essential that you practice until you can perform the physical exam without mistakes or hesitation.

As described earlier, the physical exam can take up to five minutes. Given that the history portion of the encounter is estimated to take 7–8 minutes, you should already have started the physical exam by the time you hear the announcement that you have five minutes remaining in the encounter. Bear in mind that there is no time for a complete physical exam. Instead, you should aim at conducting a focused exam to look for physical findings that can support the differential diagnosis you made after taking the history. See Figure 2-3 for an overview of the process.

Before you begin, you should inform the patient of the need for the physical exam. Then, don't forget to wash your hands with soap and water and dry them carefully. (You can wear gloves instead if you so choose.) While you are washing your hands, use the time to think about what you should examine and whether there is anything you neglected to ask the patient. You should then drape the patient if you have not already done so. The drape will be on the stool; unfold it and cover the patient from the waist down.

Ask permission before touching or uncovering the patient. Drape the patient appropriately.

Before you touch the patient, make sure your hands are warm (rub your hands together if they are cold). In a similar manner, rub the diaphragm of your stethoscope to warm it up before you use it. Do not auscultate or palpate through the patient's gown.

As you proceed, be sure to ask the patient's permission before you uncover any part of his or her body (eg, "Is it okay if I untie your gown to examine your chest?" or "Can I move the sheet down to examine your belly?"). You may also ask patients to uncover themselves. You should expose only the area you need to examine. Do not expose

FIGURE 2-3. Physical Exam Overview

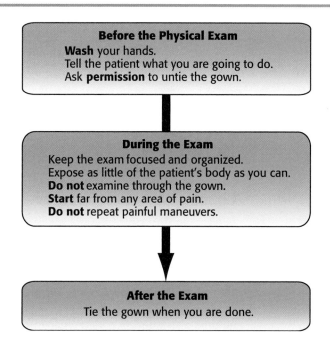

Before the Physical Exam
Wash your hands.
Tell the patient what you are going to do.
Ask **permission** to untie the gown.

During the Exam
Keep the exam focused and organized.
Expose as little of the patient's body as you can.
Do not examine through the gown.
Start far from any area of pain.
Do not repeat painful maneuvers.

After the Exam
Tie the gown when you are done.

large areas of the patient's body at once. After you have examined a given area, cover it immediately.

During the physical exam, you will be scored both for performing a given procedure and for doing so correctly. You will not get credit for conducting an extra maneuver or for examining a nonrequired system, but failure to perform a required procedure will cost you a check mark on your list. You should also bear in mind that you are not allowed to perform a corneal reflex, breast, rectal, pelvic, or genital exam. If you think any of the above-mentioned exams are indicated, you should tell the patient that you will need to do the specific exam later and then remember to add the exam to your orders on your patient note (PN). When you have concluded a given procedure, remember to say "thank you." Then explain the next step, and ask the patient for permission to proceed. The patient should always be made to feel that he or she is in control of his or her body.

In the course of the physical exam, you may ask the patient any additional questions that you feel may be pertinent to the history. It is recommended, however, that you pause the physical exam while communicating to reestablish eye contact. After the patient has answered your questions, you may resume the exam.

Finally, you should remain alert to special situations that may not unfold as they would in an ordinary physical exam. When you enter the examination room, for example, the patient may hand you an insurance form requesting that only certain systems be examined. In such cases, the patient will usually tell you that you do not need to take a history. Should this occur, simply introduce yourself, proceed to examine the systems listed, and then leave the room. No PN is required under such circumstances; instead, you are required only to fill out the form the patient gave you

> Not every patient will require an interview and a physical exam.

with the appropriate findings. In such encounters, emphasis will be placed on the correct performance of the physical exam maneuvers and on professional and appropriate interaction with the patient.

Physical Exam Review

The following is a review of the steps involved in the examination of each of the body's main systems. First, however, a special note is in order about the importance of conducting a general inspection of the patient as part of the physical exam.

Much can be learned from taking the time to step back and perform a brief inspection during the patient encounter. Many students, examinees, and residents neglect this simple but crucial task because they feel rushed. You should begin the process by telling the patient what you are doing—eg, "If you don't mind, I would like to perform a general inspection." Oftentimes a bruise, a surgical scar, a bandage, or asymmetry may be overlooked because the examiner is focusing on the tree rather than the forest.

Part of the general inspection can be done when you are greeting the patient or taking a history, but it is important to devote a few seconds to formally inspect when you can best focus on the task. The time constraints of patient encounters necessitate a targeted physical exam, but this does not mean that you should omit what is arguably its most important component. For example, examination of the cardiovascular system should begin with inspection for skin color, cigarette stains, pulsations in the neck, the appearance of labored breathing, and movement of the precordium. By following the "Look, Touch, Listen" approach, you will appear thoughtful and will often be rewarded with the discovery of unique physical findings. This important lesson should remain with you deep into your career as a physician.

Included below are samples of statements that can be used during the physical exam. Remember that it is crucial to keep the patient informed of what is going on as well as to ask for consent before each step.

1. **HEENT exam:**
   - **What to say to the patient before and during the exam:**
     - "I need to examine your sinuses, so I am going to press on your forehead and cheeks. Please tell me if you feel pain anywhere."
     - "I would like to examine your eyes now."
     - "I am going to shine this light in your eyes. Can you please look at the clock on the wall?"
     - "I need to examine your ears now."
     - "Can you please open your mouth? I need to check the inside of your mouth and your throat."
   - **What to perform during the HEENT exam:**
     - Head:
       1. Inspect the head for signs of trauma and scars.
       2. Palpate the head for tenderness or abnormalities.
     - Eyes:
       1. Inspect the sclerae and conjunctivae for color and irritation.
       2. Check the pupils for symmetry and reactivity to light.

3. Check the extraocular movements of the eyes.

4. Check visual acuity with the Snellen eye chart.

5. Perform a funduscopic exam. Remember the rule "right-right-right" (ophthalmoscope in examiner's right hand—patient's right eye—examiner's right eye) and the rule "left-left-left" (ophthalmoscope in examiner's left hand—patient's left eye—examiner's left eye).

■ Ears:

1. Conduct an external ear inspection for discharge, skin changes, or masses.

2. Palpate the external ear for pain (otitis externa); do the same for the mastoid.

3. Examine the ear canal and the tympanic membrane using an otoscope. (Don't forget to use a new speculum for each patient.)

4. Conduct the Rinne and Weber tests.

■ Nose:

1. Inspect the nose.

2. Palpate the nose and sinuses.

3. Inspect the nasal turbinates and the nasal septum with a light source.

■ Mouth and throat:

1. Inspect with a light.

2. Look for mucosal ulcers, and inspect the uvula and under the tongue for masses.

2. **Cardiovascular exam:**

■ **What to say to the patient before and during the exam:**

  ■ "I need to listen to your heart."

  ■ "Can you hold your breath, please?"

  ■ "Can you sit, please?"

  ■ "Can you turn to your left side, please?"

  ■ "I am going to examine your legs to check for fluid retention. Is that okay with you?"

  ■ "I need to check the pulse in your arms and legs now."

■ **What to perform during the cardiovascular exam:**

  ■ When examining the heart, do not lift up the patient's gown. Rather, pull the gown down the shoulder, exposing only the area to be examined.

  ■ Listen to the carotids for bruits. (Classically the bell of the stethoscope is used to listen for slow, turbulent blood flow, but the diaphragm is also acceptable in this scenario.)

  ■ Look for JVD. Remember to raise the head of the bed to 45 degrees.

  ■ Palpate the chest for the PMI, retrosternal heave, and thrills.

  ■ Listen to at least two of the four cardiac areas. (Listen to the mitral area with the patient on his left side.)

  ■ Listen to the base of the heart with the patient leaning forward.

  ■ Check for pedal edema.

  ■ Check the peripheral pulses.

  ■ Advanced techniques such as pulsus paradoxus or the Valsalva maneuver are time-consuming and unlikely to provide essential information.

3. **Pulmonary exam:**
   - **What to say to the patient before and during the exam:**
     - "I need to listen to your lungs now."
     - "Can you take a deep breath for me, please?"
     - "Can you say '99' for me, please?"
     - "I am going to tap on your back to check your lungs. Is that okay with you?"
   - **What to perform during the pulmonary exam:**
     - Inspect: Examine the shape of the chest, respiratory pattern, and deformities.
     - Palpate: Look for tenderness and tactile fremitus.
     - Percuss.
     - Auscultate for egophony, wheezes, and crackles.
     - Examine both the front and the back of the chest.
     - Don't percuss or auscultate through the patient's gown.
     - Don't percuss or auscultate over the scapula.
     - Allow a full inspiration and expiration in each area of the chest.

4. **Abdominal exam:**
   - **What to say to the patient before and during the exam:**
     - "I need to examine your belly/stomach now."
     - "I am going to listen to your belly now."
     - "I am going to press on your belly. Tell me if you feel any pain or discomfort."
     - "Now I need to tap on your belly."
     - "Do you feel any pain when I press in or when I let go? Which hurts more?"
   - **What to perform during the abdominal exam:**
     - Inspect.
     - Auscultate (always auscultate before you palpate the abdomen).
     - Percuss.
     - Palpate: Start from the point that is farthest from the pain; be gentle on the painful area, and don't try to reelicit the pain. Check for rebound tenderness, CVA tenderness, the obturator sign, the psoas sign, and Murphy's sign.
     - Check the liver span.

5. **Neurologic exam:**
   - **What to say to the patient before and during the exam—mini-mental status exam questions:**
     - "I would like to ask you some questions to test your orientation."
     - "I would like to check your memory and concentration by asking you some questions."
     - "Can you tell me your name and age?"
     - "Do you know where you are now?"
     - "Do you know the date today?"
     - Show the patient your pen and ask, "Do you know what this is?"
     - "Now I would like to ask you some questions to check your memory."
     - "I will name three objects for you, and I want you to repeat them immediately, okay? Chair, bed, and pen." (Tests immediate memory.)

- "I will ask you to repeat the names of these three objects after a few minutes." (Tests short-term memory.)
- "Do you remember what you had for lunch yesterday?" (Tests recent memory.)
- "When did you get married?" (Tests distant memory.)
- "Now can you repeat for me the names of the three objects that I mentioned to you?" (Tests short-term memory.)
- "Are you left-handed or right-handed?"
- "I will give you a piece of paper. I want you to take the paper in your right hand, fold the paper in half, and put it on the table." (Three-step command.)
- "Now I want you to write your name on the paper."
- "I want you to count backward starting with the number 100," or "Take 7 away from 100 and tell me what number you get; then keep taking 7 away until I tell you to stop." (Tests concentration.)
- "Spell *world* forward and backward." (Tests concentration.)
- "What would you do if you saw a fire coming out of a paper basket?" (Tests judgment.)

- **What to say to the patient before and during the exam—neurologic exam questions:**
  - "I am going to check your reflexes now."
  - "I am going to test the strength of your muscles now."
  - "This is up and this is down. Tell me which direction I am moving your big toe."
  - "Can you walk across the room for me, please?"

- **What to perform during the neurologic exam:**
  - Mental status examination: Orientation, memory, concentration.
  - Cranial nerves:
    1. II: Vision.
    2. III, IV, VI: Extraocular movements.
    3. V: Facial sensation, muscles of mastication.
    4. VII: "Smile, lift your brows, close your eyes and don't let me open them."
    5. IX, X: Symmetrical palate movement, gag reflex.
    6. XI: "Shrug your shoulders."
    7. XII: "Stick out your tongue."
  - Motor system:
    1. Passive motion.
    2. Active motion: Arms—flexion ("pull in"), extension ("push out"); wrists—flexion ("push down"), extension ("pull up").
    3. Hands: "Spread your fingers apart; close your fist."
    4. Legs: Knee extension ("kick out"), knee flexion ("pull in").
    5. Ankles: "Push on the gas pedal."
  - Reflexes: Biceps, triceps, brachioradialis, patellar, Achilles, Babinski.
  - Sensory system: Sharp (pin)/dull (cotton swab), vibration, position sense.
  - Cerebellum: Finger-to-nose, heel-to-shin, rapid alternating movements, Romberg's sign, gait.
  - Meningeal signs: Neck stiffness, Kernig's sign, Brudzinski's sign.

6. **Joint exam:**
   - **What to say to the patient before and during the exam:**
     - "Tell me if you feel pain anywhere."
     - "I am going to examine your knee/ankle now."
   - **What to perform during the joint exam:**
     - Inspect and compare the joint with the opposite side.
     - Palpate and check for joint tenderness.
     - Check for joint effusion.
     - Check for crepitus.
     - Check joint range of motion both by having the patient move the joint (active) and by having the examiner move it (passive).
     - Check for warmth, swelling, and redness.
     - Check for instability.
     - Check gait.
     - For the knee: Conduct a Lachman test, an anterior drawer test, a posterior drawer test, and McMurray's test, and check the stability of the medial and lateral collateral ligaments.
     - For the shoulder: Check adduction and internal rotation, abduction and external rotation, Neer's test, Hawkins' test, the drop arm test for supraspinatus tears, and O'Brien's test.
     - For the wrist: Check for Tinel's sign, Phalen's sign, signs or symptoms of Dupuytren's contracture, and Heberden's nodes.
     - For the elbow: Check for lateral and medial epicondylitis.
     - For the hip: Check abduction, adduction, flexion, and extension.
     - For the lower back: Conduct a leg raise test.
   - **Useful scales:**
     - Reflexes (0–4), with 0 being completely areflexic:
       1: Hyporeflexia
       2: Normal reflexes
       3: Hyperreflexia
       4: Hyperreflexia plus clonus (test the ankle and the knee)
     - Strength (0–5), with 0 representing an inability to move the limb:
       1: Can move limb (wiggle toes)
       2: Can lift limb against gravity
       3: Can lift limb with one-finger resistance from the examiner
       4: Can lift limb with two-finger resistance from the examiner
       5: Has full strength
     - Pulses (0–4), with 0 representing pulselessness:
       1: Weak pulse
       2: Regular pulse
       3: Increased pulse
       4: Pounding pulse

Special Challenges During the Physical Exam

During the physical exam, you may encounter any number of special problems. The following are examples of such challenges along with potential responses to each:

- **Listening to the heart in a female patient:** You can place the stethoscope anywhere around the patient's bra and between the breasts. To auscultate or palpate the PMI, if necessary ask the patient, "Can you please lift up your breast?"
- **Examining a patient who is in severe pain:** A patient in severe pain may initially seem unapproachable, refuse the physical exam, or insist that you give him something to stop his pain. In such cases, you should first ask the patient's permission to perform the physical exam. If he refuses, gently say, "I understand that you are in severe pain, and I want to help you. The physical exam that I want to do is very important in helping determine what is causing your pain. I will be as quick and gentle as possible, and once I find the reason for your pain, I should be able to give you something to make you more comfortable."
- **Examining lesions:** If you see a scar, a mole (nevus), a psoriatic lesion, or any other skin lesion during the exam, you should mention it and ask the patient about it even if it is not related to the patient's complaint.
- **Examining bruising:** Inquire about any bruises you see on the patient's body, and think about abuse as a possible cause.
- **Running out of time:** If you don't have time for a full mini-mental status exam, at least ask patients if they know their name, where they are, and what day it is.

SP Simulation of Physical Exam Findings

It bears repeating that during the physical exam it is necessary to remain cautious and attentive, as the symptoms patients exhibit during the encounter are seldom accidental and are usually reproducible. So when you notice any positive sign, take it seriously. The following are some physical signs that may be simulated by the SP:

1. **Abdomen:**
- Abdominal tenderness: The patient feels pain when you press on his abdomen. Remember that the patient is an actor. When you palpate the area, he will feel pain where he is supposed to feel pain regardless of the amount of pressure you exert. So don't try to palpate the same area again; instead, move on, and consider the pain on palpation a positive sign.
- Abdominal rigidity: The patient will contract his abdominal muscles when you try to palpate the abdomen.
- Rebound tenderness of the abdomen.
- CVA tenderness.

2. **Chest:**
- Shortness of breath.
- Wheezing: This may often sound strange, as if the patient were whistling from his mouth.
- Decreased respiratory sounds: The patient will move his chest without really inhaling any air so that you do not hear any respiratory sounds.

- Increased fremitus: The patient will say "99" in a coarse voice, creating more fremitus than usual.

3. **Nervous system:**
- Confusion.
- Dementia.
- Extensor plantar response (Babinski's sign).
- Absent or hyperactive tendon reflexes (stroke, diabetes mellitus): Eliciting the reflex in the SP is not like doing so in a real patient, where you must try more than once to ensure that you have not missed the tendon and that your strike is strong enough. In a clinical encounter, try the reflex only once; if you don't see it, it is not there. If the patient wants to show you hyperactive DTRs, he will make sure to respond with an exaggerated jerk even to the lightest and most awkward hammer hit.
- Tremor (resting, intentional).
- Facial paralysis.
- Hemiparesis.
- Gait abnormalities.
- Ataxia.
- Chorea.
- Hearing loss.
- Tinel's sign.
- Phalen's sign.
- Nuchal rigidity.
- Kernig's sign.
- Brudzinski's sign.

4. **Eyes:**
- Visual loss (central, peripheral): In a young patient, this may be multiple sclerosis.
- Photophobia: The patient will say, "I hate the light" or "I don't feel comfortable in bright light." Dim the light to make the patient feel more comfortable.
- Lid lag.
- Nystagmus.

5. **Muscles and joints:**
- Muscle weakness.
- Rigidity.
- Spasticity.
- Parkinsonism: Shuffling gait (difficulty initiating and stopping ambulation, small steps, no swinging of the arms), resting tremor, masked facies, rare blinking, cogwheel rigidity.
- Restricted range of motion of joints.

6. **Bruits and murmurs:**
- Renal artery stenosis: A patient with hypertension who is not responding to multiple antihypertensive medications. Do not be surprised if you hear an abdominal bruit.

- Thyroid bruit.
- Carotid bruit: The patient says "Hush, hush" when you place the stethoscope over his neck.
- Heart murmur: Once you place the stethoscope on the patient's heart, you will hear him saying "Hush, hush."

7. **Skin:**
- Skin lesions: You may see artificial skin discoloration (eg, painful red spots on the shin for erythema nodosum in a patient with sarcoidosis or redness over an inflamed joint in a patient with arthritis).

8. **Real physical exam findings:**
- You may see real C-section, appendectomy, cholecystectomy, or other scars. Don't overlook them. Always inquire about any scar you see.
- You may see a real nevus (mole). Ask the patient about it and advise him to check it routinely and report any change in it.
- You may see real skin lesions, such as pityriasis rosea in a Christmas-tree pattern, seborrheic dermatitis of the scalp, or acne vulgaris.
- When you listen to a patient's heart, don't be surprised to hear a real heart murmur.
- A patient with a sore throat may present with enlarged tonsils.

CLOSURE

Finishing the history and the physical exam does not mean that the patient encounter is over. To the contrary, closure is a critical part of the encounter.

The first thing you should bear in mind is that each patient encounter can be viewed as embodying one or more key questions. Most of these questions are simple and straightforward, but others may be considerably more complex. These questions should be addressed during closure.

As an example, if a patient's chief complaint is chest pain, the question that the case embodies is, What is causing the chest pain? In this instance, closure should include the formulation of a differential diagnosis consisting of the most likely causes of the patient's chest pain along with their associated workups. By contrast, if the patient has a history of diabetes mellitus and is presenting for follow-up, the case is posing two questions: First, is the patient's diabetes well controlled? And second, is the patient experiencing complications such as diabetic retinopathy or nephropathy? Here, both questions should be addressed, and the workup should aim to determine whether the diabetes is well controlled (HbA_{1c}) as well as to look for complications such as nephropathy (urine microalbuminuria).

To cite another example, if the patient is presenting following a rape, the case is posing the following questions: Are there any physical injuries? Psychological injuries? Any signs of STDs? Any signs of pregnancy? Closure should include answers to all of these questions along with a suitable workup for each.

From a broader perspective, you are expected to do several things during closure (see Figure 2-4):

- Make a transition to mark the end of your encounter.
- Summarize the chief complaint and the HPI if you have not already done so before the physical exam.
- Summarize your findings from the physical exam.
- Give your impression of the patient's clinical condition and most likely diagnosis.
- Suggest a diagnostic workup.
- Answer any questions the patient might have.
- Address the patient's concerns.
- Check to see if the patient has any more questions.
- Leave the room.

To transition into the closure, you should begin by saying something like "Thank you for letting me examine you, Mrs. Jones. Now I would like to sit down with you and give you my impression." You should then tell the patient about the possible differential diagnoses (keep to a maximum of three) and explain the meaning of any complicated medical terms you might use. You might also point out the organ or system that you think is involved and explain a simple mechanism underlying the disease. You should not, however, give the patient a definitive diagnosis at this time. Instead, tell him that you still need to run some tests to establish the final diagnosis. In some cases there will actually be no final diagnosis; instead, the case will be constructed in such a way as to be a mixture of signs and symptoms that can be construed to indicate any number of diseases.

During closure, almost every patient will have at least one challenging question to which you must respond (eg, "Do you think I have cancer, doctor?" or "Am I going to

> Leave a few minutes for closure to summarize key points to the patient.

FIGURE 2-4. Closure Overview

Counseling
Briefly summarize the history and physical findings.
Briefly discuss the diagnostic possibilities.
Do **not** give a definitive diagnosis.
Briefly explain the planned diagnostic workup.
Avoid complicated medical terms.
Ask if the patient has any questions or concerns.

Handling Challenging Questions or Concerns
Be honest but diplomatic.
Avoid giving false reassurances.

Before Leaving
Tell the patient that you will meet again with test results.
Shake the patient's hand and say goodbye.

get better?"). In answering these questions, be honest yet diplomatic. Essentially, being honest with the patient means not giving false reassurances such as "I am sure you will be cured after a week of antibiotics," or "Don't worry, I am sure it is not cancer." What you might say instead is, "Well, I cannot exclude the possibility of cancer at this point. We need to do additional testing. Regardless of the final diagnosis, however, I want to assure you that I will be available for any support you need."

If you do not know the answer to a patient's question, you should state as much. See the end of this section for examples of challenging questions patients might pose along with potential responses to each.

During closure, you should also explain to the patient the diagnostic tests you are planning to order. In doing so, you should again use nontechnical terms—for example, "We need to run some blood tests to check the function of your liver and kidneys," or "You need to have a chest x-ray and a CT scan of the head." You might further explain the latter by saying, "The CT scan is a form of x-ray imaging that gives us clear images of sections of the body." You should then add, "After we get the results of those tests, we will meet again to discuss them in detail, along with the final diagnosis and the treatment plan." Finally, you should conclude by asking the patient if he or she still has any questions.

If you find you are running out of time, do not compromise the closure. If time constraints dictate that you choose between a thorough physical exam and an appropriate closure, give priority to the execution of a proper closure.

Before you leave the room, you can finish your encounter by looking the patient in the eye and saying something like "Okay, Mr. Jones, I'll contact you when I have your test results. It was nice meeting you." You may then shake the patient's hand and leave the room. You are allowed to leave the room as soon as you think you have completed the encounter. Once you have left the encounter room, you will not be allowed to go back inside.

> You cannot reenter the examination room once you leave.

HOW TO INTERACT WITH SPECIAL PATIENTS

The following guidelines can help you deal with atypical patients and uncommon encounters.

- **The anxious patient:** Encourage the patient to talk about his feelings. Ask about the things that are causing the anxiety. Offer reasonable reassurance. You can also validate the patient's response by saying, "Any patient in your situation might react in this way, but I want you to know that I will do my best to address your concerns."
- **The angry patient:** Stay calm and don't be frightened. Remember that the patient is not really angry; he is just acting angry to test your response. Let the patient express his feelings, and inquire about the reason for his anger. You should also address the patient's anger in a reasonable way. For example, if the patient is complaining that he has been waiting for a long time, you can validate his feelings by saying, "I can understand why anyone in your situation might become

angry under the same circumstances. I am sorry I am late. The clinic is crowded, and many patients had appointments before yours." Reassure the patient that now that it is his turn, you will focus on his case and take care of him.

- **The crying patient:** Allow the crying patient to express his feelings, and wait in silence for him to finish. Offer him a tissue, and show him empathy in your facial expressions. You may also place your hand lightly on the patient's shoulder or arm and say something like "I know that you feel sad. Would you like to tell me about it?" Don't worry about time constraints in such cases. Remember that the patient is an actor and that his crying is timed. He will allow you to continue the encounter in peace if you respond correctly.

- **The patient who is in pain:** Show compassion for the patient's pain. Say something like "I know that you are in pain." Offer help by asking, "Is there anything I can do for you to help you feel more comfortable?" Do not repeat painful maneuvers. If the patient does not allow you to touch his abdomen because of the severe pain he is experiencing, tell him, "I know that you are in pain, and I want to help you. I need to examine you, though, to be able to locate the source of your pain and give you the right treatment." Reassure the patient by saying, "I will be as quick and gentle as possible."

- **The patient who can't pay for the tests or for treatment:** Reassure the patient by saying, "Not having enough money doesn't mean you can't get treatment." You might also add, "We will refer you to a social worker who can help you find resources."

- **The patient who refuses to answer your question or let you examine him:** Explain to the patient why the question or the physical exam is important. Tell him that they are necessary to allow you to understand the problem and arrive at a diagnosis. If the patient still refuses to cooperate, skip the question or the maneuver, and document his refusal and your counseling in the PN.

- **The hard-of-hearing patient:** Face the patient directly to allow him to read your lips. Speak slowly, and do not cover your mouth. Use gestures to reinforce your words. If the patient has unilateral hearing loss, sit close to the hearing side. If necessary, you can also write your question down and show it to him.

- **The patient who doesn't know the names of his medications or is taking medications whose names *you* don't recognize:** Ask the patient if he has a prescription or a written list of the medications he is currently taking. If not, ask him to bring this list with him as soon as possible.

- **The confused patient:** If the patient is forgetful or confused, he will likely answer your questions by stating, "I don't know" or "I can't remember." In such cases, ask your patient, "Is there anyone who does know about your problem, and may I contact him to obtain some information?"

- **The phone encounter:** The Step 2 CS may include a telephone encounter. As with other encounters, patient information will be posted on the door before you enter the examination room. Once you are inside, sit in front of the desk with the telephone, and push the speaker button by the yellow dot to be connected to the patient. Do not dial any numbers or touch any other buttons. You are permitted to call the SP only once. Treat this like a normal encounter and gather all the necessary information. To end the call, press the speaker button above the yellow dot. As in the pediatric encounter, there is no physical exam, so leave this portion of the PN blank.

CHALLENGING QUESTIONS AND SITUATIONS

During your encounters, every patient will ask you one or more challenging questions. Your reactions and answers to these questions will be scored. Such questions may be explicit ones that you are expected to answer directly, or they may take the form of indirect comments or statements that must be properly addressed to reveal an underlying concern. When answering the challenging questions, try to remember the following guidelines:

- Be honest and diplomatic.
- Before addressing the patient's issue, you might restate the issue back to the patient to let him know that you understand.
- Don't give the patient a final diagnosis. Instead, tell the patient about your initial impressions and about the workup you have in mind to reach a conclusive diagnosis.
- Do not give false reassurances.
- If you do not know the answer to the patient's question, tell him so, but reassure him that you will attempt to find out.

Do not give the patient a definitive diagnosis.

The following are examples of challenging questions:

Confidentiality/Ethical Issues

Challenging Question	Possible Response
A patient who needs emergent surgery says, "I can't afford the cost of staying in the hospital. I have no insurance. Just give me something to relieve the pain and I will leave."	"I know that you are concerned about medical costs, but your life will be in danger if you don't have surgery. Let our social workers help you with the cost issues."
"Should I tell my sexual partner about my venereal disease?"	"Yes. There is a chance that you have already transmitted the disease to your partner, or he or she may be the source of your infection. The most important step is to have both of you evaluated and appropriately treated."
An anxious patient who you suspect has been abused asks, "Why are you asking me these questions?"	"I am primarily concerned about your safety, and my goal is to make sure that you are in a safe environment and that you are not a victim of abuse."

Challenging Question	Possible Response
A patient recently diagnosed with HIV asks, "Do I have to tell my wife?"	"I know that it's difficult, but doing so will allow you and your wife to take the appropriate precautions to treat and prevent the transmission of the disease."
A doorway information sheet indicates that the patient is Mr. Smith and that he presents with dizziness, but when you enter the room, you find a female patient.	Begin by saying, "Excuse me, Mrs. Smith?" When the patient responds, "No, I am Mrs. Black," you can say, "Oh, I think the nurse must have given me the wrong chart. Hello, Mrs. Black. What is your problem?" You can then go on to discuss the patient's presenting complaint, but remember that the vital signs listed on the doorway information sheet are those of a different patient, so you will need to take the patient's vitals during the physical exam.
A female patient attempts to seduce her male physician by saying, "Doctor, do you have time to have dinner with me at my place?"	"I am sorry, but that would be inappropriate, since you are my patient, and it would not be permissible in the context of a doctor-patient relationship."

Patient Belief/Behavioral Issues

Challenging Question	Possible Response
An elderly male patient says, "I think that it is normal at my age to have this problem" (impotence) or "I am just getting old."	"Not necessarily. Age may play a role in the change you are experiencing in your sexual function, but your problem may have other causes that we should rule out, such as certain diseases (hypertension, diabetes) or medications. We also have medications that may improve your sexual function."
"I read in a journal that the treatment for this disease is herbal compounds."	"Herbal medicines have been suggested for many diseases. However, their safety and efficacy may not always be clear-cut. Let me know the name of the herbal medicine and I will check into its potential treatment role for this disease."

Challenging Question	Possible Response
"I am afraid of surgery."	"I understand your feelings. It is normal and very common to have these feelings before surgery. Is there anything specific that you are concerned about?"
A patient who has a serious problem (unstable angina, colon cancer) asks, "I want to go on a trip with my wife. Can we do the tests after I come back?"	"I know that you don't want to put off your trip, but you may have a serious problem that may benefit from early diagnosis and management. Also, it is possible that you could suffer complications from this problem while you are on vacation if we do not effectively deal with it before you leave."
"I did not understand your question, doctor. Could you repeat it, please?"	Repeat the question slowly. If the patient still doesn't comprehend the question, ask if there is any specific word he failed to understand, and try to explain it or use a simpler one.
"What is a bronchoscopy?" (MRI, CT, x-ray, colonoscopy)	Explain the meaning of the term using simple words. For example, "Bronchoscopy is using a thin tube connected to a camera to look into your respiratory airways and parts of your lungs," or "An MRI is a machine that uses a large magnet to obtain detailed pictures of your brain or body."
"What do you mean by *workup?*"	"It means all the tests that we are going to do to help us make the final diagnosis."
A patient who is late in seeking medical advice asks, "Do you think it is too late for recovery?"	"It is never too late to seek help, and I am glad you made the decision to pursue treatment options with me. We will do our best to help you, but next time I want you to feel comfortable coming to me as soon as you feel you might have a problem."

Challenging Question	Possible Response
A patient with pleuritic chest pain asks, "Is this a heart attack? Am I going to die?"	"On the basis of your history and my clinical exam and findings, my suspicion for a heart attack is low. It is more likely that inflammation of the membranes surrounding your lungs is causing your pain, and this is usually not a life-threatening condition. However, we still need to do some tests to confirm the diagnosis and rule out heart problems."
"Do you think I have colon cancer?" "Do you think I have a brain tumor?" "Do I have endometrial cancer?"	If the patient's chief complaint is consistent with his question, tell him, "That is one of the possibilities, but there are other explanations for your symptoms that we should rule out before making a diagnosis." However, if the chief complaint is inconsistent with his concern, say, "It is unlikely for a patient with your complaint to have this type of cancer, but if you are really worried about it, I will try to rule it out by conducting some tests."
"My friend told me that you are a very fine doctor. That's why I came to you to refill my prescription."	"I am happy that you came to see me, but since this is your first visit, I can't give you a refill without first reviewing your history to better understand your need for this medication. I will also need to do a physical exam and perhaps order some tests."
"Will my insurance cover the expenses of this test?"	"I'm not sure, but I can refer you to a social worker who does have that information. If necessary, I can write a note to your insurance company indicating the importance of this test."
A person who wants to return to work at a job that can negatively affect his health asks, "Can I go back to work?"	"Unfortunately, work may actually worsen your condition. Therefore, I would prefer that you stay at home for now. I can write a letter to your employer explaining your situation."
"Do you think that this tumor I have could become malignant?"	"We really won't know until we remove the tumor and get a pathology report on it. We will keep you informed as soon as we get any information."

Challenging Question	Possible Response
"Since I stopped smoking, I have gained weight. I want to go back to smoking in order to lose weight."	"There are healthier ways to lose weight than smoking, such as exercise and diet. Smoking will increase your risk of cancer, heart problems, and lung disease."
A patient with a shoulder injury says, "I am afraid of losing my job if my shoulder doesn't get better."	"We will do our best to help you recover from your shoulder injury. With your permission, I will communicate the situation to your employer."
"Will I ever feel better, doctor?"	The answer depends on the prognosis of the disease and can vary from "Yes, most people with this disease are completely cured" to "A complete cure may be difficult to achieve at this advanced stage, but we have a lot to offer in terms of controlling the symptoms and improving your quality of life."
A person who has a broken arm asks, "Doctor, do you think I will be able to move my arm again like before?"	"It is hard to tell right now, but these fractures usually heal well, and with physical therapy you should regain the normal range of motion of your arm."
"I think that life is full of misery. Why do we have to live?"	"Life can certainly be challenging. Is there something in particular that is bothering you? Have you thought of ending your life?" You can then continue screening for depression.
A young man with multiple sexual partners and a recent-onset skin rash says, "I am afraid that I might have AIDS."	"Having multiple sexual partners does put you at risk for STDs, including HIV infection, but this rash may be due to many other causes. I agree that we should do an HIV test on you in addition to a few other tests."
A patient who needs hospitalization says, "My child is at home alone. I have to leave now."	"I understand your concern about your child, but right now staying in the hospital is in your best interests. With your permission, one of our social workers can make some phone calls to arrange for child care."

Challenging Question	Possible Response
"Do you have anything that will make me feel better? Please, doctor, I am in pain."	"I know that you are in pain, but I need to know what is causing your pain in order to give you the appropriate treatment. After I am done with my evaluation, we can decide on the best way to help manage your pain."
A patient you believe is pretending (malingering) says, "Please, doctor, I need a week off from work. The pain in my back is terrible."	"I know that you are uncomfortable, but after examining you, I don't find disability significant enough to keep you out of work. I plan to prescribe pain medication and exercises, but a large part of your recovery will involve continuing your normal daily activities."
"Stop asking me all these stupid questions and just give me something for this pain."	"I know that you're in pain, but I need to determine the cause of the pain if I am to give you the right treatment. After I am done with my evaluation, we will give you the appropriate treatment."
"So what's the plan, doctor?"	"After we get the results of your tests, we will meet again. At that time, I will try to answer any questions you might have."
"Do you think I will need surgery?"	"I will try to manage your problem medically, but if that doesn't work, you may need surgery. We can see how things go and then try to make that decision together in the future."
A female patient has only one sexual partner, and she is diagnosed with an STD. She asks you, "Could he possibly be cheating on me?"	"You most likely contracted this infection from your partner. It would be best to talk to your partner about this to clear things up. He needs to be tested and treated, or else you risk becoming reinfected."
A patient is shouting angrily, "Where have you been, doctor? I have been waiting here for the whole day."	"I am sorry you had to wait so long. We had some unexpected delays this morning. But I'm here now, and I will focus on you and your concerns and spend as much time with you as you need."

Challenging Question	Possible Response
A bleeding patient reacts angrily when you mention that she may need a blood transfusion and states that she refuses to be given any blood.	First determine the reason for the patient's reaction, and then respond accordingly. For example: ■ "I have a religious objection to receiving blood." You say, "I respect your opinion and will make sure you do not receive a blood transfusion until we have explained its benefits and have obtained your permission." ■ "My brother died following a blood transfusion, and I'm afraid the same thing will happen to me." You respond, "I am sorry for your loss, but I want you to know that it is rare for patients to die as a result of a blood transfusion. I will take all necessary precautions before giving you any blood." ■ "I have had a blood transfusion before, and I had a serious reaction." You say, "Thank you for telling me this. I will determine the reason you had this reaction and will treat it before giving you any blood."
A patient is wandering around the room ignoring you and is not answering your questions or listening to you.	"I can only imagine how any patient in your situation might feel, but if you don't speak with me, I will not be able to help you. So please have a seat and help me determine what is going on."
A patient repeats your questions before answering them.	The patient may have a problem understanding or hearing you. Ask the patient why he is repeating your questions. If the problem relates to comprehension and you are not a native English speaker, ask him to stop you whenever he has difficulty understanding what you are saying. If the problem relates to his hearing, draw closer to him.

Challenging Question	Possible Response
A patient asks you a question while you are washing your hands.	Tell him that you would like to give him your full attention. Make sure you establish eye contact when you respond to him.
During the encounter, a patient asks if he can take a bathroom break.	Do not force him to stay in the examination room, and offer him your assistance.
A patient wants to be examined by another doctor.	Find out why. You can say, "It is certainly your right to choose another provider, but I want to reassure you that I am a well-qualified doctor and can help you if you will allow me to address your concerns. If we still need another opinion, I would be happy to help you select another doctor who might be a better fit for you."
A patient with auditory hallucinations asks if you think he is crazy.	"There is no such diagnosis in medicine. I think you may have a physiological problem or a disorder in your mood, and there is a good chance that we can address it."
A patient asks you if his previous doctor made a mistake in his treatment.	If the patient indicates that the previous doctor's findings or treatment differs from yours, you can say, "Although your previous doctor may have had a different treatment plan, we have to do our best to make a decision on the basis of what we have discovered today. I'm sorry if this may be frustrating for you, but we want to give you the treatment that we think will be most effective and safe for you."
A patient wants to know how to deal with a son who is gay.	Ask the patient if she or her son has any guilt or confused feelings about his sexual orientation. If so, encourage her or her son to seek guidance from a mental health professional.

Disease-Related Issues

Challenging Question	Possible Response
An educated 58-year-old woman asks, "I read in a scientific journal that hormonal replacement therapy causes breast cancer. What do you think of that, doctor?"	"Studies do in fact show a slight increase in the risk of developing breast cancer after more than four years of combination estrogen and progesterone use for hormonal replacement therapy. The current recommendations are to use hormonal replacement therapy solely for the relief of hot flashes, and only for a limited period of time."
"Did I have a stroke?"	"We don't know yet. Your symptoms could be explained by a small stroke, but we need to wait for the results of your MRI."
"Do I have lung cancer?"	"We do not know at this point. It is a possibility, but we still need to do additional tests."
An African American man with sickle cell anemia presents with back and chest pain and says, "Please, doctor, I need some Demerol now or I will die from pain."	"I know that you are in pain, but I need to ask you a few questions first to better understand your pain. Then we will get you some medications to help ease your discomfort."
A patient with symptoms of a common cold says, "I think I need antibiotics, doctor."	"It appears that you have a common cold, which is caused by a virus. Antibiotics do not treat viruses, and they have adverse effects that could make you feel worse. We should focus on treating your symptoms."
"My mother had breast cancer. What is the possibility that I will have breast cancer too?"	"You are at increased risk, but it doesn't mean that you will get it. There are other risk factors that need to be considered, and regular screening tests will be very important."
A 55-year-old man says, "I had a colonoscopy six years ago, and they removed a polyp. Do you think that I have to repeat the colonoscopy?"	"Yes, it should be repeated. We need to screen for more polyps, and in this way we hope to prevent the development of colon cancer."
A patient with headache or confusion asks, "Do you think I have Alzheimer's disease?"	"I don't know. Alzheimer's disease is one of several possible causes that we will investigate."

Challenging Question	Possible Response
"Can I get pregnant even though my tubes are tied?"	"There is no single contraceptive method that is 100% effective. The risk of pregnancy after tubal ligation is less than 1%, but on rare occasions it does occur. There is a high probability that if such a pregnancy occurs, it will be an ectopic pregnancy."
A woman who is in her first trimester of pregnancy with vaginal bleeding asks, "Do you think I am losing my pregnancy?"	"Bleeding early in pregnancy increases your risk of losing the pregnancy, but at the same time, most women who have bleeding carry the pregnancy to term without any problems."
"My brother has colon cancer. What are the chances that I will develop colon cancer as well?"	"Some types of colon cancer are hereditary, and you may be at increased risk, but it doesn't mean that you will get colon cancer for sure. I need to get more information about your personal and family history to determine your level of risk."
A patient with palpitations says, "My mother had a thyroid problem; do you think it is my thyroid?"	"That is a possibility. We always check a thyroid blood test, but we will also consider many other possible causes of palpitations."
"Obesity runs in my family. Do you think that is why I am overweight?"	"Genes play an important role in obesity, but lifestyle, diet, and daily habits are also major factors influencing weight. These factors can be used in a way that can help you lose weight."
A young man with dysuria asks, "Do you think I have an STD?"	"That is one of the possibilities. We will do some cultures to find out for sure, and we will also check a urine sample, since your symptoms may be due to a urinary tract infection."
"I am drinking a lot of water, doctor. What do you think the reason is?"	"This may simply be due to dehydration, or it may be a sign of a disease such as diabetes. We need to do some tests to determine the cause."
A patient with COPD asks, "Will I get better if I stop smoking?"	"Most patients with your condition who stop smoking will experience a gradual improvement in their symptoms, in addition to a significantly decreased risk of lung cancer in the future."

Challenging Question	Possible Response
A patient with possible appendicitis asks for a cup of water to drink.	"I am sorry, but I can't give you anything to eat or drink right now. You may need emergent surgery, and anesthesia is much safer if your stomach is completely empty."
A patient with infectious mononucleosis asks, "Can I go back to school, doctor?"	"Now that you have recovered from the acute stage of the disease, you can go back to school, but I want you to stay away from any strenuous exercise or contact sports, as you may rupture your spleen."
A very thin patient with weight loss asks, "Doctor, do you think I am too fat?"	Even if the patient appears to be thin, do not state as much. Instead, respond by saying, "I cannot tell right now. First I need to determine your height and weight and calculate your body mass index, and then we can let the numbers tell us if you are at a healthy weight."

COUNSELING

During at least one of your encounters, you are likely to find a patient who smokes, drinks, or has another habit that may adversely affect his or her health. Although these behaviors may or may not be relevant to your primary diagnosis, it is important that they be addressed in a rapid yet caring manner. Here are some examples of conversations you might have with your patient. Try to practice saying some of these aloud, making sure to change them to fit your personality and style.

The Smoker

Examinee: Do you smoke cigarettes?
SP: Yes, I have smoked one pack a day for 20 years.
Examinee: Have you ever tried to quit?
SP: Yes, but it never works.
Examinee: Well, I strongly recommend that you quit smoking. Smoking is a major cause of cancer and heart disease. Are you interested in trying to quit now?
SP1: Yes. (If the answer is "no," see below.)
Examinee: I would be happy to help you quit smoking. We have many tools to help you do that, and I will be with you every step of the way. Let's set up an appointment for two weeks from today, and we can get started on it then. Is that okay with you?
SP2: No, I don't want to quit.
Examinee: I understand that you aren't ready to quit smoking yet, but I want to assure you that whenever you are ready, I will be here to help you.

> The **5 A's** are recommended guidelines to help patients quit smoking.
> 1. **Ask** the patient about tobacco use.
> 2. **Advise** him or her to quit.
> 3. **Assess** the patient's willingness to make an attempt to quit.
> 4. **Assist** in the quit attempt.
> 5. **Arrange** for follow-up.

The Alcoholic

Examinee: How many drinks do you have in a week?

SP: It is hard to say. Too many.

Examinee: How many drinks do you have per day?

SP: Oh, maybe five or so.

Examinee: Have you ever felt the need to **cut down** on your drinking? Have you ever felt **annoyed** by criticism of your drinking? Have you ever felt **guilty** about drinking? Have you ever had to take a morning **eye opener?** (In general, any patient who admits to many drinks per week should receive the CAGE questionnaire. A "yes" answer to any one of the questions in the CAGE questionnaire should raise suspicion and prompt further questioning.)

SP: All of these things apply.

Examinee: I am concerned about your drinking. It can lead to liver disease, cause problems with bleeding, or even predispose you to early dementia. Are you interested in cutting down or quitting?

SP1: Yes. (If the answer is "no," see below.)

Examinee: I am glad you want to quit. A variety of resources are available to help you quit drinking, and I would like to discuss them with you. Let's make an appointment later this week to talk about your options. In the meantime, I have printed up a list of resources, and my office assistant will bring it to you.

SP2: No, I am not ready to quit.

Examinee: I realize that you are not ready to quit drinking, but I want to assure you that if you do decide to try, I will be here for you. Okay?

The Patient with Uncontrolled Diabetes

Examinee: According to your blood glucose readings, your diabetes is not adequately controlled. How often do you forget to take your medication? (Check for noncompliance.)

SP1: Taking all these medications just gets so confusing. I can never remember when to take them.

Examinee: Diabetes can certainly be a challenge to manage. Do you have someone who could help you take your medications? If not, we have a social worker who might be able to arrange for a nurse to come to your home. Are you interested in that?

SP2: I have been taking my medications exactly as they were prescribed to me.

Examinee: Tell me about your diet. (Check for dietary management.)

SP2: I eat regular meals, but I really like to drink soda. Diet soda tastes awful!

Examinee: You must be very careful about your sugar consumption. It is prudent to keep your blood sugar within normal limits. Persistently high blood sugar can cause damage to your eyes, kidneys, and nerves. You will also be at higher risk for developing infections, heart attacks, and strokes. Fortunately, we have a diabetes educator who may be able to help you. Are you interested in meeting with her?

The Sexually Promiscuous Patient

Examinee: Are you currently in a sexual relationship?

SP: Yes.

Examinee: Can you tell me about your partner or partners?

SP: I have a girlfriend, but I also see a couple of other women on the side.

Examinee: Are you using any type of protection with these partners?

SP: My girlfriend is on the pill, but I don't use anything with the other women I see.

Examinee: Condoms reduce the risk of sexually transmitted infections. Do you think you could try to use condoms?

SP: I tried them, but I just don't like them.

Examinee: I understand that you may not like to use condoms, but I am concerned that you may be putting yourself and your partners at risk for STDs. You could contract HIV, herpes, chlamydia, or any of a number of other STDs. The complications of these diseases include infertility, painful infections, or even death. If anyone with whom you have sexual contact has an STD, you could share it among all of them, including your girlfriend. I hope you will consider using a condom in the future. Do you have any questions for me?

The Depressed Patient

Examinee: Do you have problems **sleeping?** Have you lost **interest** in things that used to interest you? Do you feel **guilty?** Do you lack your usual **energy?** Has it been difficult for you to **concentrate?** Has your **appetite** changed? Have you felt agitated or lethargic? (**Psychomotor** disturbances.) Do you feel as though you want to hurt yourself or someone else or commit **suicide?** (If you suspect depression, ask the questions posed in the mnemonic **SIG E CAPS.**)

SP: (Answers affirmatively to many of these questions.)

Examinee: You answered "yes" to many of my questions. I believe that you may be depressed. Depression is a common disease; it is due to a chemical imbalance in the brain that causes many of the symptoms you have described to me. Fortunately, we have medications that can help; however, these medications work best when they are combined with counseling. I can write you a prescription and also give you a referral to see a therapist. Is this something you are interested in?

The Patient with an STD (Trichomoniasis)

Examinee: Your symptoms are due to an infection called trichomoniasis, a sexually transmitted infection that has been given to you by one of your sexual partners. This infection responds well to treatment with antibiotics and is curable. You will also need to be tested for all other STDs. Your partner needs to be informed and treated as well; otherwise you will be at risk of contracting the infection again. Unless you use condoms, you should avoid sexual intercourse until you finish the course of antibiotics and your partner gets treated.

THE PATIENT NOTE

Once you have completed an encounter, your final task will be to compose a PN (see Figure 2-5 for a detailed overview of the clinical encounter and PN). Toward this goal, you will find a desk with a computer on it immediately outside the encounter

FIGURE 2-5. Summary Overview of the Patient Encounter

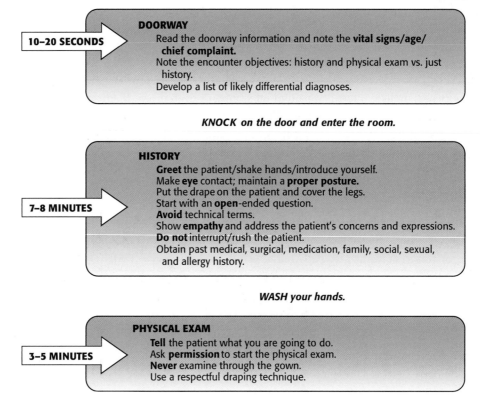

First announcement:
"Examinees, you may enter the room."

10–20 SECONDS

DOORWAY
Read the doorway information and note the **vital signs/age/ chief complaint.**
Note the encounter objectives: history and physical exam vs. just history.
Develop a list of likely differential diagnoses.

KNOCK on the door and enter the room.

7–8 MINUTES

HISTORY
Greet the patient/shake hands/introduce yourself.
Make **eye** contact; maintain a **proper posture.**
Put the drape on the patient and cover the legs.
Start with an **open**-ended question.
Avoid technical terms.
Show **empathy** and address the patient's concerns and expressions.
Do not interrupt/rush the patient.
Obtain past medical, surgical, medication, family, social, sexual, and allergy history.

WASH your hands.

3–5 MINUTES

PHYSICAL EXAM
Tell the patient what you are going to do.
Ask **permission** to start the physical exam.
Never examine through the gown.
Use a respectful draping technique.

(continued)

room. **Remember that all examinees taking the Step 2 CS will now be required to type, not handwrite, the PN.** You will be given 10 minutes to type the PN and will be notified when two minutes remain. If you leave the encounter room before the end of the 15-minute period allotted for your patient encounter, you can devote the extra time you have to typing the PN. You are allowed to review the doorway information while you are typing the PN.

The PN screen located outside the encounter room will have your identification information and fields for History, Physical Exam, Differential Diagnosis, and Diagnostic Workup. Each field can accommodate only a certain number of characters: The character limits are 950 for History, 950 for Physical Exam, and 100 for each of the fields in Differential Diagnosis and Diagnostic Workup. One benefit of the computer note is that it allows you to delete extraneous information in favor of more pertinent portions of your note if you run out of space, so use this to your advantage, and use the space wisely.

FIGURE 2-5. Summary Overview of the Patient Encounter *(continued)*

Second announcement:
*"Examinees, you have **five minutes left** for this encounter."*
*By this time you should be **halfway** through your exam.*

2–3 MINUTES

CLOSURE
Explain your diagnostic possibilities/workups.
Avoid complicated medical terms.
Ask if the patient has any concerns.
Be prepared to handle **challenging questions.**
Avoid giving false reassurances.
Do the **counseling.**
Say goodbye, thank the patient, and leave the encounter.

Third announcement:
*"This encounter is now **finished."***

10 MINUTES

TYPED PATIENT NOTE
Document **key** CC, HPI, PMH, meds, PSH, SH, ROS, FH.
Document **key** physical findings.
Include **pertinent positives** and **negatives.**
Give up to **three** possible diagnoses with supporting history
   and physical findings.
Order up to **eight** diagnostic tests.
Do **not** consult, hospitalize, or treat the patient.
Order **rectal, pelvic, genital,** or **breast** exams if needed.

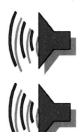

Fourth announcement:
"You have two minutes left."

Fifth announcement:
"Your time is now finished."

Before you start typing the PN, take a few seconds to review the history, including the chief complaint, how it started, its progression, and the main symptoms. Then take a deep breath and try to relax. If you get nervous and try to rush, your thoughts may become garbled, and you will risk losing the point of your story.

Note that you will not be able to render diagrams such as the neurology stick figure for reflexes. You can simulate typing the PN online at the USMLE Web site.

Writing the Patient Note

You will be required to fill out four main sections in your PN: the history, physical exam, differential diagnosis, and initial diagnostic workup.

Summarizing the history. In writing the history, be clear, direct, and concise, and avoid long and complex phrases. Make sure the history flows in a logical sequence. Also bear in mind that it is not necessary to write a detailed, all-inclusive history.

The components that should be included are as follows:

- Chief complaint (CC)
- History of present illness (HPI)
- Review of systems (ROS)
- Past medical history (PMH)
- Past surgical history (PSH)
- Social history (SH)
- Family history (FH)

When you are summarizing the history, you need to be efficient with your time. One way to save time is to make ample use of abbreviations. Train yourself to use the abbreviations that are listed in the USMLE Step 2 CS orientation materials. You will find a copy of this list on each desk. You are allowed to use any abbreviations that are commonly used in U.S. hospitals. If you are unsure of the correct abbreviation, it is better to spell out the word or phrase.

In general, two styles of writing—narrative and "bullet"—are acceptable as long as your history is both comprehensive and coherent. Two examples can be found in the candidate orientation manual, and multiple examples of both styles are included in this book's sample cases.

Outlining the physical exam. To summarize the physical exam, write a list of the systems that you examined, outlining all the relevant positive and negative findings. If you did not perform a maneuver that you think was necessary, it is better not to lie and pretend that you did. Be honest and list only the items you examined. For example, do not claim that you saw diabetic retinopathy in a patient with diabetes mellitus if you did not even get to see the eye fundus. See Figure 2-6 for some examples of how to document physical exam findings.

Developing a differential. In writing the differential, you should use three of the following tables to list your three possible diagnoses and the historical and physical exam data that support them.

Diagnosis	
History Finding(s):	**Physical Exam Finding(s):**

You are not required to list that many if two diagnoses suffice, but in general any common chief complaint will have at least three possible etiologies. It is preferable that your diagnoses be listed in order of probability, from the most to the least probable. Below each diagnosis, you need to list historical and physical findings that support why your diagnosis is likely. You do not need to list three findings for each, and in

FIGURE 2-6. Examples of How to Document Physical Exam Findings

- **HEENT:**
  - Head: Atraumatic, normocephalic.
  - Eyes: EOMI, PERRLA, normal eye fundus.
  - Nose: No nasal congestion.
  - Throat: No tonsillar erythema, exudates, or enlargement.
  - Mouth: Moist mucous membranes, good dentition, no lesions.

- **Neck:** Supple, no JVD, normal thyroid, no cervical LAD.

- **Nervous System:**
  - Mental status: Alert and oriented x 3, good concentration.
  - Cranial nerves II–XII grossly intact.
  - Motor: Strength 5/5 in all muscle groups.
  - DTRs: 2+ intact and symmetric, Babinski ⊖.
  - Sensation: Intact to sharp and dull.
  - Cerebellum: ⊖ Romberg sign, intact finger to nose.

- **Chest/Lung:**
  - Clear to auscultation bilaterally.
  - No rales, rhonchi, wheezing, or rubs.
  - No tenderness to palpation.
  - Tactile fremitus WNL.

- **Heart:**
  - PMI not displaced.
  - Regular rate and rhythm.
  - Normal S1, S2.
  - No murmurs, rubs, or gallops.

- **Abdomen:**
  - Soft, nontender, nondistended, BS ⊕, no hepatosplenomegaly.

- **Extremities:**
  - No clubbing, cyanosis, or edema.

- **Mental Status Exam:**
  - Patient speaks slowly.
  - No hostile behavior toward the interviewer.
  - Blunt affect with poor eye contact.
  - Inattentive to interviewer.
  - 3/3 registration, 3/3 recall at 3 minutes.
  - Distant memories are impaired.
  - Oriented to person, date, and place.
  - Completed three-step command.
  - Right-handed.
  - 1/5 on serial 7s.
  - Poor judgment.

some cases, such as telephone interactions, you will not have any physical exam data at all.

Specifying the initial diagnostic workup. In summarizing your workup, list a maximum of eight tests that would help confirm or rule out the diagnoses you listed on your differential. It is best to start with the "forbidden" physical exam maneuvers (eg, rectal exam, pelvic exam) if you feel that such procedures are indicated. Then state the required laboratory and radiologic tests, starting with the most simple and straightforward tests and ending with the most complex. Do not include referrals, treatments, hospitalizations, or consults, as these will not be scored.

> Tests in the diagnostic workup should be specific.

Be specific in your orders. Instead of "chem 7," "thyroid panel," or "liver function tests," you should specify "Na, K," "TSH and total T_4," and "AST and ALT." You may, however, order electrolytes. Each group of related tests (blood tests, x-rays) should be listed together.

Scoring the Patient Note

The PN will be scored by a physician on the basis of its organization, quality of information, and interpretation of data. The final score will represent the average PN score of all 10 scored encounters.

How to Prepare

The cardinal rule for preparing to write a PN is to practice, practice, and practice. Imagine that you are in the actual exam, and try to type the PN within 10 minutes. When using the cases presented in this book, try to write your PN and then compare your note with ours. Ask yourself the following questions:

- Is the history complete?
- Does it make sense?
- Are the physical exam results complete?
- Is the differential diagnosis correct?
- Are the tests correct and in the right order?

There are two styles you can use both to document the physical exam and to compose the PN. So choose a method, memorize it, and stick with it. In this book, we will give you samples of bullet-style and traditional narrative-style formats so that you can familiarize yourself with both.

If you are running out of time, start from the bottom of the PN. Write down the differential diagnosis, the tests conducted, the physical exam, and then the history and the review of systems (listing only the positives first).

Minicases

In this section, we will attempt to cover most of the clinical cases that you are likely to encounter on the Step 2 CS. The main title of each case represents a chief complaint that you may see on the doorway information sheet before you enter the examination room or a complaint that you may have to elicit from the standardized patient. After each chief complaint, key points pertinent to the history and physical exam are reviewed. Each clinical case consists of three components:

- **Presentation:** A brief clinical vignette with some pertinent positives and negatives.
- **Differential:** An appropriate differential diagnosis; the most likely diagnosis appears in boldface. The supporting history and physical findings for each diagnosis are not provided.
- **Workup:** The main diagnostic tests that should be considered for each disease. Note that the diagnostic tests in the third column are generally listed in rough order of priority. In clinical practice, many tests may be performed at the same time or not at all.

The sum of the **Differential** column will give you a wide differential diagnosis for the chief complaint, whereas the sum of the **Workup** column will give you a pool of tests from which to choose in the exam.

If you are studying by yourself, we suggest that you read the vignette and then try to figure out the diagnosis and workup. Think through the supporting history and physical findings for each diagnosis. If you are studying with a partner or in a group, we suggest that you take turns reading the vignette aloud and allow each other to figure out the differential diagnosis and workup.

HEADACHE

Key History

Onset (acute vs. chronic), location (unilateral vs. bilateral), quality (dull vs. stabbing), intensity (is it the "worst headache of their life"?), duration, timing (does it disturb sleep?), presence of associated neurologic symptoms (paresthesias, visual stigmata, weakness, numbness, ataxia, photophobia, dizziness, auras, neck stiffness); nausea/vomiting, jaw claudication, recent trauma, dental surgery, sinusitis symptoms; exacerbating factors (stress, fatigue, menses, exercise, certain foods) and alleviating factors (rest, medications); patient and family history of headache; history of trauma.

Key Physical Exam

Vital signs; inspection and palpation of entire head; ENT inspection; complete neurologic exam, including funduscopic exam.

Presentation	Differential	Workup
21 yo F presents with several episodes of throbbing left temporal pain that last for 2–3 hours. Before onset, she sees flashes of light in her right visual field and feels weakness and numbness on the right side of her body for a few minutes. Her headaches are often associated with nausea and vomiting. She has a family history of migraine.	**Migraine (complicated)** Tension headache Cluster headache Pseudotumor cerebri CNS vasculitis Partial seizure Intracranial neoplasm	CBC ESR CT—head MRI—brain LP—CSF analysis
26 yo M presents with severe right temporal headaches associated with ipsilateral rhinorrhea, eye tearing, and redness. Episodes have occurred at the same time every night for the past week and last for 45 minutes.	**Cluster headache** Migraine Tension headache Intracranial neoplasm Pseudotumor cerebri	CBC CT—head MRI—brain LP—CSF analysis ESR
65 yo F presents with severe, intermittent right temporal headache, fever, blurred vision in her right eye, and pain in her jaw when chewing.	**Temporal arteritis (giant cell arteritis)** Migraine Cluster headache Tension headache Meningitis Carotid artery dissection Pseudotumor cerebri Trigeminal neuralgia Intracranial neoplasm Temporomandibular joint (TMJ) disorder	ESR CBC CRP Temporal artery biopsy Doppler U/S—carotid MRI—brain LP—CSF analysis

Presentation	Differential	Workup
■ 30 yo F presents with frontal headache, fever, and nasal discharge. There is pain on palpation of the frontal and maxillary sinuses. She has a history of allergies.	**Sinusitis** Migraine Tension headache Meningitis Intracranial neoplasm	CBC XR—sinus CT—sinus LP—CSF analysis
■ 50 yo F presents with recurrent episodes of bilateral squeezing headaches that occur 3–4 times a week, typically toward the end of her work day. She is experiencing significant stress in her life and recently decreased her intake of caffeine.	**Tension headache** Migraine Depression Caffeine or analgesic withdrawal Hypertension Cluster headache Pseudotumor cerebri Intracranial neoplasm	CBC Electrolytes ESR CT—head LP—CSF analysis

■ 35 yo M presents with sudden severe headache, vomiting, confusion, left hemiplegia, and nuchal rigidity.	**Subarachnoid
	   hemorrhage**
	Migraine
	Meningitis/encephalitis
	Intracranial hemorrhage
	Vertebral artery dissection
	Intracranial venous
	   thrombosis
	Acute hypertension
	Intracranial neoplasm
		Noncontrast CT—head
		LP—CSF analysis
		CBC
		PT/PTT/INR
		Urine toxicology

■ 25 yo M presents with high fever, severe headache, confusion, photophobia, and nuchal rigidity.	**Meningitis**
	Migraine
	Subarachnoid hemorrhage
	Sinusitis/encephalitis
	Intracranial or epidural
	   abscess
		CBC
		CT—head
		MRI—brain
		LP—CSF analysis (cell
		   count, protein, glucose,
		   Gram stain, PCR for
		   specific pathogens,
		   culture)

■ 18 yo obese F presents with a pulsatile headache, vomiting, and blurred vision for the past 2–3 weeks. She is taking OCPs.	**Pseudotumor cerebri**
	Tension headache
	Migraine
	Cluster headache
	Meningitis
	Intracranial venous
	   thrombosis
	Intracranial neoplasm
		Urine hCG
		CBC
		CT—head
		LP—opening pressure and
		   CSF analysis

MINICASES

Presentation	Differential	Workup
■ 57 yo M c/o daily pain in the right cheek for the past month. The pain is electric and stabbing in character and occurs while he is shaving. Each episode lasts 2–4 minutes.	**Trigeminal neuralgia** Tension headache Migraine Cluster headache TMJ disorder Intracranial neoplasm	CBC ESR MRI—brain

CONFUSION/MEMORY LOSS

Key History

Must include history from family members/caregivers when available. Detailed time course of cognitive deficits (acute vs. chronic/gradual onset); associated symptoms (constitutional, incontinence, ataxia, hypothyroid symptoms, depression); screen for delirium (waxing/waning level of alertness); falls, medications (and recent medication changes); history of stroke or other atherosclerotic vascular disease, syphilis, HIV risk factors, alcohol use, or vitamin B_{12} deficiency; family history of Alzheimer's disease or other neurologic disorders.

Key Physical Exam

Vital signs; complete neurologic exam, including mini-mental status exam and gait; general physical exam, including ENT, heart, lungs, abdomen, and extremities.

Presentation	Differential	Workup
■ 81 yo M presents with progressive confusion for the past several years accompanied by forgetfulness and clumsiness. He has a history of hypertension, diabetes mellitus, and 2 strokes with residual left hemiparesis. His mental status has worsened after each stroke (stepwise decline in cognitive function).	**Vascular ("multi-infarct") dementia** Alzheimer's disease Normal pressure hydrocephalus Chronic subdural hematoma Intracranial neoplasm Depression B_{12} deficiency Neurosyphilis Hypothyroidism	CBC VDRL/RPR Serum B_{12} TSH MRI—brain CT—head LP—CSF analysis

Presentation	Differential	Workup
■ 84 yo F brought by her son c/o forgetfulness (eg, forgets phone numbers, loses her way back home) and difficulty performing some of her daily activities (eg, bathing, dressing, managing money, using the phone). The problem has progressed gradually over the past few years.	**Alzheimer's disease** Vascular dementia Depression Hypothyroidism Chronic subdural hematoma Normal pressure hydrocephalus Intracranial neoplasm B_{12} deficiency Neurosyphilis	CBC VDRL/RPR Serum B_{12} TSH MRI—brain (preferred) CT—head LP—CSF analysis
■ 72 yo M presents with memory loss, gait disturbance, and urinary incontinence for the past 6 months.	**Normal pressure hydrocephalus** Alzheimer's disease Vascular dementia Chronic subdural hematoma Intracranial neoplasm Depression B_{12} deficiency Neurosyphilis Hypothyroidism	CT—head MRI—brain LP—opening pressure and CSF analysis Serum B_{12} VDRL/RPR TSH
■ 55 yo M presents with a rapidly progressive change in mental status, inability to concentrate, and memory impairment for the past 2 months. His symptoms are associated with myoclonus, ataxia, and a startle response.	**Creutzfeldt-Jakob disease** Vascular dementia Lewy body dementia Wernicke's encephalopathy Normal pressure hydrocephalus Chronic subdural hematoma Intracranial neoplasm Depression Delirium B_{12} deficiency Neurosyphilis	CBC Electrolytes, calcium Serum B_{12} VDRL/RPR MRI—brain (preferred) CT—head EEG LP—CSF analysis Brain biopsy

MINICASES

CONFUSION/MEMORY LOSS (cont'd)

Presentation	Differential	Workup
■ 70 yo insulin-dependent diabetic M presents with episodes of confusion, dizziness, palpitations, diaphoresis, and weakness.	**Hypoglycemia** Transient ischemic attack Arrhythmia Delirium Angina	Glucose CBC Electrolytes CPK-MB, troponin Echocardiography ECG MRI—brain Doppler U/S—carotid
■ 55 yo F presents with gradual altered mental status and headache. Two weeks ago she slipped, hit her head on the ground, and lost consciousness for 2 minutes.	**Subdural hematoma** SIADH (causing hyponatremia) Creutzfeldt-Jakob disease Intracranial neoplasm	CT—head CBC Electrolytes MRI—brain LP—CSF analysis

LOSS OF VISION

Key History

Acute vs. chronic, progression, ability to see light; associated symptoms (eye pain, discharge, itching, tearing, photophobia, redness, headache, weakness, numbness, floaters, sparks); history of cardiac, rheumatic, thrombotic, autoimmune, or neurologic disorders; jaw claudication, medications, trauma.

Key Physical Exam

Vital signs; cardiovascular, HEENT, funduscopic, and neurologic exams.

Presentation	Differential	Workup
■ 73 yo M presents with acute loss of vision in his left eye, palpitations, and shortness of breath. He has a history of atrial fibrillation and cataracts in his right eye. He has no eye pain, discharge, redness, or photophobia. He has not experienced headache, weakness, or numbness.	**Retinal artery occlusion** Retinal vein occlusion Acute angle-closure glaucoma Retinal detachment Temporal arteritis (giant cell arteritis)	Fluorescein angiogram Echocardiography Doppler U/S—carotid Intraocular tonometry ESR Temporal artery biopsy CBC

DEPRESSED MOOD

Key History

Onset, duration; sleep patterns; appetite and weight change; drug and alcohol use; life stresses, excessive guilt, suicidality, social function, decreased interest (anhedonia), decreased energy, decreased concentration, psychomotor agitation or retardation; family history of mood disorders; prior episodes; medications.

Key Physical Exam

Vital signs; head and neck exam; neurologic exam; mental status exam, including documentation of appearance, behavior, speech, mood, affect, thought process, thought content, cognition (measured by the 30-point mini-mental status exam), insight, and judgment.

Presentation	Differential	Workup
68 yo M presents with a 2-month history of crying spells, excessive sleep, poor hygiene, and a 15-lb (6.8-kg) weight loss, all following his wife's death. He cannot enjoy time with his grandchildren and admits to thinking he has seen his dead wife in line at the supermarket or standing in the kitchen making dinner.	**Normal bereavement** Adjustment disorder with depressed mood Major depressive disorder with psychotic features Schizoaffective disorder Depressive disorder not otherwise specified	Physical exam TSH CBC Urine toxicology Beck Depression Inventory
42 yo F presents with a 4-week history of excessive fatigue, insomnia, and anhedonia. She states that she thinks constantly about death. She has suffered 5 similar episodes in the past, the first in her 20s, and has made 2 previous suicide attempts. She further admits to increased alcohol use in the past month.	**Major depressive disorder** Substance-induced mood disorder Dysthymic disorder	Physical exam Mental status exam Beck Depression Inventory Blood alcohol level TSH CBC Urine toxicology
26 yo F presents with a 6.5-lb (2.9-kg) weight loss in the past 2 months, accompanied by early-morning awakening, excessive guilt, and psychomotor retardation. She does not identify a trigger for the depressive episode but reports several weeks of increased energy, sexual promiscuity, irresponsible spending, and racing thoughts approximately 6 months before her presentation.	**Bipolar I disorder** Bipolar II disorder Cyclothymic disorder Major depressive disorder Schizoaffective disorder	Physical exam Mental status exam Urine toxicology

PSYCHOSIS

Key History

Positive symptoms (delusions, hallucinations, disorganized thoughts, disorganized or catatonic behavior), negative symptoms (blunted affect, social withdrawal, decreased motivation, decreased speech/thought), cognitive symptoms (disorganized speech or thought patterns, paranoia); age at first symptoms and/or hospitalization; previous psychiatric medications; alcohol and substance use.

Key Physical Exam

Vital signs; mental status exam; during physical exam, pay particular attention to general appearance (eg, poor grooming, odd or poorly fitting clothing).

Presentation	Differential	Workup
■ 19 yo M c/o receiving messages from his television set. He reports that he did not have many friends in high school. In college, he started to suspect his roommate of bugging the phone. He stopped going to classes because he felt that his professors were saying horrible things about him that no one else noticed. He rarely showered or left his room and has recently been hearing a voice from his television set telling him to "guard against the evil empire."	**Schizophrenia** Schizoid or schizotypal personality disorder Schizophreniform disorder Psychotic disorder due to a general medical condition Substance-induced psychosis Depression with psychotic features	Mental status exam Urine toxicology TSH CBC Electrolytes
■ 28 yo F c/o seeing bugs crawling on her bed for the past 2 days and hearing loud voices when she is alone in her room. She has never experienced anything similar in the past. She recently ingested an unknown substance.	**Substance-induced psychosis** Brief psychotic disorder Schizophreniform disorder Schizophrenia Psychotic disorder due to a general medical condition	Urine toxicology Mental status exam TSH CBC Electrolytes, BUN/Cr AST/ALT
■ 48 yo F presents with a 1-week history of auditory hallucinations that state, "I am worthless" and "I should kill myself." She also reports a 2-week history of weight loss, early-morning awakening, decreased motivation, and overwhelming feelings of guilt.	**Schizoaffective disorder** Mood disorder with psychotic features Schizophrenia Schizophreniform disorder Psychotic disorder due to a general medical condition	Mental status exam Beck Depression Inventory TSH CBC Electrolytes

DIZZINESS

Key History

Lightheadedness vs. vertigo, ± auditory symptoms (hearing loss, tinnitus), duration of episodes, context (occurs with positioning, following head trauma); other associated symptoms (visual disturbance, URI, nausea); neck pain or injury; medications; history of atherosclerotic vascular disease.

Key Physical Exam

Vital signs; complete neurologic exam, including Romberg test, nystagmus, tilt test (eg, Dix-Hallpike maneuver), gait, hearing, and Weber and Rinne tests; ENT exam; cardiovascular exam.

Presentation	Differential	Workup
35 yo F presents with intermittent episodes of vertigo, tinnitus, nausea, and hearing loss within the past week.	**Ménière's disease** Vestibular neuronitis Labyrinthitis Benign positional vertigo Acoustic neuroma	CBC VDRL/RPR (syphilis is a cause of Ménière's disease) MRI—brain Dix-Hallpike maneuver
55 yo F c/o dizziness for the past day. She feels faint and has severe diarrhea that started 2 days ago. She takes furosemide for hypertension.	**Orthostatic hypotension due to dehydration (diarrhea, diuretic use)** Vestibular neuronitis Labyrinthitis Benign positional vertigo Vertebrobasilar insufficiency	Orthostatic vital signs CBC Electrolytes Rectal exam, stool for occult blood Stool leukocytes
65 yo M presents with postural dizziness and unsteadiness. He has hypertension and was started on hydrochlorothiazide 2 days ago.	**Drug-induced orthostatic hypotension** Vestibular neuronitis Labyrinthitis Benign positional vertigo Brain stem or cerebellar tumor Acute renal failure	Orthostatic vital signs CBC Electrolytes Echocardiography MRI—brain
44 yo F c/o dizziness on moving her head to the left. She feels that the room is spinning around her head. A tilt test results in nystagmus and nausea.	**Benign positional vertigo** Vestibular neuronitis Labyrinthitis Ménière's disease	Dix-Hallpike maneuver MRI—brain Audiogram

Presentation	Differential	Workup
■ 55 yo F c/o dizziness that started this morning. She is nauseated and has vomited once in the past day. She had a URI 2 days ago and has experienced no hearing loss.	**Vestibular neuronitis** Labyrinthitis Ménière's disease Benign positional vertigo Vertigo associated with cervical spine disease or injury Vertebrobasilar insufficiency	CBC Electrolytes Electronystagmography MRI/MRA—brain
■ 55 yo F c/o dizziness that started this morning and of "not hearing well." She feels nauseated and has vomited once in the past day. She had a URI 2 days ago.	**Labyrinthitis** Vestibular neuronitis Ménière's disease Acoustic neuroma Vertebrobasilar insufficiency	Audiogram Electronystagmography MRI/MRA—brain

LOSS OF CONSCIOUSNESS

Key History

Presence or absence of preceding symptoms (nausea, diaphoresis, palpitations, pallor, lightheadedness), context (exertional, postural, traumatic; stressful, painful, or claustrophobic experience; dehydration); associated tongue biting or incontinence, tonic-clonic movements, prolonged confusion; dyspnea or pulmonary embolism risk factors; history of heart disease, arrhythmia, hypertension, or diabetes; alcohol and drug use.

Key Physical Exam

Vital signs, including orthostatics; complete neurologic exam; carotid and cardiac exam; lung exam; exam of the lower extremities.

Presentation	Differential	Workup
■ 26 yo M presents after falling and losing consciousness at work. He had rhythmic movements of the limbs, bit his tongue, and lost control of his bladder. He was subsequently confused after regaining consciousness (as witnessed by his colleagues).	**Generalized tonic-clonic seizure** Convulsive syncope Substance abuse/overdose Malingering Hypoglycemia	CBC Electrolytes, glucose Urine toxicology EEG MRI—brain CT—head LP—CSF analysis ECG

Presentation	Differential	Workup
■ 55 yo M c/o falling after feeling dizzy and unsteady. He experienced transient loss of consciousness. His past medical history is significant for hypertension and diabetes mellitus.	**Drug-induced orthostatic hypotension (causing syncope)** Hypoglycemia Cardiac arrhythmia Syncope (vasovagal, other causes) Stroke MI Pulmonary embolism	Orthostatic vital signs CBC Electrolytes, glucose Echocardiography CT—head ECG V/Q scan CTA—chest with IV contrast D-dimer
■ 65 yo M presents after falling and losing consciousness for a few seconds. He had no warning before passing out but recently had palpitations. His history includes a coronary artery bypass graft.	**Cardiac arrhythmia (causing syncope)** Severe aortic stenosis Syncope (other causes) Seizure Pulmonary embolism	ECG Holter monitoring CBC Electrolytes, glucose Echocardiography CT—head

NUMBNESS/WEAKNESS

Key History

Distribution (unilateral, bilateral, proximal, distal), duration, ± progression, pain (especially headache, neck or back pain); constitutional symptoms, other neurologic symptoms; history of diabetes, alcoholism, atherosclerotic vascular disease.

Key Physical Exam

Vital signs; neurologic and musculoskeletal exams; relevant vascular exam.

Presentation	Differential	Workup
■ 68 yo M presents following a 20-minute episode of slurred speech, right facial drooping and numbness, and right hand weakness. His symptoms had totally resolved by the time he got to the emergency department. He has a history of hypertension, diabetes mellitus, and heavy smoking.	**Transient ischemic attack (TIA)** Hypoglycemia Seizure Stroke Facial nerve palsy	CT—head CBC Electrolytes, glucose Fasting lipid panel ECG MRI—brain Doppler U/S—carotid Echocardiography EEG

Presentation	Differential	Workup
■ 68 yo M presents with slurred speech, right facial drooping and numbness, and right hand weakness. Babinski's sign is present on the right. He has a history of hypertension, diabetes mellitus, and heavy smoking.	**Stroke** TIA Seizure Intracranial neoplasm Subdural or epidural hematoma	CT—head CBC Electrolytes PT/PTT/INR Fasting lipid panel MRI—brain Doppler U/S—carotid Echocardiography ECG
■ 33 yo F presents with ascending loss of strength in her lower legs over the past 2 weeks. She had a recent URI.	**Guillain-Barré syndrome** Multiple sclerosis Polymyositis Myasthenia gravis Peripheral neuropathy Tumor in the vertebral canal	CBC Electrolytes CPK LP—CSF analysis MRI—spine EMG Nerve conduction studies Tensilon (edrophonium) test Serum B_{12}
■ 30 yo F presents with weakness, loss of sensation, and tingling in her left leg that started this morning. She is also experiencing right eye pain, decreased vision, and double vision. She reports feeling "electric shocks" down her spine upon flexing her head.	**Multiple sclerosis** Stroke Conversion disorder Malingering CNS tumor Neurosyphilis Syringomyelia CNS vasculitis	CBC ESR VDRL/RPR MRI—brain, spine LP—CSF analysis Retinal evoked potentials
■ 55 yo M presents with tingling and numbness in his hands and feet (glove-and-stocking distribution) for the past 2 months. He has a history of diabetes mellitus, hypertension, and alcoholism. There is decreased soft touch, vibratory, and position sense in the feet.	**Diabetic peripheral neuropathy** Alcoholic peripheral neuropathy B_{12} deficiency Hypocalcemia Hyperventilation Paraproteinemia/myeloma	HbA_{1c} ESR Calcium Serum B_{12} UA Serum and urine protein electrophoresis

MINICASES

Presentation	Differential	Workup
■ 40 yo F presents with occasional double vision and droopy eyelids at night with normalization by morning.	**Myasthenia gravis** Horner's syndrome Multiple sclerosis Intracranial neoplasm compressing CN III, IV, or VI Amyotrophic lateral sclerosis	Tensilon (edrophonium) test Serum ACh receptor antibodies CXR CT—chest MRI—brain EMG
■ 25 yo M presents with hemiparesis after a tonic-clonic seizure that resolved within a few hours.	**Todd's paralysis** TIA Stroke Complicated migraine Malingering	CBC Electrolytes EEG MRI—brain Doppler U/S—carotid
■ 56 yo obese F c/o tingling and numbness of her thumb, index finger, and middle finger for the past 5 months. Her symptoms are constant, have progressively worsened, and are relieved with rest. She works as a secretary. She has a history of fatigue and a 20-lb (9-kg) weight gain over the same period.	**Carpal tunnel syndrome secondary to hypothyroidism** Overuse injury of median nerve Medial epicondylitis	Phalen's maneuver and Tinel's sign Nerve conduction studies TSH CBC

FATIGUE AND SLEEPINESS

Key History

Duration; sleep hygiene, snoring, waking up choking/gasping, witnessed apnea; overexertion; stress, depression, or other emotional problems; lifestyle changes, shift changes at work; diet, weight changes; other constitutional symptoms; symptoms of thyroid disease; history of bleeding or anemia; medications; alcohol, caffeine, and drug use.

Key Physical Exam

Vital signs; ENT exam (conjunctival pallor, oropharynx/palate, lymphadenopathy, thyroid exam); heart, lung, abdominal, neurologic, and extremity (pallor, coolness at distal extremities) exams; consider rectal exam and occult blood testing.

Presentation	Differential	Workup
■ 40 yo F c/o feeling tired, hopeless, and worthless and of having suicidal thoughts. She lost her job and has been having fights with her husband about money.	**Depression** Adjustment disorder Hypothyroidism Anemia	CBC TSH HIV/STD testing Beck Depression Inventory

Presentation	Differential	Workup
■ 44 yo M presents with fatigue, insomnia, and nightmares about a murder that he witnessed in a mall 1 year ago. Since then, he has avoided the mall and has not gone out at night.	**Posttraumatic stress disorder** Depression Generalized anxiety disorder Psychotic or delusional disorder Hypothyroidism	CBC TSH Urine toxicology Beck Depression Inventory
■ 55 yo M presents with fatigue, weight loss, and constipation. He has a family history of colon cancer.	**Colon cancer** Hypothyroidism Renal failure Hypercalcemia Depression	Rectal exam, stool for occult blood CBC Electrolytes, BUN/Cr, calcium AST/ALT TSH Colonoscopy Barium enema CT—abdomen/pelvis
■ 40 yo F presents with fatigue, weight gain, sleepiness, cold intolerance, constipation, and dry skin.	**Hypothyroidism** Depression Diabetes Anemia	TSH, FT_3, FT_4 CBC Fasting glucose HbA_{1c}
■ 50 yo obese F presents with fatigue and daytime sleepiness. She snores heavily and naps 3–4 times per day but never feels refreshed. She also has hypertension.	**Obstructive sleep apnea** Hypothyroidism Chronic fatigue syndrome Narcolepsy	CBC TSH Nocturnal pulse oximetry Polysomnography ECG
■ 20 yo M presents with fatigue, thirst, increased appetite, and polyuria.	**Diabetes mellitus** Atypical depression Primary polydipsia Diabetes insipidus	Glucose tolerance test HbA_{1c} UA CBC Electrolytes, BUN/Cr, glucose
■ 35 yo M policeman c/o feeling tired and sleepy during the day. He changed to the night shift last week.	**Shift work sleep disorder** Sleep apnea Depression Anemia	CBC Nocturnal pulse oximetry Polysomnography

NIGHT SWEATS

Key History

Onset, duration, severity, frequency, timing, patterns (escalating, waxing, waning), precipitants (eg, food, medications); associated diseases and symptoms (fever, recent URIs, associated cough, hemoptysis, pleuritic chest pain); lymphadenopathy, rash, malaise, weight loss, itching, diarrhea, nausea/vomiting, early satiety, anorexia; presence of significant risk factors (eg, traveling to areas with endemic infections, IV drug use); alcohol history, sexual exposure, sick contacts, exposure to high-risk populations such as prisoners or homeless people; menstrual history, menopausal status, travel history.

Key Physical Exam

Vital signs; HEENT exam, including inspection of the throat and other areas for lymphadenopathy; heart and lung exam; abdominal exam for hepatosplenomegaly; skin exam; musculoskeletal exam for joint pain.

Presentation	Differential	Workup
▪ 30 yo M presents with night sweats, cough, and swollen glands of 1 month's duration. He recently emigrated from the African subcontinent.	**Tuberculosis** Acute HIV infection Lymphoma Leukemia Hyperthyroidism	PPD/QuantiFERON Gold CBC CXR Sputum Gram stain, acid-fast stain, and culture HIV antibody TSH, FT$_4$
▪ 45 yo F presents with excessive sweating, unintentional weight loss, palpitations, diarrhea, and shortness of breath.	**Hyperthyroidism** Pheochromocytoma Carcinoid syndrome Tuberculosis	TSH, FT$_4$ 24-hour urinary catecholamines 5-HIAA CBC PPD

INSOMNIA

Key History

Primary vs. secondary, duration, description (trouble falling asleep vs. multiple awakenings vs. early-morning awakening); daytime sleepiness; other medical problems keeping patient awake at night, such as arthritis (pain) or diabetes (polyuria); evidence of a common sleep disorder (eg, sleep apnea, restless leg syndrome); associated symptoms, including loud snoring, nightmares, and depression; caffeine, alcohol, medication, and recreational drug use; work or lifestyle (jet lag or shift work), stressors, sleep hygiene; presence of psychiatric symptoms (eg, grandiose delusions, irritability).

INSOMNIA *(cont'd)*

Key Physical Exam

Vital signs; mental status exam; thyroid exam.

Presentation	Differential	Workup
■ 25 yo F presents with a 3-week history of difficulty falling asleep. She sleeps 7 hours per night without nightmares or snoring. She recently began college and is having trouble with her boyfriend. She drinks 3–4 cups of coffee a day.	**Stress-induced insomnia** Caffeine-induced insomnia Insomnia with circadian rhythm sleep disorder Insomnia related to major depressive disorder	Polysomnography Mental status exam Urine toxicology CBC TSH
■ 55 yo obese M presents with several months of poor sleep, daytime fatigue, and morning headaches. His wife reports that he snores loudly.	**Obstructive sleep apnea** Daytime fatigue in primary hypersomnia Insomnia with circadian rhythm sleep disorder Insomnia related to major depressive disorder	CBC TSH Polysomnography ECG
■ 33 yo F c/o 3 weeks of fatigue and trouble sleeping. She states that she falls asleep easily but wakes up at 3 A.M. and cannot return to sleep. She also reports an unintentional weight loss of 8 lbs (3.6 kg) and an inability to enjoy the things she once liked to do.	**Insomnia related to major depressive disorder** Primary hypersomnia Insomnia with circadian rhythm sleep disorder	Mental status exam TSH CBC Polysomnography

SORE THROAT

Key History

Duration, fever, other ENT symptoms (ear pain, nasal or sinus congestion), odynophagia, swollen glands, ± cough, rash; sick contacts, HIV risk factors.

Key Physical Exam

Vital signs; ENT exam, including oral thrush, tonsillar exudate, and lymphadenopathy; lung, abdominal (focusing on splenomegaly), and skin exams.

SORE THROAT *(cont'd)*

Presentation	Differential	Workup
■ 26 yo F presents with sore throat, fever, severe fatigue, and loss of appetite for the past week. She also reports epigastric and LUQ discomfort. She has cervical lymphadenopathy and a rash. Her boyfriend recently experienced similar symptoms.	**Infectious mononucleosis** Hepatitis Viral or bacterial pharyngitis Acute HIV infection Secondary syphilis	CBC with peripheral smear Monospot test Throat culture AST/ALT/bilirubin/ alkaline phosphatase HIV antibody and viral load Anti-EBV antibodies VDRL/RPR
■ 26 yo M presents with sore throat, fever, rash, and weight loss. He has a history of IV drug abuse and sharing needles.	**HIV, acute retroviral syndrome** Infectious mononucleosis Hepatitis Viral pharyngitis Streptococcal tonsillitis/ scarlet fever Secondary syphilis	CBC with peripheral smear HIV antibody and viral load CD4 count Monospot test Throat culture VDRL/RPR AST/ALT/bilirubin/ alkaline phosphatase
■ 46 yo F presents with fever and sore throat.	**Pharyngitis (bacterial or viral)** *Mycoplasma* pneumonia Acute HIV infection Infectious mononucleosis	Throat swab for culture and rapid streptococcal antigen Monospot test CBC Serologic test (cold agglutinin titer) for *Mycoplasma* HIV antibody and viral load

COUGH/SHORTNESS OF BREATH

Key History

Acute/subacute vs. chronic, increased frequency of cough if chronic, timing; presence/description of sputum, presence of hemoptysis; associated symptoms (constitutional, URI, postnasal drip, dyspnea, wheezing, chest pain, heartburn); exacerbating and alleviating factors, exposures; smoking history; history of lung disease, posttussive emesis, or heart failure; allergies; medications (especially ACE inhibitors).

Key Physical Exam

Vital signs ± pulse oximetry; exam of nasal mucosa, oropharynx, heart, lungs, lymph nodes, and extremities (clubbing, cyanosis, edema).

Presentation	Differential	Workup
30 yo M presents with shortness of breath, cough, and wheezing that worsen in cold air. He has had several such episodes in the past 4 months.	**Asthma** GERD Bronchitis Pneumonitis Foreign body	CBC CXR Peak flow measurement PFTs Methacholine challenge test
56 yo F presents with shortness of breath and a productive cough that has lasted for at least 3 months each year over the past 2 years. She is a heavy smoker.	**COPD—chronic bronchitis** Bronchiectasis Lung cancer Tuberculosis	CBC Sputum Gram stain and culture CXR PFTs CT—chest PPD
58 yo M presents with 1 week of pleuritic chest pain, fever, chills, and cough with purulent yellow sputum. He is a heavy smoker with COPD.	**Pneumonia** COPD exacerbation (bronchitis) Lung abscess Lung cancer Tuberculosis Pericarditis	CBC Sputum Gram stain and culture CXR CT—chest ECG PPD
25 yo F presents with 2 weeks of nonproductive cough. Three weeks ago she had a sore throat and a runny nose.	**Atypical pneumonia** Reactive airway disease URI-associated cough ("postinfectious") Postnasal drip GERD	CBC Induced sputum Gram stain and culture CXR IgM detection for *Mycoplasma pneumoniae* Urine *Legionella* antigen
65 yo M presents with worsening cough for the past 6 months accompanied by hemoptysis, dyspnea, weakness, and weight loss. He is a heavy smoker.	**Lung cancer** Tuberculosis Lung abscess COPD Vasculitis (eg, Wegener's granulomatosis) Interstitial lung disease CHF	CBC Sputum Gram stain, culture, and cytology CXR CT—chest PPD ANCA Bronchoscopy Echocardiography

MINICASES

Presentation	Differential	Workup
■ 55 yo M presents with increased dyspnea and sputum production for the past 3 days. He has COPD and stopped using his inhalers last week. He stopped smoking 2 days ago.	**COPD exacerbation (bronchitis)** Lung cancer Pneumonia URI CHF	CBC CXR ABG PFTs Sputum Gram stain and culture CT—chest Echocardiography
■ 34 yo F nurse presents with worsening cough of 6 weeks' duration accompanied by weight loss, fatigue, night sweats, and fever. She has a history of contact with tuberculosis patients at work.	**Tuberculosis** Pneumonia Lung abscess Vasculitis Lymphoma Metastatic cancer HIV/AIDS Sarcoidosis	CBC PPD/QuantiFERON Gold Sputum Gram stain, acid-fast stain, and culture CXR CT—chest Bronchoscopy HIV antibody Lymph node biopsy
■ 35 yo M presents with shortness of breath and cough. He has had unprotected sex with multiple sexual partners and was recently exposed to a patient with active tuberculosis.	**Tuberculosis** Pneumonia (including *Pneumocystis jiroveci*) Bronchitis Asthma Acute HIV infection CHF (cardiomyopathy)	CBC PPD/QuantiFERON Gold Sputum Gram stain, acid-fast stain, silver stain, and culture CXR HIV antibody Echocardiography
■ 50 yo M presents with a cough that is exacerbated by lying down at night and improved by propping up on 3 pillows. He also reports exertional dyspnea.	**CHF** Cardiac valvular disease GERD Pulmonary fibrosis COPD Postnasal drip	CBC CXR ECG Echocardiography PFTs BNP CT—chest
■ 60 yo M presents with worsening dyspnea of 6 hours' duration and a cough that is accompanied by pink, frothy sputum.	**Pulmonary edema** CHF Mitral valve stenosis Arrhythmia Asthma Pneumonia	ECG CXR CBC ABG PFTs BNP

CHEST PAIN

Key History

Location, quality, severity, radiation, duration, context (exertional, postprandial, positional, cocaine use, trauma); associated symptoms (sweating, nausea, dyspnea, palpitations, sense of doom, fever); exacerbating and alleviating factors (especially medications); history of similar symptoms; known heart or lung disease or history of diagnostic testing; cardiac risk factors (hypertension, hyperlipidemia, smoking, family history of early MI); pulmonary embolism risk factors (history of DVT, coagulopathy, malignancy, recent immobilization).

Key Physical Exam

Vital signs ± BP in both arms; complete cardiovascular exam (JVD, PMI, chest wall tenderness, heart sounds, pulses, edema); lung and abdominal exams; lower extremity exam (inspection for signs of DVT).

Presentation	Differential	Workup
■ 60 yo M presents with sudden onset of substernal heavy chest pain that has lasted for 30 minutes and radiates to the left arm. The pain is accompanied by dyspnea, diaphoresis, and nausea. He has a history of hypertension, hyperlipidemia, and smoking.	**Myocardial infarction (MI)** GERD Angina Costochondritis Aortic dissection Pericarditis Pulmonary embolism Pneumothorax	ECG CPK-MB, troponin × 3 CXR CBC Electrolytes Echocardiography Cardiac catheterization D-dimer Helical CT
■ 20 yo African American F presents with acute onset of severe chest pain for a few hours. She has a history of sickle cell disease and multiple hospitalizations for pain and anemia management.	**Sickle cell disease—acute chest syndrome** Pulmonary embolism Pneumonia MI Pneumothorax Aortic dissection	CBC with reticulocyte count and peripheral smear LDH ABG D-dimer CXR CPK-MB, troponin ECG CTA—chest with IV contrast
■ 45 yo F presents with a retrosternal burning sensation that occurs after heavy meals and when lying down. Her symptoms are relieved by antacids.	**GERD** Esophagitis Peptic ulcer disease Esophageal spasm MI Angina	ECG Barium swallow Upper endoscopy Esophageal pH monitoring

Presentation	Differential	Workup
■ 55 yo M presents with retrosternal squeezing pain that lasts for 2 minutes and occurs with exercise. It is relieved by rest and is not related to food intake.	**Stable angina** Esophageal spasm Esophagitis	ECG CPK-MB, troponin CXR CBC Electrolytes Exercise stress test Upper endoscopy/pH monitor Cardiac catheterization
■ 34 yo F presents with retrosternal stabbing chest pain that improves when she leans forward and worsens with deep inspiration. She had a URI 1 week ago.	**Pericarditis** Aortic dissection MI Costochondritis GERD Esophageal rupture	ECG CPK-MB, troponin CXR Echocardiography CBC Upper endoscopy ESR
■ 33 yo F presents with stabbing chest pain that worsens with deep inspiration and is relieved by aspirin. She had a URI 1 week ago. Chest wall tenderness is noted.	**Costochondritis** Pneumonia MI Pulmonary embolism Pericarditis Pleurisy Muscle strain	ECG CPK-MB, troponin CXR CBC
■ 70 yo F presents with acute onset of shortness of breath at rest and pleuritic chest pain. She also presents with tachycardia, hypotension, tachypnea, and mild fever. She is recovering from hip replacement surgery.	**Pulmonary embolism** Pneumonia Costochondritis MI CHF Aortic dissection	D-dimer ECG CXR ABG CPK-MB, troponin CBC Electrolytes, BUN/Cr, glucose CTA—chest with IV contrast Doppler U/S—legs

MINICASES

Presentation	Differential	Workup
■ 55 yo M presents with sudden onset of severe chest pain that radiates to his back. He has a history of uncontrolled hypertension.	**Aortic dissection** MI Pericarditis Esophageal rupture Esophageal spasm GERD Pancreatitis Fat embolism	ECG CPK-MB, troponin CXR CBC Amylase, lipase CTA—chest with IV contrast Transesophageal echocardiography (TEE) MRI/MRA—aorta Aortic angiography Upper endoscopy

PALPITATIONS

Key History

Gradual vs. acute onset/offset, context (exertion, caffeine, anxiety); associated symptoms (lightheadedness, loss of consciousness, chest pain, dyspnea, fever, sweating, pale skin, flushing, diarrhea); hyperthyroid symptoms; history of bleeding or anemia; history of heart disease, hypertension, or diabetes.

Key Physical Exam

Vital signs; endocrine/thyroid exam, including exophthalmos, lid retraction, lid lag, gland size, bruit, and tremor; complete cardiovascular exam.

Presentation	Differential	Workup
■ 70 yo diabetic M presents with episodes of palpitations and diaphoresis. He is on insulin.	**Hypoglycemia** Cardiac arrhythmia Angina Hyperthyroidism Hyperventilation episodes Panic attack Pheochromocytoma Carcinoid syndrome	Glucose CBC Electrolytes TSH ECG Holter monitor 24-hour urinary catecholamines 5-HIAA

Presentation	Differential	Workup
■ 35 yo M presents with several episodes of palpitations, sweating, and rapid breathing. Episodes occur unexpectedly, and he does not recall any triggers. He has had 4–5 episodes per month for several months. Each episode lasts 2–3 minutes. He does not have any history of psychiatric illness except for separation anxiety as a child.	**Panic attack** Generalized anxiety disorder Acute stress disorder Specific phobia Hyperthyroidism Agoraphobia Substance abuse/ dependence Mitral valve prolapse Pheochromocytoma	CBC Electrolytes TSH, FT_4 ECG Echocardiography Urine toxicology 24-hour urinary catecholamines
■ 19 yo F presents with episodic palpitations, especially during presentations in front of her class. Episodes include heart pounding, facial blushing, and hand tremor. She also experiences excessive sweating and rapid breathing. She complains of intense worry and trouble sleeping for days or weeks before an upcoming social situation. Now she avoids all social events because she is afraid of humiliating herself.	**Social phobia** Avoidant personality disorder Agoraphobia/specific phobia Panic attack Generalized anxiety disorder Substance abuse/ dependence Hyperthyroidism	CBC Electrolytes ECG Echocardiography TSH, FT_4 Mental status exam
■ 34 yo F presents with episodic palpitations accompanied by lightheadedness and sharp, atypical chest pain.	**Mitral valve prolapse** Cardiac arrhythmia Panic attack Pheochromocytoma	ECG Echocardiography Holter monitor 24-hour urinary catecholamines

WEIGHT LOSS

Key History

Amount, duration, ± intention; diet and exercise history; body image, anxiety or depression; other constitutional symptoms; hyperthyroid symptoms (palpitations, tremor, diarrhea); family history of thyroid disease; HIV risk factors; tobacco, alcohol, and drug use; medications; history of cancer; blood in urine or stool.

Key Physical Exam

Vital signs; complete physical.

Presentation	Differential	Workup
▪ 42 yo F presents with a 15.5-lb (7-kg) weight loss within the past 2 months. She has a fine tremor, and her pulse is 112.	**Hyperthyroidism** Cancer HIV infection Dieting/diet drugs Anorexia nervosa Malabsorption	TSH, FT$_4$ CBC Electrolytes HIV antibody Urine toxicology

WEIGHT GAIN

Key History

Amount, duration, timing (relation to medication changes, smoking cessation, depression); diet history; hypothyroid symptoms (fatigue, constipation, skin/hair/nail changes); menstrual irregularity, hirsutism; medical history; alcohol and drug use.

Key Physical Exam

Vital signs; complete exam, including signs of Cushing's syndrome (hypertension, central obesity, moon face, buffalo hump, supraclavicular fat pads, purple abdominal striae); edema resulting from water retention in renal disease.

Presentation	Differential	Workup
▪ 44 yo F presents with a weight gain of > 25 lbs (11.3 kg) within the past 2 months. She quit smoking 3 months ago and is on amitriptyline for depression. She also reports cold intolerance and constipation.	**Smoking cessation** Drug side effect Hypothyroidism Cushing's syndrome Polycystic ovary syndrome Diabetes mellitus Atypical depression	CBC Electrolytes, glucose TSH 24-hour urine free cortisol Dexamethasone suppression test

▪ 30 yo F presents with weight gain over the past 3 months. She also reports tremor, palpitations, anxiety, and hunger that is relieved by eating. She exhibits proximal muscle weakness and easy bruising.	**Insulinoma**
	Reactive postprandial
	  hypoglycemia
	Cushing's syndrome
		Blood glucose and plasma
		  insulin
		Glucose tolerance test
		24-hour urine free cortisol

DYSPHAGIA

Key History

Solids or liquids vs. both solids and liquids, ± progression, occurring at the beginning or middle of swallow; constitutional symptoms (especially weight loss); hoarseness, drooling, regurgitation of liquids vs. undigested food, odynophagia, GERD symptoms; medications; HIV risk factors; history of anxiety, smoking, Raynaud's phenomenon.

Key Physical Exam

Vital signs; head and neck exam; heart, lung, and abdominal exams; skin exam (for signs of scleroderma/CREST).

Presentation	Differential	Workup
75 yo M presents with dysphagia that started with solids and progressed to liquids. He is an alcoholic and a heavy smoker. He has had an unintentional weight loss of 15 lbs (6.8 kg) within the past 4 months.	**Esophageal cancer** Achalasia Esophagitis Systemic sclerosis Esophageal stricture Amyotrophic lateral sclerosis	CBC CXR Upper endoscopy with biopsy Barium swallow CT—chest
45 yo F presents with dysphagia for 2 weeks accompanied by mouth and throat pain, fatigue, and a craving for ice and clay.	**Plummer-Vinson syndrome** Esophageal cancer Esophagitis Achalasia Systemic sclerosis Mitral valve stenosis	CBC Serum iron, ferritin, TIBC Barium swallow Upper endoscopy Video fluoroscopy
48 yo F presents with dysphagia for both solids and liquids that has slowly progressed in severity within the past year. It is associated with difficulty belching and regurgitation of undigested food, especially at night. She has lost 5.5 lbs (2.5 kg) in the past 2 months.	**Achalasia** Plummer-Vinson syndrome Esophageal cancer Esophagitis Systemic sclerosis Mitral valve stenosis Esophageal stricture Zenker's diverticulum	CXR Upper endoscopy Barium swallow Esophageal manometry XR—neck
38 yo M presents with dysphagia and pain on swallowing solids more than liquids. Exam reveals oral thrush.	**Esophagitis (CMV, HSV, HIV, pill-induced)** Systemic sclerosis GERD Esophageal stricture Zenker's diverticulum	CBC Upper endoscopy Barium swallow HIV antibody and viral load CD4 count

MINICASES

NECK MASS

Key History

Onset, size, location, mobility, pain, movement with swallowing; obstructive symptoms (dysphagia, shortness of breath); other masses; associated symptoms (constitutional, hematologic, GI, endocrine, pulmonary); ill contacts.

Key Physical Exam

Vital signs; HEENT exam; exam of lymph nodes, spleen, and tonsils; heart, lung, and abdominal exams.

Presentation	Differential	Workup
■ 39 yo F presents with a single 2-cm mass on the right side of her neck along with night sweats, fever, weight loss, loss of appetite, and early satiety. The mass is painless and movable and has not changed in size. She does not report heat intolerance, tremor, palpitations, hoarseness, cough, difficulty breathing, difficulty swallowing, or abdominal pain. Her husband was recently discharged from prison, and her mother has a history of gastric cancer.	**Hodgkin's/non-Hodgkin's lymphoma** Tuberculosis Thyroid nodule Gastric carcinoma	CBC with differential Electrolytes ESR, CRP Lymph node biopsy PPD CXR TSH U/S—thyroid Upper endoscopy

NAUSEA/VOMITING

Key History

Acuity of onset, ± abdominal pain, relation to meals, sick contacts, possible food poisoning, possible pregnancy; neurologic symptoms (headache, stiff neck, vertigo, focal numbness or weakness); urinary symptoms; other associated symptoms (GI, chest pain); exacerbating and alleviating factors; medications; history of prior abdominal surgery.

Key Physical Exam

Vital signs; ENT; consider funduscopic exam (increased intracranial pressure); complete abdominal exam; consider heart, lung, and rectal exams.

Presentation	Differential	Workup
■ 20 yo F presents with nausea, vomiting (especially in the morning), fatigue, and polyuria. Her last menstrual period was 6 weeks ago, and her breasts are full and tender. She is sexually active with her boyfriend, and they occasionally use condoms for contraception.	**Pregnancy** Gastritis Hypercalcemia Diabetes mellitus UTI Depression	Urine hCG Pelvic exam U/S—pelvis CBC Electrolytes, calcium, glucose UA, urine culture HIV antibody

ABDOMINAL PAIN

Key History

Location, quality, intensity, duration, radiation, timing (relation to meals); associated symptoms (constitutional, GI, cardiac, pulmonary, renal, pelvic); exacerbating and alleviating factors; history of similar symptoms; history of abdominal surgeries, trauma, gallstones, renal stones, atherosclerotic vascular disease; medications (eg, NSAIDs, corticosteroids); alcohol and drug use; domestic violence, stress/anxiety, sexual history, pregnancy history.

Key Physical Exam

Vital signs; heart and lung exams; abdominal exam, including tenderness, guarding, rebound, Murphy's sign, psoas and obturator signs, and CVA percussion; bowel sounds, aortic bruits; rectal exam; pelvic exam (women).

Presentation	Differential	Workup
45 yo M presents with sudden onset of colicky right-sided flank pain that radiates to the testicles, accompanied by nausea, vomiting, hematuria, and CVA tenderness.	**Nephrolithiasis** Renal cell carcinoma Pyelonephritis GI etiology (eg, appendicitis)	UA, urine culture and sensitivity, urine cytology BUN/Cr CT—abdomen U/S—renal KUB IVP Blood culture
60 yo M presents with dull epigastric pain that radiates to the back, accompanied by weight loss, dark urine, and clay-colored stool. He is a heavy drinker and smoker. He appears jaundiced on exam.	**Pancreatic cancer** Cholangiocarcinoma Acute viral hepatitis Acute alcoholic hepatitis Chronic pancreatitis Cholecystitis/ choledocholithiasis Abdominal aortic aneurysm Peptic ulcer disease	CBC Electrolytes Amylase, lipase AST/ALT/bilirubin/ alkaline phosphatase CT—abdomen U/S—abdomen
56 yo M presents with severe midepigastric abdominal pain that radiates to the back and improves when he leans forward. He also reports anorexia, nausea, and vomiting. He is an alcoholic and has spent the past 3 days binge drinking.	**Acute pancreatitis** Peptic ulcer disease Cholecystitis/ choledocholithiasis Gastritis Abdominal aortic aneurysm Mesenteric ischemia Alcoholic hepatitis Boerhaave syndrome	CBC Electrolytes, BUN/Cr Amylase, lipase AST/ALT/bilirubin/ alkaline phosphatase U/S—abdomen CT—abdomen Upper endoscopy ECG

MINICASES

Presentation	Differential	Workup
■ 41 yo obese F presents with RUQ abdominal pain that radiates to the right scapula and is associated with nausea, vomiting, and a fever of 101.5°F. The pain started after she ate fatty food. She has had similar but less intense episodes that lasted a few hours. Exam reveals a positive Murphy's sign.	**Acute cholecystitis** Choledocholithiasis Hepatitis Ascending cholangitis Peptic ulcer disease Fitz-Hugh–Curtis syndrome Acute subhepatic appendicitis	CBC AST/ALT/bilirubin/ alkaline phosphatase U/S—abdomen CT—abdomen Blood culture
■ 43 yo obese F presents with RUQ abdominal pain, fever, and jaundice. She was diagnosed with asymptomatic gallstones 1 year ago. She is found to be hypotensive on exam.	**Ascending cholangitis** Acute gallstone cholangitis Acute cholecystitis Hepatitis Sclerosing cholangitis Fitz-Hugh–Curtis syndrome	CBC AST/ALT/bilirubin/ alkaline phosphatase Blood culture Viral hepatitis serologies U/S—abdomen MRCP ERCP
■ 25 yo M presents with RUQ pain, fever, anorexia, nausea, and vomiting. He has dark urine and clay-colored stool.	**Acute hepatitis** Acute cholecystitis Ascending cholangitis Choledocholithiasis Pancreatitis Acute glomerulonephritis	CBC Amylase, lipase AST/ALT/bilirubin/ alkaline phosphatase Viral hepatitis serologies UA U/S—abdomen
■ 35 yo M presents with burning epigastric pain that starts 2–3 hours after meals. The pain is relieved by food and antacids.	**Peptic ulcer disease** Gastritis GERD Cholecystitis Chronic pancreatitis Mesenteric ischemia	Rectal exam, stool for occult blood Amylase, lipase, lactate AST/ALT/bilirubin/ alkaline phosphatase Upper endoscopy (including H pylori testing) Upper GI series

Presentation	Differential	Workup

37 yo M presents with severe epigastric pain, nausea, vomiting, and mild fever. He appears toxic. He has a history of intermittent epigastric pain that is relieved by food and antacids. He also smokes heavily and takes aspirin on a daily basis.	**Perforated peptic ulcer**
	Acute pancreatitis
	Hepatitis
	Cholecystitis
	Gallstone cholangitis
	Mesenteric ischemia
		Rectal exam
		CBC
		Electrolytes
		Amylase, lipase, lactate
		AST/ALT/bilirubin/
		   alkaline phosphatase
		CXR
		KUB
		CT—abdomen
		Upper endoscopy
		   (including *H pylori*
		   testing)
		Blood culture

18 yo M boxer presents with severe LUQ abdominal pain that radiates to the left scapula. He had infectious mononucleosis 3 weeks ago.	**Splenic rupture**
	Kidney stone
	Rib fracture
	Pneumonia
	Perforated peptic ulcer
	Splenic infarct
		CBC
		Electrolytes
		CXR
		CT—abdomen
		U/S—abdomen (if
		   hemodynamically
		   unstable)

40 yo M presents with crampy abdominal pain, vomiting, abdominal distention, and inability to pass flatus or stool. He has a history of multiple abdominal surgeries.	**Intestinal obstruction**
	Small bowel or colon
	   cancer
	Volvulus
	Gastroenteritis
	Food poisoning
	Ileus
	Hernia
		Rectal exam
		CBC
		Electrolytes
		AXR
		CT—abdomen/pelvis with
		   contrast
		Colonoscopy

70 yo F presents with acute onset of severe, crampy abdominal pain. She recently vomited and had a massive dark bowel movement. She has a history of CHF and atrial fibrillation, for which she has received digitalis. Her pain is out of proportion to the exam.	**Mesenteric ischemia/** **infarction** Diverticulitis Peptic ulcer disease Gastroenteritis Acute pancreatitis Cholecystitis	Rectal exam CBC Amylase, lipase, lactate ECG AXR CT—abdomen Mesenteric angiography Barium enema

MINICASES

Presentation	Differential	Workup
■ 21 yo F presents with acute onset of severe RLQ pain, nausea, and vomiting. She has no fever, urinary symptoms, or vaginal bleeding and has never taken OCPs. Her last menstrual period was regular, and she has no history of STDs. She has been told that she had a cyst on her right ovary.	**Ovarian torsion** Appendicitis Nephrolithiasis Ectopic pregnancy Ruptured ovarian cyst Pelvic inflammatory disease Bowel infarction or perforation	Pelvic exam Urine hCG Doppler U/S—pelvis Rectal exam UA CBC CT—abdomen Laparoscopy Chlamydia and gonorrhea testing, VDRL/RPR
■ 68 yo M presents with LLQ abdominal pain, fever, and chills for the past 3 days. He also reports recent onset of alternating diarrhea and constipation. He consumes a low-fiber, high-fat diet.	**Diverticulitis** Crohn's disease Ulcerative colitis Gastroenteritis Abscess	Rectal exam CBC Electrolytes CXR AXR CT—abdomen Blood culture
■ 20 yo M presents with severe RLQ abdominal pain, nausea, and vomiting. His discomfort started yesterday as a vague pain around the umbilicus. As the pain worsened, it became sharp and migrated to the RLQ. McBurney's and psoas signs are positive.	**Acute appendicitis** Gastroenteritis Diverticulitis Crohn's disease Nephrolithiasis Volvulus or other intestinal obstruction Perforation Acute cholecystitis	CBC Electrolytes CT—abdomen AXR U/S—abdomen Blood culture
■ 30 yo F presents with periumbilical pain for 6 months. The pain never awakens her from sleep. It is relieved by defecation and worsens when she is upset. She has alternating constipation and diarrhea but no nausea, vomiting, weight loss, or anorexia.	**Irritable bowel syndrome** Crohn's disease Celiac disease Chronic pancreatitis GI parasitic infection (amebiasis, giardiasis) Endometriosis	Rectal exam, stool for occult blood Pelvic exam Urine hCG CBC Electrolytes Colonoscopy CT—abdomen/pelvis Stool for ova and parasitology, *Entamoeba histolytica* antigen

MINICASES

Presentation	Differential	Workup
▪ 24 yo F presents with bilateral lower abdominal pain that started with the first day of her menstrual period. The pain is associated with fever and a thick, greenish-yellow vaginal discharge. She has had unprotected sex with multiple sexual partners.	**Pelvic inflammatory disease** Endometriosis Dysmenorrhea Vaginitis Cystitis Spontaneous abortion Pyelonephritis	Pelvic exam Urine hCG Cervical cultures CBC ESR UA, urine culture U/S—pelvis

CONSTIPATION/DIARRHEA

Key History

Frequency, color, odor, and volume of stools; presence of mucus or flatulence; whether stools float in bowl; duration of change in bowel habits; associated symptoms (constitutional, abdominal pain, bloating, tenesmus, sense of incomplete evacuation, melena or hematochezia); thyroid disease symptoms (eg, feeling hot, palpitations, weight loss); diet (especially fiber and fluid intake); medications (including recent antibiotics); sick contacts, travel, camping, HIV risk factors; history of abdominal surgeries, diabetes, pancreatitis; alcohol and drug use; family history of colon cancer.

Key Physical Exam

Vital signs; relevant thyroid/endocrine exam; abdominal and rectal exams; ± female pelvic exam.

Presentation	Differential	Workup
▪ 67 yo M presents with alternating diarrhea and constipation, decreased stool caliber, and blood in the stool for the past 8 months. He also reports unintentional weight loss. He is on a low-fiber diet and has a family history of colon cancer. His last colonoscopy was 12 years ago.	**Colorectal cancer** Irritable bowel syndrome Diverticulosis GI parasitic infection (ascariasis, giardiasis) Inflammatory bowel disease	Rectal exam, stool for occult blood CBC Electrolytes AST/ALT/bilirubin/ alkaline phosphatase Colonoscopy Barium enema CT—abdomen/pelvis
▪ 28 yo M presents with constipation (hard stool) for the past 3 weeks. Since his mother died 2 months ago, he and his father have eaten only junk food.	**Low-fiber diet** Depression Substance abuse (eg, heroin) Irritable bowel syndrome Hypothyroidism	Rectal exam TSH Electrolytes Urine toxicology

MINICASES

Presentation	Differential	Workup
■ 30 yo F presents with alternating constipation and diarrhea accompanied by abdominal pain that is relieved by defecation. She has no nausea, vomiting, weight loss, or blood in her stool.	**Irritable bowel syndrome** Inflammatory bowel disease Celiac disease Chronic pancreatitis GI parasitic infection (ascariasis, giardiasis) Lactose intolerance	Rectal exam, stool for occult blood CBC Electrolytes Colonoscopy Stool for ova and parasitology CT—abdomen/pelvis
■ 33 yo M presents with watery diarrhea, vomiting, and diffuse abdominal pain that began yesterday. He also reports feeling hot. Several of his coworkers are also ill.	**Infectious diarrhea (gastroenteritis)—** bacterial, viral, parasitic, protozoal Food poisoning	Rectal exam, stool for occult blood Stool leukocytes and culture CBC Electrolytes CT—abdomen/pelvis
■ 40 yo F presents with watery diarrhea and abdominal cramps. Last week she was on antibiotics for a UTI.	**Pseudomembranous (*Clostridium difficile*) colitis** Gastroenteritis Cryptosporidiosis Food poisoning Inflammatory bowel disease	Stool for *C difficile* toxin Rectal exam, stool for occult blood Stool leukocytes and culture CBC Electrolytes
■ 25 yo M presents with watery diarrhea and abdominal cramps. He was recently in Mexico.	**Traveler's diarrhea** Giardiasis Amebiasis Food poisoning Hepatitis A	Rectal exam Stool leukocytes, culture, *Giardia* antigen, *Entamoeba histolytica* antigen CBC Electrolytes AST/ALT/bilirubin/ alkaline phosphatase Viral hepatitis serologies
■ 30 yo F presents with watery diarrhea, abdominal cramping, and bloating. Her symptoms are aggravated by milk ingestion and are relieved by fasting.	**Lactose intolerance** Gastroenteritis Inflammatory bowel disease Irritable bowel syndrome Hyperthyroidism	Rectal exam Stool leukocytes and culture Hydrogen breath test TSH

MINICASES

Presentation	Differential	Workup
■ 33 yo M presents with watery diarrhea, diffuse abdominal pain, and weight loss within the past 3 weeks. He has a history of aphthous ulcers. He has not responded to antibiotics.	**Crohn's disease** Gastroenteritis Ulcerative colitis Celiac disease Pseudomembranous colitis Hyperthyroidism Small bowel lymphoma Carcinoid syndrome	Rectal exam, stool for occult blood Stool leukocytes and culture CBC Electrolytes Colonoscopy CT—abdomen TSH Small bowel series 5-HIAA

UPPER GI BLEEDING

Key History

Amount, duration, context (after severe vomiting, alcohol ingestion, nosebleed); associated symptoms (constitutional, nausea, abdominal pain, dyspepsia); medications (especially blood thinners, NSAIDs, and corticosteroids); history of peptic ulcer disease, liver disease, abdominal aortic aneurysm repair, easy bleeding.

Key Physical Exam

Vital signs, including orthostatics; ENT, heart, lung, abdominal, and rectal exams.

Presentation	Differential	Workup
■ 45 yo F presents with coffee-ground emesis for the past 3 days. Her stool is dark and tarry. She has a history of intermittent epigastric pain that is relieved by food and antacids.	**Bleeding peptic ulcer** Gastritis Gastric cancer Esophageal varices	Rectal exam CBC, type and cross Electrolytes AST/ALT/bilirubin/ alkaline phosphatase INR Upper endoscopy (including *H pylori* testing if ulcer is confirmed)
■ 40 yo F presents with epigastric pain and coffee-ground emesis. She has a history of rheumatoid arthritis that has been treated with NSAIDs. She is an alcoholic.	**Gastritis** Bleeding peptic ulcer Gastric cancer Esophageal varices Mallory-Weiss tear	Rectal exam CBC, type and cross Electrolytes AST/ALT/bilirubin/ alkaline phosphatase INR Upper endoscopy

BLOOD IN STOOL

Key History

Melena vs. bright red blood; amount, duration; associated symptoms (constitutional, abdominal or rectal pain, tenesmus, constipation/diarrhea); menstrual cycle; trauma; history of similar symptoms; prior colonoscopy; medications (especially blood thinners); history of easy bleeding or atherosclerotic vascular disease, renal disease, aortic valve disease, liver disease, alcoholism, or abdominal aortic aneurysm repair; family history of colon cancer.

Key Physical Exam

Vital signs ± orthostatics; abdominal and rectal exams.

Presentation	Differential	Workup
■ 67 yo M presents with blood in his stool, weight loss, and constipation. He has a family history of colon cancer.	**Colorectal cancer** Anal fissure Hemorrhoids Diverticulosis Ischemic bowel disease Angiodysplasia Upper GI bleeding Inflammatory bowel disease	Rectal exam CBC AST/ALT/bilirubin/ alkaline phosphatase INR Colonoscopy CEA CT—abdomen/pelvis
■ 33 yo F presents with rectal bleeding and diarrhea for the past week. She has had lower abdominal pain and tenesmus for several months.	**Ulcerative colitis** Crohn's disease Proctitis Anal fissure Hemorrhoids Diverticulosis Dysentery	Rectal exam CBC PT/PTT Colonoscopy CT—abdomen/pelvis
■ 58 yo M presents with painless bright red blood per rectum and chronic constipation. He consumes a low-fiber diet.	**Diverticulosis** Anal fissure Hemorrhoids Angiodysplasia Colorectal cancer	Rectal exam CBC, type and cross PT/PTT Electrolytes Colonoscopy Tagged RBC scan CT—abdomen/pelvis

HEMATURIA

Key History

Amount, duration, ± clots; associated symptoms (constitutional, renal colic, dysuria, irritative voiding symptoms); point along the stream (initial vs. terminal vs. throughout); medications; history of vigorous exercise, trauma, smoking, stones, cancer, or easy bleeding; skin bruising (purpura).

Key Physical Exam

Vital signs; lymph nodes; abdominal exam; genitourinary and rectal exams; extremities.

Presentation	Differential	Workup
65 yo M presents with painless hematuria. He is a heavy smoker and works as a painter.	**Bladder cancer** Renal cell carcinoma Nephrolithiasis Acute glomerulonephritis Prostate cancer Coagulation disorder (ie, factor VIII antibodies)	Genitourinary exam UA, urine cytology BUN/Cr PSA CBC PT/PTT Cystoscopy U/S—renal/bladder CT—abdomen/pelvis Prostate biopsy
35 yo M presents with painless hematuria. He has a family history of kidney disease.	**Polycystic kidney disease** Nephrolithiasis Acute glomerulonephritis (eg, IgA nephropathy) UTI Coagulation disorder Bladder cancer	Genitourinary exam UA, urine cytology BUN/Cr PSA CBC PT/PTT U/S—renal CT—abdomen/pelvis
55 yo M presents with flank pain and blood in his urine without dysuria. He has experienced weight loss and fever over the past 2 months. Exam reveals a flank mass.	**Renal cell carcinoma** Bladder cancer Nephrolithiasis Acute glomerulonephritis Pyelonephritis Prostate cancer	Genitourinary, rectal exams UA, urine cytology BUN/Cr PSA CBC PT/PTT U/S—renal CT—abdomen/pelvis Cystoscopy

OTHER URINARY SYMPTOMS

Key History

Duration, obstructive symptoms (hesitancy, diminished stream, sense of incomplete bladder emptying, straining, postvoid dribbling, leakage with cough or sneeze, incontinence), irritative symptoms (urgency, frequency, nocturia), constitutional symptoms; bone pain; medications; history of UTIs, urethral stricture, or urinary tract instrumentation; stones, diabetes, alcoholism.

Key Physical Exam

Vital signs; abdominal exam (including suprapubic percussion to assess for a distended bladder); genital and rectal exams; focused neurologic exam.

Presentation	Differential	Workup
60 yo M presents with nocturia, urgency, weak stream, and terminal dribbling. He denies any weight loss, fatigue, or bone pain. He has had 2 episodes of urinary retention that required catheterization.	**Benign prostatic hypertrophy (BPH)** Prostate cancer UTI Bladder stones	Rectal exam UA CBC BUN/Cr Alkaline phosphatase U/S—prostate (transrectal) PSA
71 yo M presents with nocturia, urgency, a weak stream, terminal dribbling, hematuria, and lower back pain for the past 4 months. He has also experienced weight loss and fatigue.	**Prostate cancer** BPH Renal cell carcinoma UTI Bladder stones	Rectal exam UA CBC BUN/Cr PSA U/S—prostate (transrectal) Prostate biopsy Alkaline phosphatase CT—pelvis MRI—spine
18 yo M presents with a burning sensation during urination and urethral discharge. He recently had unprotected sex with a new partner.	**Urethritis** Cystitis Prostatitis	Genital, rectal exams UA, urine culture Gram stain and culture of urethral discharge Chlamydia and gonorrhea PCR
45 yo diabetic F presents with dysuria, urinary frequency, fever, chills, and nausea for the past 3 days. There is left CVA tenderness on exam.	**Acute pyelonephritis** Nephrolithiasis Lower UTI (cystitis, urethritis) Renal cell carcinoma	UA, urine culture and sensitivity Blood culture CBC BUN/Cr U/S—renal CT—abdomen

MINICASES

Presentation	Differential	Workup
■ 55 yo F presents with urinary leakage after exercise. She loses a small amount of urine when she coughs, laughs, or sneezes. She also complains of vague low back pain. She has a history of multiple vaginal deliveries, and her mother had the same problem after the onset of menopause.	**Stress incontinence** Mixed incontinence Urge incontinence Overflow incontinence Functional incontinence UTI Diabetes mellitus	UA, urine culture BUN/Cr Urodynamic testing IVP Cystourethroscopy
■ 33 yo F presents with urinary leakage. She is unable to suppress the urge to urinate and loses large amounts of urine without warning. She has a history of UTIs and a family history of diabetes mellitus. She drinks 8 cups of coffee per day. She has been under stress since her sister passed away a few months ago.	**Urge incontinence** Mixed incontinence Stress incontinence Overflow incontinence Functional incontinence UTI Diabetes mellitus	CBC Electrolytes, BUN/Cr, glucose UA, urine culture Urodynamic testing IVP Cystourethroscopy

ERECTILE DYSFUNCTION (ED)

Key History

Duration, severity, ± nocturnal erections, libido, stress or depression, trauma, associated incontinence; gynecomastia or loss of body hair; medications (and recent changes); medical history (hypertension, diabetes, high cholesterol, known atherosclerotic vascular disease, prior prostate surgery, liver disease, thyroid disease, neurologic disease); smoking, alcohol, and drug use.

Key Physical Exam

Vital signs; cardiovascular exam; genital and rectal exams.

Presentation	Differential	Workup
■ 47 yo M presents with impotence that started 3 months ago. He has hypertension and was started on atenolol 4 months ago. He also has diabetes and is on insulin.	**Drug-related ED** ED caused by hypertension ED caused by diabetes mellitus Psychogenic ED Peyronie's disease	Genital exam Rectal exam Glucose CBC Testosterone level

AMENORRHEA

Key History

Primary vs. secondary, duration, possible pregnancy; associated symptoms (headache, decreased peripheral vision, galactorrhea, hirsutism, virilization, hot flashes, vaginal dryness, symptoms of thyroid disease); history of anorexia nervosa, excessive dieting, vigorous exercise, pregnancies, D&Cs, uterine infections; drug use; medications.

Key Physical Exam

Vital signs; breast exam; complete pelvic exam.

Presentation	Differential	Workup
40 yo F presents with amenorrhea, morning nausea and vomiting, fatigue, and polyuria. Her last menstrual period was 6 weeks ago, and her breasts are full and tender. She uses the rhythm method for contraception.	**Pregnancy** Anovulatory cycle Hyperprolactinemia UTI Hypothyroidism	Urine hCG U/S—abdomen/pelvis Pelvic exam CBC UA, urine culture Prolactin, TSH Baseline Pap smear, cervical cultures, rubella antibody, HIV antibody, hepatitis B surface antigen, VDRL/RPR
23 yo obese F presents with amenorrhea for 6 months, facial hair, and infertility for the past 3 years.	**Polycystic ovary syndrome** Thyroid disease Hyperprolactinemia Pregnancy Ovarian or adrenal malignancy Premature ovarian failure	Urine hCG LH/FSH, TSH, prolactin Pelvic exam Testosterone, DHEAS
35 yo F presents with amenorrhea, galactorrhea, visual field defects, and headaches for the past 6 months.	**Amenorrhea secondary to prolactinoma** Pregnancy Thyroid disease Premature ovarian failure Pituitary tumor	Urine hCG LH/FSH, TSH, prolactin MRI—brain Pelvic and breast exams

Presentation	Differential	Workup
■ 48 yo F presents with amenorrhea for the past 6 months accompanied by hot flashes, night sweats, emotional lability, and dyspareunia.	**Menopause** Pregnancy Pituitary tumor Thyroid disease	Urine hCG LH/FSH, TSH, prolactin Testosterone, DHEAS Pelvic exam CBC MRI—brain
■ 35 yo F presents with amenorrhea, cold intolerance, coarse hair, weight loss, and fatigue. She has a history of abruptio placentae followed by hypovolemic shock and failure of lactation 2 years ago.	**Sheehan's syndrome** Premature ovarian failure Pituitary tumor Thyroid disease Asherman's syndrome	Urine hCG LH/FSH, prolactin CBC Pelvic exam TSH, FT_4 ACTH MRI—brain Hysteroscopy
■ 18 yo F presents with amenorrhea for the past 4 months. She is 5 feet, 6 inches (167.6 cm) and weighs 90 lbs (40.9 kg). She has a history of exercise and heat intolerance.	**Anorexia nervosa** Pregnancy Hyperthyroidism	Urine hCG CBC TSH, FT_4 LH/FSH
■ 29 yo F presents with amenorrhea for the past 6 months. She has a history of occasional palpitations and dizziness. She lost her fiancé in a car accident in which she was a passenger.	**Anxiety-induced amenorrhea** Posttraumatic stress disorder Depression Hyperthyroidism	CBC TSH, FT_4 Urine cortisol level Progesterone challenge test LH/FSH, estradiol levels

VAGINAL BLEEDING

Key History

Pre- vs. postmenopausal status, duration, amount; menstrual history and relation to last menstrual period; associated discharge, pelvic or abdominal pain, or urinary symptoms; trauma; medications (especially blood thinners, contraceptives); history of easy bleeding or bruising; history of abnormal Pap smears.

Key Physical Exam

Vital signs; abdominal exam; complete pelvic exam.

MINICASES

Presentation	Differential	Workup
17 yo F presents with prolonged, excessive menstrual bleeding occurring irregularly within the past 6 months.	**Dysfunctional uterine bleeding** Coagulation disorder (eg, von Willebrand's disease, hemophilia) Cervical cancer Molar pregnancy Hypothyroidism Diabetes mellitus	Urine hCG Pelvic exam Cervical culture Pap smear CBC ESR Glucose PT/PTT LH/FSH, TSH, prolactin U/S—pelvis
61 yo obese F presents with profuse vaginal bleeding for the past month. Her last menstrual period was 10 years ago. She has a history of hypertension and diabetes mellitus. She is nulliparous.	**Endometrial cancer** Cervical cancer Atrophic endometrium Endometrial hyperplasia Endometrial polyps Atrophic vaginitis	Pelvic exam Pap smear Endometrial biopsy Endometrial curettage U/S—pelvis Colposcopy Hysteroscopy
45 yo G5P5 F presents with postcoital bleeding. She is a cigarette smoker and takes OCPs.	**Cervical cancer** Endometrial cancer Cervical polyp Cervicitis Trauma (eg, cervical laceration)	Pelvic exam Pap smear Colposcopy and biopsy HPV testing Endometrial biopsy
28 yo F who is 8 weeks pregnant presents with lower abdominal pain and vaginal bleeding.	**Spontaneous abortion** Ectopic pregnancy Molar pregnancy	Urine hCG Quantitative serum hCG U/S—abdomen/pelvis Pelvic exam CBC PT/PTT
32 yo F presents with sudden onset of left lower abdominal pain that radiates to the scapula and back and is associated with vaginal bleeding. Her last menstrual period was 5 weeks ago. She has a history of pelvic inflammatory disease and unprotected intercourse.	**Ectopic pregnancy** Ruptured ovarian cyst Ovarian torsion Pelvic inflammatory disease	Urine hCG Quantitative serum hCG U/S—abdomen/pelvis Pelvic exam Cervical cultures

MINICASES

125

VAGINAL DISCHARGE

Key History

Amount, color, consistency, odor, duration; associated vaginal burning, pain, or pruritus; recent sexual activity; onset of last menstrual period; use of contraceptives, tampons, and douches; history of similar symptoms; history of STDs.

Key Physical Exam

Vital signs; abdominal exam; complete pelvic exam.

Presentation	Differential	Workup
■ 28 yo F presents with a thin, grayish-white, foul-smelling vaginal discharge.	**Bacterial vaginosis** Vaginitis—candidal Vaginitis—trichomonal Cervicitis (chlamydia, gonorrhea)	Pelvic exam Wet mount, KOH prep, "whiff test" pH of vaginal fluid Cervical cultures
■ 30 yo F presents with a thick, white, cottage cheese–like, odorless vaginal discharge and vaginal itching.	**Vaginitis—candidal** Bacterial vaginosis Vaginitis—trichomonal	Pelvic exam Wet mount, KOH prep, "whiff test" pH of vaginal fluid Cervical cultures
■ 35 yo F presents with a malodorous, profuse, frothy, greenish vaginal discharge with intense vaginal itching and discomfort.	**Vaginitis—trichomonal** Vaginitis—candidal Bacterial vaginosis Cervicitis (chlamydia, gonorrhea)	Pelvic exam Wet mount, KOH prep, "whiff test" pH of vaginal fluid Cervical cultures

DYSPAREUNIA

Key History

Duration, timing; associated symptoms (vaginal discharge, rash, painful menses, GI symptoms, hot flashes); adequacy of lubrication, menopausal status, libido; sexual history, history of sexual trauma or domestic violence; history of endometriosis, pelvic inflammatory disease, or prior abdominal/pelvic surgeries.

Key Physical Exam

Vital signs; abdominal exam; complete pelvic exam.

DYSPAREUNIA *(cont'd)*

Presentation	Differential	Workup
■ 54 yo F c/o painful intercourse. Her last menstrual period was 9 months ago. She has hot flashes.	**Atrophic vaginitis** Endometriosis Cervicitis Depression Domestic violence	Pelvic exam LH/FSH Wet mount, KOH prep Cervical cultures
■ 37 yo F presents with dyspareunia, inability to conceive, and dysmenorrhea.	**Endometriosis** Cervicitis Vaginismus Vulvodynia Pelvic inflammatory disease Depression Domestic violence	Pelvic exam Wet mount, KOH prep Cervical cultures U/S—pelvis Laparoscopy Endometrial biopsy

ABUSE

Key History

Establish confidentiality; directly question about physical, sexual, or emotional abuse and about fear, safety, backup plan; history of frequent accidents/injuries, mental illness, drug use; firearms in the home.

Key Physical Exam

Vital signs; complete exam ± pelvic exam.

Presentation	Differential	Workup
■ 28 yo F c/o multiple facial and bodily injuries. She claims that she fell on the stairs. She was hospitalized for physical injuries 7 months ago. She presents with her husband.	**Domestic violence** Osteogenesis imperfecta Substance abuse Consensual violent sexual behavior	XR—skeletal survey CT—maxillofacial Urine toxicology CBC

ABUSE *(cont'd)*

Presentation	Differential	Workup
■ 30 yo F presents with multiple facial and physical injuries. She states that she was attacked and raped by 2 men.	**Rape** Domestic violence	Forensic exam (sexual assault forensic evidence [SAFE] collection kit) Pelvic exam Urine hCG Wet mount, KOH prep Cervical cultures Chlamydia and gonorrhea testing XR—skeletal survey CBC HIV antibody Viral hepatitis serologies

JOINT/LIMB PAIN

Key History

Location, quality, intensity, duration, pattern (small vs. large joints; number involved; swelling, redness, warmth); associated symptoms (constitutional, red eye, oral or genital ulceration, diarrhea, dysuria, rash, focal numbness/weakness, morning stiffness); exacerbating and alleviating factors; trauma (including vigorous exercise); medications; DVT risk factors; alcohol and drug use; family history of rheumatic disease.

Key Physical Exam

Vital signs; HEENT and musculoskeletal exams; relevant neurovascular exam.

Presentation	Differential	Workup
■ 30 yo F presents with wrist pain and a black eye after tripping, falling, and hitting her head on the edge of a table. She looks anxious and gives an inconsistent story.	**Domestic violence** Factitious disorder Substance abuse	XR—wrist CT—head Urine toxicology

Presentation	Differential	Workup
■ 30 yo F secretary presents with wrist pain and a sensation of numbness and burning in her palm and the first, second, and third fingers of her right hand. The pain worsens at night and is relieved by loose shaking of the hand. There is sensory loss in the same fingers. Exam reveals a positive Tinel's sign.	**Carpal tunnel syndrome** Median nerve compression in the forearm or arm Radiculopathy of nerve roots C6 and C7 in the cervical spine De Quervain's tenosynovitis	Phalen's maneuver and Tinel's sign Finkelstein's test Nerve conduction studies EMG
■ 28 yo F presents with pain in the interphalangeal joints of her hands accompanied by hair loss and a rash on her face.	**Systemic lupus erythematosus (SLE)** Rheumatoid arthritis Psoriatic arthritis Parvovirus B19 infection	ANA, anti-dsDNA, ESR, C3, C4, RF, CCP CBC XR—hands UA Antibody titers for parvovirus B19
■ 28 yo F presents with pain in the metacarpophalangeal joints of both hands. Her left knee is also painful and red. She has morning joint stiffness that lasts for an hour. Her mother had rheumatoid arthritis.	**Rheumatoid arthritis** SLE Disseminated gonorrhea Arthritis associated with inflammatory bowel disease	XR—hands, left knee ANA, anti-dsDNA, ESR, RF, CCP CBC Cervical culture Arthrocentesis and synovial fluid analysis
■ 18 yo M presents with pain in the interphalangeal joints of both hands. He also has scaly, salmon-pink lesions on the extensor surface of his elbows and knees.	**Psoriatic arthritis** Rheumatoid arthritis SLE Gout	ANA, ESR, RF, CCP CBC XR—hands XR—pelvis/sacroiliac joints Uric acid
■ 65 yo F presents with inability to use her left leg or bear weight on it after tripping on a carpet. Onset of menopause was 20 years ago, and she did not receive HRT or calcium supplements. Her left leg is externally rotated, shortened, and adducted, and there is tenderness in her left groin.	**Hip fracture** Hip dislocation Pelvic fracture	XR—hip/pelvis CT or MRI—hip CBC, type and cross Serum calcium and vitamin D Bone density scan (DEXA)

Presentation	Differential	Workup
■ 40 yo M presents with pain in the right groin after a motor vehicle accident. His right leg is flexed at the hip, adducted, and internally rotated.	**Hip dislocation— traumatic** Hip fracture	XR—hip CT or MRI—hip CBC, type and cross PT/PTT Urine toxicology and blood alcohol level
■ 56 yo obese F presents with right knee stiffness and pain that increases with movement. Her symptoms have gradually worsened over the past 10 years. She has noticed swelling and deformity of the joint and is having difficulty walking.	**Osteoarthritis** Pseudogout Gout Meniscal or ligament damage	XR—knee CBC ESR Knee arthrocentesis and synovial fluid analysis (cell count, Gram stain, culture, crystals) Uric acid MRI—knee
■ 45 yo M presents with fevers and right knee pain with swelling and redness.	**Septic arthritis** Gout Pseudogout Lyme arthritis Trauma Reiter's syndrome (reactive arthritis)	CBC Knee arthrocentesis and synovial fluid analysis (cell count, Gram stain, culture, crystals) Blood, urethral cultures XR—knee Uric acid Lyme titers—IgG and IgM
■ 65 yo M presents with right foot pain. He has been training for a marathon.	**Stress fracture** Plantar fasciitis Foot sprain or strain	XR—foot Bone scan—foot MRI—foot
■ 65 yo M presents with pain in the heel of the right foot that is most notable with his first few steps and then improves as he continues walking. He has no known trauma.	**Plantar fasciitis** Heel fracture Splinter/foreign body	XR—heel Bone scan—foot
■ 55 yo M presents with pain in the elbow when he plays tennis. His grip is impaired as a result of the pain. There is tenderness over the lateral epicondyle as well as pain on resisted wrist dorsiflexion (Cozen's test) with the elbow in extension.	**Tennis elbow (lateral epicondylitis)** Stress fracture	XR—arm Bone scan MRI—elbow

Presentation	Differential	Workup
■ 27 yo F presents with painful wrists and elbows, a swollen and hot knee joint that is painful on flexion, a rash on her limbs, and vaginal discharge. She is sexually active with multiple partners and occasionally uses condoms.	**Disseminated gonorrhea** Rheumatoid arthritis SLE Reiter's syndrome (reactive arthritis)	Knee arthrocentesis and synovial fluid analysis (cell count, Gram stain, culture) ANA, anti-dsDNA, ESR, RF, CCP CBC Blood, cervical cultures XR—knee
■ 60 yo F presents with pain in both legs that is induced by walking and is relieved by rest. She had cardiac bypass surgery 6 months ago and continues to smoke heavily.	**Peripheral vascular disease (intermittent claudication)** Leriche syndrome (aortoiliac occlusive disease) Lumbar spinal stenosis (pseudoclaudication) Osteoarthritis	Ankle-brachial index Doppler U/S—lower extremity Angiography MRI—L-spine
■ 45 yo F presents with right calf pain. Her calf is tender, warm, red, and swollen compared to the left side. She was started on OCPs 2 months ago for dysfunctional uterine bleeding.	**DVT** Baker's cyst rupture Myositis Cellulitis Superficial venous thrombosis	Doppler U/S—right leg CBC D-dimer
■ 60 yo F c/o left arm pain that started while she was swimming and was relieved by rest.	**Angina/MI** Tendinitis Osteoarthritis	ECG CBC XR—shoulder CXR Echocardiography Stress test
■ 50 yo M presents with right shoulder pain after falling onto his outstretched hand while skiing. He noticed deformity of his shoulder and had to hold his right arm.	**Shoulder dislocation** Fracture of the humerus Rotator cuff injury	XR—shoulder XR—arm MRI—shoulder

Presentation	Differential	Workup
■ 55 yo M presents with crampy bilateral thigh and calf pain, fatigue, and dark urine. He is on simvastatin and clofibrate for hyperlipidemia.	**Rhabdomyolysis due to statins** Polymyositis Inclusion body myositis	CBC Phosphate, potassium, BUN/Cr, glucose, calcium, uric acid CPK Aldolase UA Urine myoglobin

LOW BACK PAIN

Key History

Location, quality, intensity, radiation, context (moving furniture, bending/twisting, trauma), timing (disturbs sleep); associated symptoms (especially constitutional, incontinence); exacerbating and alleviating factors; history of cancer, recurrent UTIs, diabetes, renal stones, IV drug use, smoking.

Key Physical Exam

Vital signs; neurologic exam (especially L4–S1 nerve roots); back palpation and range of motion (although rarely of diagnostic utility); hip exam (can refer pain to the back); consider rectal exam.

Presentation	Differential	Workup
■ 45 yo F presents with low back pain that radiates to the lateral aspect of her left foot. The straight leg raise is positive. The patient is unable to tiptoe.	**Disk herniation** Lumbar muscle strain Tumor in the vertebral canal	XR—L-spine MRI—L-spine
■ 45 yo F presents with low back pain that started after she cleaned her house. The pain does not radiate, and there is no sensory deficit or weakness in her legs. Paraspinal muscle tenderness and spasm are also noted.	**Lumbar muscle strain** Disk herniation Vertebral compression fracture	XR—L-spine MRI—L-spine
■ 45 yo M presents with pain in the lower back and legs during prolonged standing and walking. The pain is relieved by sitting and leaning forward (eg, pushing a grocery cart).	**Lumbar spinal stenosis** Lumbar muscle strain Tumor in the vertebral canal Peripheral vascular disease	MRI—L-spine (preferred) XR—L-spine CT—L-spine Ankle-brachial index

Presentation	Differential	Workup
■ 17 yo M presents with low back pain that radiates to the left leg and began after he fell on his knee during gym class. He also describes areas of loss of sensation in his left foot. The pain and sensory loss do not match any known distribution. He insists on requesting a week off from school because of his injury.	**Malingering** Lumbar muscle strain Disk herniation Knee or leg fracture Ankylosing spondylitis	XR—L-spine/knee MRI—L-spine

CHILD WITH FEVER

No child will be present; the mother will relate the story. When you enter the examination room, you may see a telephone with instructions to pick up the handset. Upon doing so, you will be speaking to the parent of the child.

Key History

Severity, duration; associated localizing symptoms such as rash, wheezing, cough, and ear discharge; poor appetite, convulsions, lethargy, sleepiness; sick contacts, day care, immunizations.

Key Physical Exam

Vital signs; HEENT, neck, heart, lung, abdominal, and skin exams.

Presentation	Differential	Workup
■ 20-day-old M presents with fever, decreased breast-feeding, and lethargy. He was born at 36 weeks as a result of premature rupture of membranes.	**Neonatal sepsis** Meningitis Pneumonia Pyelonephritis	Physical exam CBC Electrolytes Blood culture LP—CSF analysis CXR UA, urine culture
■ 3 yo M presents with a 2-day history of fever and pulling on his right ear. He is otherwise healthy, and his immunizations are up to date. His older sister recently had a cold. The child attends a day care center.	**Acute otitis media** URI Meningitis Pyelonephritis	Physical exam (including pneumatic otoscopy) CBC Blood culture Tympanocentesis culture LP—CSF analysis UA, urine culture

Presentation	Differential	Workup
▪ 12-month-old M presents with fever for the past 2 days accompanied by a maculopapular rash on his face and body. He has not yet received the MMR vaccine.	**Measles (or other viral exanthem)** Rubella Roseola Fifth disease Varicella Scarlet fever Meningitis	Physical exam CBC Viral antibodies/titers Throat swab for culture LP—CSF analysis
▪ 4 yo M presents with diarrhea, vomiting, lethargy, weakness, and fever. The child attends a day care center where several children have had similar symptoms.	**Gastroenteritis (viral, bacterial, parasitic)** Food poisoning UTI URI Volvulus Intussusception	Physical exam Stool exam and culture CBC Electrolytes UA, urine culture AXR

CHILD WITH GI SYMPTOMS

No child will be present; only the parent will relate the story, either in person or by telephone.

Key History

Onset, location, quality, intensity, duration, radiation, timing (relation to meals); associated symptoms (constitutional, GI, cardiac, pulmonary, renal, pelvic); changes in weight, skin rash, bloody/mucoid stools, change in stool color; exacerbating and alleviating factors; history of similar symptoms; history of abdominal surgeries; medications; sick contacts, day care, immunizations.

Key Physical Exam

Vital signs; exam for signs of dehydration (BP, heart rate, skin turgor); heart and lung exams; abdominal exam; rectal exam; pelvic exam (women).

Presentation	Differential	Workup
■ 1-month-old F is brought in because she has been spitting up her milk for the last 10 days. The vomiting episodes have increased in frequency and forcefulness. Emesis is nonbloody and nonbilious. The episodes usually occur immediately after breastfeeding. She has stopped gaining weight.	**Pyloric stenosis** Partial duodenal atresia GERD Gastroenteritis Hepatitis UTI Otitis media	Physical exam CBC Electrolytes U/S—abdomen Barium swallow pH probe Endoscopy AST/ALT/bilirubin/ alkaline phosphatase UA, urine culture Tympanocentesis culture
■ 3 yo M presents with constipation. The child has had 1 bowel movement per week since birth despite the use of stool softeners. At birth, he did not pass meconium for 48 hours. He has poor weight gain. There is a family history of this problem.	**Hirschsprung's disease** Low-fiber diet Anal stenosis Hypothyroidism Lead poisoning	Physical exam Rectal exam Stool exam and culture Barium enema Suction rectal biopsy Anorectal manometry TSH, FT_4 CBC Electrolytes Serum lead level
■ 8-month-old F presents with sudden-onset colicky abdominal pain with vomiting. The episodes are 20 minutes apart, and the child is completely well between episodes. She had loose stools several hours before the pain, but her stools are now bloody.	**Intussusception** Appendicitis Meckel's diverticulum Volvulus Gastroenteritis Enterocolitis Blunt abdominal trauma	Physical exam Rectal exam, stool for occult blood CBC Electrolytes Contrast enema U/S—abdomen CT—abdomen
■ 7 yo M presents with abdominal pain that is generalized, crampy, worse in the morning, and seemingly less prominent during weekends and holidays. He has missed many school days because of the pain. Growth and development are normal. His parents recently divorced.	**Somatoform disorder** Malingering Irritable bowel syndrome Lactose intolerance Child abuse	Physical exam CBC Electrolytes U/S—abdomen CT—abdomen Amylase, lipase Stool exam

MINICASES

135

CHILD WITH GI SYMPTOMS (cont'd)

Presentation	Differential	Workup
■ 2-month-old M presents with persistent crying for 2 weeks. The episodes subside after passing flatus or eructation. There is no change in appetite, weight, or growth. There is no vomiting, constipation, or fever.	**Colic** Formula allergy GERD Lactose intolerance Strangulated hernia Testicular torsion Gastroenteritis	Physical exam Rectal exam, stool for occult blood U/S—abdomen U/S—testicular

CHILD WITH RED EYE

No child will be present; only the parent will relate the story, either in person or by telephone.

Key History

Onset, location, duration, affecting one or both eyes; eye discharge, itching, pain, photophobia, tearing; associated symptoms (constitutional, dermatologic, GI, cardiac, pulmonary, renal, pelvic, rheumatologic); exacerbating and alleviating factors; medications; sick contacts, day care, immunizations; history of similar symptoms.

Key Physical Exam

Vital signs; HEENT exam.

Presentation	Differential	Workup
■ 3 yo F presents with a 3-day history of "pink eye." It began in the right eye but now involves both eyes. She has mucoid discharge, itching, and difficulty opening her eyes in the morning. Her mother had the flu last week. She has a history of asthma and atopic dermatitis.	**Bacterial conjunctivitis** Viral conjunctivitis Keratitis Seasonal allergies Uveitis	Physical exam Ophthalmoscopic eye exam CBC Electrolytes Discharge cultures Slit lamp exam

CHILD WITH SHORT STATURE

No child will be present; only the parent will relate the story, either in person or by telephone.

Key History

Associated symptoms (constitutional, GI, cardiac, pulmonary, renal, pelvic, endocrine); medications; prenatal and birth history, growth history; past medical history; family history; cognitive abilities, school performance.

Key Physical Exam

Vital signs; height, weight; HEENT, heart, lung, abdominal, and neurologic exams.

Presentation	Differential	Workup
■ 14 yo M presents with short stature and lack of sexual development. His birth weight and length were normal, but he is the shortest child in his class. His father and uncles had the same problem when they were young, but they are now of normal stature.	**Constitutional short stature** Growth hormone (GH) deficiency Hypothyroidism Chronic renal insufficiency Genetic causes Cystic fibrosis	Physical exam CBC Electrolytes GH stimulation test IGF-1, IGFBP-3 levels TSH, FT$_4$ XR—hand U/S—renal and cardiac Sweat chloride testing BUN/Cr Karyotype

BEHAVIORAL PROBLEMS IN CHILDHOOD

No child will be present; only the parent will relate the story, either in person or by telephone.

Key History

Onset, severity, duration, triggers; physical violence or use of weapons; substance use, developmental history, changes in environment or school performance; change in personality, anhedonia.

Key Physical Exam

Vital signs; neurologic exam.

Presentation	Differential	Workup
■ 9 yo M presents with a 2-year history of angry outbursts both in school and at home. His mother complains that he runs around "as if driven by a motor." His teacher reports that he cannot sit still in class, regularly interrupts his classmates, and has trouble making friends.	**Attention-deficit hyperactivity disorder (ADHD)** Oppositional defiant disorder Manic episode Conduct disorder Hyperthyroidism	Physical exam Mental status exam TSH, FT$_4$ EEG

Presentation	Differential	Workup
12 yo F presents with a 2-month history of fighting in school, truancy, and breaking curfew. Her parents recently divorced, and she just started school in a new district. Before her parents divorced, she was an average student with no behavioral problems.	**Adjustment disorder** Substance intoxication, abuse, or dependence Manic episode Oppositional defiant disorder Conduct disorder	Physical exam Mental status exam Urine toxicology
15 yo M presents with a 1-year history of failing grades, school absenteeism, and legal problems, including shoplifting. His parents report that he spends most of his time alone in his room, adding that when he does go out, it is with a new set of friends.	**Substance abuse** Conduct disorder Oppositional defiant disorder Adjustment disorder	Urine toxicology Mental status exam Physical exam
5 yo M presents with a 6-month history of temper tantrums that last 5–10 minutes and immediately follow a disappointment or a discipline. He has no trouble sleeping, has had no change in appetite, and does not display these behaviors when he is at day care.	**Age-appropriate behavior** ADHD Oppositional defiant disorder	Physical exam Mental status exam

Practice Cases

This section consists of 44 commonly encountered cases that approximate those you might find on the actual USMLE Step 2 CS exam. Each case consists of four parts:

1. **Doorway information sheet:** Designed to simulate the actual information that you will find on the doorway of each examination room, this sheet contains the opening scenario, vital signs, and the tasks you are required to perform during the exam. You should read this sheet just before starting the 15-minute encounter.

2. **Checklist/SP sheet:** This sheet outlines information that standardized patients (SPs) will use to guide them during the interview and lists questions SPs might ask you, along with potential responses to these questions. It also includes a sample checklist that SPs will use to evaluate your performance in the areas of entrance, history taking, diagnosis, closure, and follow-up recommendations, as well as your ability to conduct a patient-centered interview.

3. **Blank patient note:** A blank form is supplied on which you can write your own note after you complete the patient encounter. In accordance with recent exam changes, this form includes blank matrices that you can use to outline the three most likely differential diagnoses; the history and exam findings that support each; and the initial testing modalities that you have proposed to establish a definitive diagnosis.

4. **Sample patient note and discussion:** This sheet includes a sample patient note for you to review after you have written your own, as well as a discussion of reasonable differential diagnoses and diagnostic tests to consider in each case.

Because the cases in this section are designed to simulate the actual exam, you will derive the most benefit by practicing them with a friend who can act as an SP. To maximize the effectiveness of these practice cases, you should also time each encounter in accordance with the guidelines provided in Sections 1 and 2 and compare each of your patient notes with those provided in the text.

For a quicker self-review, you can try to formulate a patient note after reviewing the doorway sheet and the SP checklist, and then compare your note with the sample note provided.

CASE 1
DOORWAY INFORMATION

Opening Scenario

Joseph Short, a 46-year-old male, comes to the ED complaining of chest pain.

Vital Signs

BP: 165/85 mm Hg

Temp: 98.6°F (37°C)

RR: 22/minute

HR: 90/minute, regular

Examinee Tasks

1. Take a focused history.
2. Perform a focused physical exam (do not perform rectal, genitourinary, or female breast exam).
3. Explain your clinical impression and workup plan to the patient.
4. Write the patient note after leaving the room.

Checklist/SP Sheet

Patient Description

Patient is a 46 yo M.

Notes for the SP

- Lie on the bed and exhibit pain.
- Place your hands in the middle of your chest.
- Exhibit difficulty breathing.
- If ECG is mentioned by the examinee, ask, "What is an ECG?"

Challenging Questions to Ask

"Is this a heart attack? Am I going to die?"

Sample Examinee Response

"As you suspect, your symptoms are of significant concern. We need to learn more about what's going on to know if your pain is life threatening."

Examinee Checklist

Building the Doctor-Patient Relationship

Entrance

☐ Examinee knocked on the door before entering.

☐ Examinee introduced self by name.

☐ Examinee identified his/her role or position.

☐ Examinee correctly used patient's name.

☐ Examinee made eye contact with the SP.

Reflective Listening

☐ Examinee asked an open-ended question and actively listened to the response.

☐ Examinee asked the SP to list his/her concerns and listened to the response without interrupting.

☐ Examinee summarized the SP's concerns, often using the SP's own words.

Information Gathering

☐ Examinee elicited data efficiently and accurately.

☑ Question	Patient Response
☐ Chief complaint	Chest pain.
☐ Onset	Forty minutes ago.
☐ Precipitating events	Nothing; I was asleep and woke up at 5:00 in the morning having this pain.
☐ Progression	Constant severity.
☐ Severity on a scale	7/10.
☐ Location	Middle of the chest. It feels as if it's right underneath the bone.
☐ Radiation	To my neck, upper back, and left arm.
☐ Quality	Pressure. Like something sitting on my chest.
☐ Alleviating/exacerbating factors	Nothing.
☐ Shortness of breath	Yes.
☐ Nausea/vomiting	I feel nauseated, but I didn't vomit.
☐ Sweating	Yes.
☐ Associated symptoms (cough, wheezing, abdominal pain, diarrhea/constipation)	None.
☐ Previous episodes of similar pain	Yes, but not exactly the same.
☐ Onset	The past 3 months.
☐ Severity	Less severe.
☐ Frequency	I have had 2–3 episodes a week, each lasting 5–10 minutes.
☐ Precipitating events	Walking up the stairs, strenuous work, and heavy meals.
☐ Alleviating factors	Antacids.
☐ Associated symptoms	None.
☐ Current medications	Maalox, diuretic.

☑ Question	Patient Response
☐ Past medical history	Hypertension for 5 years, treated with a diuretic. High cholesterol, managed with diet; I have not been very compliant with the diet. GERD 10 years ago, treated with antacids.
☐ Past surgical history	None.
☐ Family history	My father died of lung cancer at age 72. My mother is alive and has a peptic ulcer. No early heart attacks.
☐ Occupation	Accountant.
☐ Alcohol use	Once in a while.
☐ Illicit drug use	Cocaine, once a week.
☐ Duration of cocaine use	Ten years.
☐ Last time of cocaine use	Yesterday afternoon.
☐ Tobacco	Stopped 3 months ago.
☐ Duration	Twenty-five years.
☐ Amount	One pack a day.
☐ Sexual activity	Well, doctor, to be honest, I haven't had sex with my wife for the past 3 months because I get this pain in my chest during sex.
☐ Exercise	No.
☐ Diet	My doctor gave me a strict diet last year to lower my cholesterol, but I always cheat.
☐ Drug allergies	No.

Connecting with the Patient

☐ Examinee recognized the SP's emotions and responded with PEARLS.

Physical Examination

☐ Examinee washed his/her hands.

☐ Examinee asked permission to start the exam.

☐ Examinee used respectful draping.

☐ Examinee did not repeat painful maneuvers.

☑ Exam Component	Maneuver
☐ Neck exam	Looked for JVD, carotid auscultation
☐ CV exam	Inspection, auscultation, palpation
☐ Pulmonary exam	Auscultation, palpation, percussion
☐ Abdominal exam	Auscultation, palpation, percussion
☐ Extremities	Checked peripheral pulses, checked blood pressure in both arms, looked for edema and cyanosis

Closure

☐ Examinee discussed initial diagnostic impressions.

☐ Examinee discussed initial management plans:

  ☐ Follow-up tests.

  ☐ Lifestyle modification (diet, exercise).

☐ Examinee asked if the SP had any other questions or concerns.

Sample Closure

Mr. Short, the source of your pain can be a cardiac problem such as a heart attack or angina, or it may be due to acid reflux, lung problems, or disorders related to the large blood vessels in your chest. It is crucial that we perform some tests to identify the source of your problem. We will start with an ECG and some blood work, but more complex tests may be needed as well. In the meantime, I strongly recommend that you stop using cocaine, since use of this drug can lead to a variety of medical problems, including heart attacks. Do you have any questions for me?

Patient Note

History

Physical Examination

Patient Note

Differential Diagnosis

Diagnosis #1

History Finding(s):   Physical Exam Finding(s):

Diagnosis #2

History Finding(s):   Physical Exam Finding(s):

Diagnosis #3

History Finding(s):   Physical Exam Finding(s):

Diagnostic Workup

Patient Note

History

HPI: 46 yo M c/o substernal chest pain. The pain started 40 minutes before the patient presented to the ED. The pain woke the patient from sleep at 5:00 A.M. with a steady 7/10 pressure sensation in the middle of his chest that radiated to the left arm, upper back, and neck. Nothing makes it worse or better. Nausea, sweating, and dyspnea are also present. Similar episodes have occurred during the past 3 months, 2–3 times/week. These episodes were precipitated by walking up the stairs, strenuous work, sexual intercourse, and heavy meals. Pain during these episodes was less severe, lasted for 5–10 minutes, and disappeared spontaneously or after taking antacids.

ROS: Negative except as above.

Allergies: NKDA.

Medications: Maalox, diuretic.

PMH: Hypertension for 5 years, treated with a diuretic. High cholesterol, managed with diet. GERD 10 years ago, treated with antacids.

SH: 1 PPD for 25 years; stopped 3 months ago. Occasional EtOH, occasional cocaine for 10 years (last used yesterday afternoon). No regular exercise; poorly adherent to diet.

FH: Father died of lung cancer at age 72. Mother has peptic ulcers. No early coronary disease.

Physical Examination

Patient is in severe pain.

VS: BP 165/85 mm Hg (both arms), RR 22/minute.

Neck: No JVD, no bruits.

Chest: No tenderness, clear symmetric breath sounds bilaterally.

Heart: Apical impulse not displaced; RRR; normal S1/S2; no murmurs, rubs, or gallops.

Abdomen: Soft, nondistended, nontender, ⊕ BS, no hepatosplenomegaly.

Extremities: No edema, peripheral pulses 2+ and symmetric.

Differential Diagnosis

Diagnosis #1: Myocardial ischemia or infarction	
History Finding(s):	**Physical Exam Finding(s):**
Pressure-like substernal chest pain	
Pain radiates to left arm, upper back, and neck	
Pain awakens patient at night	

Diagnosis #2: Cocaine-induced myocardial ischemia	
History Finding(s):	**Physical Exam Finding(s):**
History of cocaine use	
Last used yesterday afternoon	
Pressure-like substernal chest pain	

Diagnosis #3: GERD

History Finding(s):	Physical Exam Finding(s):
Pain in midchest	
Previous pain was relieved by antacids	
Previous pain occurred after heavy meals	

Diagnostic Workup

ECG
Cardiac enzymes (CPK, CPK-MB, troponin)
Transthoracic echocardiography
Upper endoscopy
Urine toxicology

CASE DISCUSSION

Patient Note Differential Diagnoses

- **Myocardial ischemia or infarction:** The patient has multiple cardiac risk factors, including smoking, hypertension, and hyperlipidemia, and his symptoms are classic for cardiac ischemia.

- **Cocaine-induced myocardial ischemia:** Cocaine can predispose to premature atherosclerosis and can induce myocardial ischemia and infarction either by causing coronary artery vasoconstriction or by increasing myocardial energy requirements.

- **GERD:** Severe chest pain is atypical but not uncommon for GERD and may worsen with recumbency overnight. Other atypical symptoms include chronic cough, wheezing, and dysphagia. The classic symptom of GERD is heartburn, which may be exacerbated by meals.

Additional Differential Diagnoses

- **Aortic dissection:** With the sudden onset of severe chest pain, aortic dissection should be suspected given the high potential for death if missed (and the potential for harm if mistaken for acute MI and treated with thrombolytic therapy). However, the patient's pain is not the classic sudden, tearing chest pain that radiates to the back. In addition, his peripheral pulses and blood pressures are not diminished or unequal, and there is no aortic regurgitant murmur (although physical exam findings have poor sensitivity and specificity to diagnose aortic dissection).

- **Pericarditis:** The absence of pain that changes with position or respiration and the absence of a pericardial friction rub make pericarditis less likely.

- **Pneumothorax:** This diagnosis should be considered in a patient with acute chest pain and difficulty breathing, but it is less likely in this case given that breath sounds are symmetric.

- **Pulmonary embolism:** As above, this is on the differential for acute chest pain and difficulty breathing, but this patient has no apparent risk factors for pulmonary embolism.

- **Costochondritis (or other musculoskeletal chest pain):** This is more typically associated with pain on palpation or pleuritic pain.

Diagnostic Workup

- **ECG:** Acute myocardial ischemia, infarction, and pericarditis have characteristic changes on ECG.

- **Cardiac enzymes (CPK, CPK-MB, troponin):** Specific tests for myocardial tissue necrosis that can turn positive as early as 4–6 hours after onset of pain.

- **Transthoracic echocardiography (TTE):** Can demonstrate segmental wall motion abnormalities in suspected acute MI (infarction is unlikely in the absence of wall motion abnormalities).

- **Upper endoscopy:** Can be used to document tissue damage characteristic of GERD. However, it can be normal in up to one-half of symptomatic patients; esophageal probe (pH and manometry measurements) together with endoscopic visualization constitutes an effective diagnostic technique.

- **Urine toxicology:** To help confirm the patient's history of recent cocaine use.

- **Cardiac catheterization:** Can diagnose and treat coronary artery disease.

- **Transesophageal echocardiography (TEE):** Highly specific and sensitive for aortic dissection, and can be done rapidly at the bedside.

- **CXR:** A widened mediastinum suggests aortic dissection and may reveal other causes of chest pain, including pneumothorax and pneumonia.

- **CT—chest with IV contrast:** Another rapidly available diagnostic study that can rule out aortic dissection or pulmonary embolism.

- **Cholesterol panel:** Can identify a critical risk factor for cardiovascular disease.

Opening Scenario

Carl Fisher, a 57-year-old male, comes to the ED complaining of bloody urine.

Vital Signs

BP: 130/80 mm Hg

Temp: 98.5°F (36.9°C)

RR: 13/minute

HR: 72/minute, regular

Examinee Tasks

1. Take a focused history.

2. Perform a focused physical exam (do not perform rectal, genitourinary, or female breast exam).

3. Explain your clinical impression and workup plan to the patient.

4. Write the patient note after leaving the room.

Checklist/SP Sheet

Patient Description

Patient is a 57 yo M.

Notes for the SP

- Show pain when the examinee checks for CVA tenderness on the right.
- If the examinee mentions prostate disease, ask, "What's prostate disease?"

Challenging Questions to Ask

"They told me that having blood in my urine is because of my old age. Is that true?"

Sample Examinee Response

"No. Bloody urine is rarely normal. We will need to run a few more tests to determine the cause of this finding."

Examinee Checklist

Building the Doctor-Patient Relationship

Entrance

☐ Examinee knocked on the door before entering.

☐ Examinee introduced self by name.

☐ Examinee identified his/her role or position.

☐ Examinee correctly used patient's name.

☐ Examinee made eye contact with the SP.

Reflective Listening

☐ Examinee asked an open-ended question and actively listened to the response.

☐ Examinee asked the SP to list his/her concerns and listened to the response without interrupting.

☐ Examinee summarized the SP's concerns, often using the SP's own words.

Information Gathering

☐ Examinee elicited data efficiently and accurately.

☑ Question	Patient Response
☐ Chief complaint	I have blood in my urine, doctor.
☐ How did he know it was blood?	It was bright red and later had some clots.
☐ Onset	Yesterday morning.
☐ Progression	That was the only time it has ever happened; my urine is back to normal.
☐ Pain/burning on urination	None.
☐ Fever	None.
☐ Abdominal/flank pain	None.
☐ Polyuria, frequency	Yes. I have to go to the bathroom every 2–3 hours now.
☐ Straining during urination	Yes.
☐ Nocturia	Yes.
☐ Weak stream	Yes.
☐ Dribbling	Yes.
☐ Onset of the previous symptoms	Two years ago. They told me I am getting old; am I?
☐ History of renal stones	No.
☐ Associated symptoms (nausea/vomiting, diarrhea/constipation)	None.
☐ Constitutional symptoms (weight loss, appetite changes, night sweats)	None.
☐ Previous similar episodes	No.
☐ Current medications	Allopurinol.
☐ Past medical history	Gout.
☐ Past surgical history	Appendectomy at age 23.
☐ Family history	My father died at age 80 because of a kidney problem. My mother is alive and healthy.
☐ Occupation	Painter.
☐ Alcohol use	A couple of beers after work, 2–3 times a week.
☐ Illicit drug use	No.
☐ Tobacco	Yes, I have smoked a pack a day for 30 years.

☑ Question	Patient Response
☐ Sexual activity	I have a girlfriend; I met her 2 years ago through a mutual friend.
☐ Sexual orientation	Women only.
☐ Use of condoms	Regularly.
☐ History of STDs	None.
☐ Drug allergies	No.

Connecting with the Patient

☐ Examinee recognized the SP's emotions and responded with PEARLS.

Physical Examination

☐ Examinee washed his/her hands.

☐ Examinee asked permission to start the exam.

☐ Examinee used respectful draping.

☐ Examinee did not repeat painful maneuvers.

☑ Exam Component	Maneuver
☐ CV exam	Auscultation
☐ Pulmonary exam	Auscultation
☐ Abdominal exam	Auscultation, palpation, percussion, checked for CVA tenderness
☐ Extremities	Inspection

Closure

☐ Examinee discussed initial diagnostic impressions.

☐ Examinee discussed initial management plans:

    ☐ Follow-up tests: Examinee mentioned the need for a genital exam and a rectal exam for the prostate.

☐ Examinee asked if the SP had any other questions or concerns.

Sample Closure

Mr. Fisher, the blood in your urine could be caused by a variety of factors, so I would like to do a few tests to elicit an answer. First I will draw some blood, and then I will perform a genital exam as well as a rectal exam to assess your prostate. I will then order a urine test to look for signs of infection. Depending on the results we obtain, I may also order some imaging studies to determine if there is a stone in your kidneys, an anatomic abnormality, or a tumor. Do you have any questions for me?

USMLE STEP 2 CS **Patient Note**

History

Physical Examination

PRACTICE CASES

Patient Note

Differential Diagnosis

Diagnosis #1

History Finding(s):   **Physical Exam Finding(s):**

Diagnosis #2

History Finding(s):   **Physical Exam Finding(s):**

Diagnosis #3

History Finding(s):   **Physical Exam Finding(s):**

Diagnostic Workup

Patient Note

History

HPI: *57 yo male c/o 1 episode of painless hematuria yesterday morning. He has no fever, no abdominal or flank pain, and no dysuria. No history of renal stones. He has a 2-year history of straining on urination, polyuria, nocturia, weak urinary stream, and dribbling. No nausea, vomiting, diarrhea, or constipation. No change in appetite or weight loss. No previous similar episodes.*

ROS: *Negative except as above.*

Allergies: *NKDA.*

Medications: *Allopurinol.*

PMH: *Gout.*

PSH: *Appendectomy, age 23.*

SH: *1 PPD for 30 years, 2 beers 2–3 times/week, no illicit drugs. Works as a painter. Heterosexual, has a partner, and uses condoms regularly.*

FH: *Father died from kidney disease at age 80.*

Physical Examination

Patient is in no acute distress.

VS: *WNL.*

Chest: *Clear breath sounds bilaterally.*

Heart: *RRR; normal S1/S2; no murmurs, rubs, or gallops.*

Abdomen: *Soft, nondistended, nontender, ⊕ BS, no hepatosplenomegaly. Mild right CVA tenderness.*

Extremities: *No edema.*

Differential Diagnosis

Diagnosis #1: Bladder cancer

History Finding(s):	Physical Exam Finding(s):
Hematuria	
Straining on urination	
Weak urinary stream and dribbling	
Works as painter (exposure to industrial solvents)	
History of smoking 1 PPD × 30 years	

Diagnosis #2: Urolithiasis

History Finding(s):	Physical Exam Finding(s):
Hematuria	CVA tenderness
Straining on urination	

Diagnosis #3: Benign prostatic hypertrophy	
History Finding(s):	*Physical Exam Finding(s):*
Polyuria, nocturia	
Weak urinary stream and dribbling	
Straining on urination	

Diagnostic Workup

Genital exam
Rectal exam
Cystoscopy
U/S—renal
UA
CT—abdomen/pelvis
PSA

CASE DISCUSSION

Patient Note Differential Diagnoses

A useful mnemonic for the differential diagnosis of hematuria is **HITTERS**—etiologies include **H**ematologic or coagulation disorders, **I**nfection, **T**rauma, **T**umor, **E**xercise, **R**enal disorders, and **S**tones. Gynecologic sources may need to be excluded in women. The passage of clots often localizes the source of bleeding to the lower urinary tract. Gross hematuria in adults represents malignancy until proven otherwise.

- **Bladder cancer:** Hematuria and irritative voiding symptoms are consistent with this diagnosis, and the patient's cigarette smoking and possible occupational exposure to industrial solvents are risk factors. However, the finding of right CVA tenderness is unusual and could be a sign of upper urinary tract disease.

- **Urolithiasis:** Despite the presence of hematuria and CVA tenderness, this very common diagnosis is unlikely in the absence of sudden, severe colicky flank pain. Pain may migrate to the groin and is not alleviated by changes in position.

- **Benign prostatic hypertrophy (BPH):** The patient's urinary symptoms are classic for this diagnosis except that hematuria (if present) is usually microscopic. Again, CVA tenderness may signal upper urinary tract pathology.

Additional Differential Diagnoses

- **Prostate cancer:** As above, this diagnosis is plausible but is hard to reconcile with the presence of CVA tenderness (could postulate metastasis to a right posterior rib).

- **Renal cell carcinoma:** The classic triad is hematuria, flank pain, and a palpable mass. Constitutional symptoms may be prominent. The patient's other urinary symptoms may be due to coexisting BPH.

- **Glomerulonephritis:** The absence of hypertension or signs of volume overload (eg, edema) argues against intrinsic renal disease. However, remember that IgA nephropathy is the most common acute glomerulonephritis and most often presents with an episode of gross hematuria. Presentation is usually concurrent with URI, GI symptoms, or a flulike illness.

- **UTI:** This can cause hematuria but is uncommon in males. The patient has no other symptoms to suggest acute infection.

Diagnostic Workup

- **Genital exam:** To exclude a urologic source of bleeding in men.
- **Rectal exam:** To detect masses as well as prostatic enlargement or nodules.
- **Cystoscopy:** The gold standard for the diagnosis of bladder cancer.
- **U/S—renal:** Can detect bladder and renal masses and stones, but is operator dependent and less sensitive in detecting ureteral disease.
- **UA:** To assess hematuria, pyuria, bacteriuria, and the like. Dysmorphic RBCs or casts are signs of glomerular disease.
- **CT—abdomen/pelvis:** To evaluate the urinary tract. Can identify neoplasms and a variety of benign conditions, such as stones.
- **PSA:** The serum level correlates with the volume of both benign and malignant prostatic tissue. It can be normal in about 20% of patients with nonmetastatic prostate cancer.

- **Urine culture:** To exclude UTI.

- **Urine cytology:** Has variable sensitivity in detecting bladder cancers, depending on the grade and stage of the tumor. Three voided samples should be examined to maximize sensitivity.

- **BUN/Cr:** To evaluate kidney function.

- **IVP:** Provides an assessment of the kidneys, ureters, and bladder. IVP has generally been replaced by CT urography to circumvent the need for contrast administration.

Opening Scenario

Rick Meyer, a 51-year-old male construction worker, comes to the office complaining of back pain.

Vital Signs

BP: 120/85 mm Hg

Temp: 98.2°F (36.8°C)

RR: 20/minute

HR: 80/minute, regular

Examinee Tasks

1. Take a focused history.

2. Perform a focused physical exam (do not perform rectal, genitourinary, or female breast exam).

3. Explain your clinical impression and workup plan to the patient.

4. Write the patient note after leaving the room.

Checklist/SP Sheet

Patient Description

Patient is a 51 yo M who lives with his girlfriend.

Notes for the SP

- Pretend that you have paraspinal lower back tenderness when examined.
- Show normal reflexes, sensation, and strength in both lower extremities.
- Lean forward slightly when walking.

Challenging Questions to Ask

"I don't think I can go to work, doctor. Can you write a letter to my boss so that I can have some time off?"

Sample Examinee Response

"You're right; heavy construction work can worsen your back pain or cause it to heal more slowly. I will ask your boss to reassign you to light duty for a while."

Examinee Checklist

Building the Doctor-Patient Relationship

Entrance

☐ Examinee knocked on the door before entering.

☐ Examinee introduced self by name.

☐ Examinee identified his/her role or position.

☐ Examinee correctly used patient's name.

☐ Examinee made eye contact with the SP.

Reflective Listening

☐ Examinee asked an open-ended question and actively listened to the response.

☐ Examinee asked the SP to list his/her concerns and listened to the response without interrupting.

☐ Examinee summarized the SP's concerns, often using the SP's own words.

Information Gathering

☐ Examinee elicited data efficiently and accurately.

☑ Question	Patient Response
☐ Chief complaint	Pain in my back.
☐ Onset	One week ago.
☐ Associated/precipitating events	I was lifting some heavy boxes; then my back started hurting right away.
☐ Progression	It has been the same.
☐ Severity on a scale	8/10.
☐ Location	The middle of my lower back.
☐ Radiation	It radiates to my left thigh and sometimes reaches my left foot.
☐ Quality	Sharp.
☐ Alleviating factors	Lying still in bed.
☐ Exacerbating factors	Walking, sitting for a long time, coughing.
☐ Weakness/numbness	None.
☐ Difficulty urinating	I noticed that over the past 6 months I have had to strain in order to urinate. Sometimes I feel as if I haven't emptied my bladder fully.
☐ Urinary or fecal incontinence	No.
☐ Fever, night sweats, weight loss	No.
☐ History of back pain in the past	Well, for the past year I have been having back pain on and off, mainly when I walk. It is usually accompanied by pain in my legs. That pain goes away when I stop walking and sit down.
☐ Current medications	I take ibuprofen. It helps, but the pain is still there.
☐ Past medical history	None.
☐ Past surgical history	None.
☐ Family history	My father died of a heart attack at age 65, and my mother is healthy.
☐ Occupation	Construction worker.
☐ Alcohol use	Yes, a couple of beers on the weekends.
☐ CAGE questions	No (to all 4).
☐ Illicit drug use	Never.

☑ Question	Patient Response
☐ Tobacco	Yes, a pack a day for the past 18 years.
☐ Drug allergies	Penicillin gives me a rash.

Connecting with the Patient

☐ Examinee recognized the SP's emotions and responded with PEARLS.

Physical Examination

☐ Examinee washed his/her hands.

☐ Examinee asked permission to start the exam.

☐ Examinee used respectful draping.

☐ Examinee did not repeat painful maneuvers.

☑ Exam Component	Maneuver
☐ Back exam	Inspection, palpation, range of motion
☐ Extremities	Inspection, palpation of peripheral pulses, hip exam
☐ Neurologic exam	Motor, DTRs, Babinski's sign, gait (including toe and heel walking), passive straight leg raising, sensory exam

Closure

☐ Examinee discussed initial diagnostic impressions.

☐ Examinee discussed initial management plans:

    ☐ Follow-up tests: Examinee mentioned the need for a rectal exam.

☐ Examinee asked if the SP had any other questions or concerns.

Sample Closure

Mr. Meyer, I am concerned about your difficulty urinating, so I would like to do a rectal exam and assess your prostate for benign growths or cancer. I would also like to run some blood tests and order an x-ray and possibly an MRI of your back so that I can better determine the cause of your pain. In the meantime, as we discussed, I will write a note to your employer requesting that you be given only light duties while you are at work. Do you have any questions for me?

USMLE STEP 2 CS **Patient Note**

History

Physical Examination

Patient Note

Differential Diagnosis

Diagnosis #1

History Finding(s):   Physical Exam Finding(s):

Diagnosis #2

History Finding(s):   Physical Exam Finding(s):

Diagnosis #3

History Finding(s):   Physical Exam Finding(s):

Diagnostic Workup

Patient Note

History

HPI: 51 yo M construction worker c/o low back pain that started after he lifted heavy boxes 1 week ago. The pain is 8/10 and sharp, and it radiates to the left thigh and sometimes to the left foot. Pain worsens with movement, cough, and sitting for a long time. It is relieved by lying still and partially by ibuprofen. He denies urinary/stool incontinence or weakness/loss of sensation in the lower extremities. No fever, night sweats, or weight loss. He does report difficulty urinating and incomplete emptying of the bladder for 6 months as well as a 1-year history of intermittent low back pain. The pain is exacerbated by sitting for long periods but is relieved by sitting after ambulation.

ROS: Negative except as above.

Allergies: Penicillin, causes rash.

Medications: Ibuprofen.

PMH: None.

PSH: None.

SH: 1 PPD for 18 years, 1–2 beers on weekends, CAGE 0/4.

FH: Noncontributory.

Physical Examination

Patient is in mild distress due to back pain.

VS: WNL.

Back: Mild paraspinal muscle tenderness bilaterally, normal range of motion, no warmth or erythema.

Extremities: 2+ popliteal, dorsalis pedis, and posterior tibial pulses bilaterally. Hips normal, nontender range of motion bilaterally.

Neuro: Motor: Strength 5/5 throughout, including left great toe dorsiflexion. DTRs: 2+ symmetric, ⊖ Babinski bilaterally. Gait: Normal (including toe and heel walking), although he walks with back slightly bent forward. Straight leg raising ⊖ bilaterally. Sensation: Intact.

Differential Diagnosis

Diagnosis #1: Disk herniation	
History Finding(s):	**Physical Exam Finding(s):**
Low back pain	
Pain started after lifting heavy boxes	
Pain radiates to left thigh and foot	
Pain worsens with movement and is relieved by lying still	

Diagnosis #2: Lumbar spinal stenosis

History Finding(s):	Physical Exam Finding(s):
History of intermittent low back pain and leg pain with ambulation	Walks with back slightly bent forward
Pain resolves with sitting	

Diagnosis #3: Metastatic prostate cancer

History Finding(s):	Physical Exam Finding(s):
Difficulty urinating	
Incomplete emptying of the bladder	
Low back pain	

Diagnostic Workup

XR—L-spine
MRI—L-spine
Rectal exam
PSA

CASE DISCUSSION

Patient Note Differential Diagnoses

- **Disk herniation:** Low back pain radiating down the buttock and below the knee suggests nerve root irritation due to disk herniation. However, this pattern is nonspecific and can also be caused by sacroiliitis, facet joint degenerative arthritis, spinal stenosis, or other causes of sciatica. Most disk herniations occur at the L4–L5 or L5–S1 vertebral levels. These nerve roots are quickly assessed by checking the knee-jerk reflex (L4), great toe dorsiflexion (L5), and ankle-jerk reflex (S1). Ipsilateral straight leg raising that produces radicular symptoms (with the leg raised < 60 degrees) is highly sensitive but nonspecific in herniations at these levels. This patient may have disk herniation but has no objective evidence of neurologic compromise at this point.

- **Lumbar spinal stenosis:** This is most often seen in patients older than 60 years of age. They present with gradual onset of back pain that radiates to the buttocks and legs with or without leg numbness and weakness. Pain usually occurs with walking or prolonged standing and subsides with sitting or leaning forward (as in this case).

- **Metastatic prostate cancer:** The most common cancers leading to vertebral body metastases are prostate, breast, lung, multiple myeloma, and lymphoma. In metastatic disease, patients complain of gradual-onset back pain (or occasionally acute pain in the case of pathologic fracture) with or without neurologic symptoms. Pain may be worse at night and unrelieved by rest. This patient's urinary symptoms and low back pain may be signs of prostatic disease.

Additional Differential Diagnoses

- **Lumbar muscle strain:** This often follows strenuous or unusual exertion, but pain usually does not radiate to the extremities. Paraspinal muscle tenderness is often present.

- **Degenerative arthritis:** Degenerative back diseases are common, and classically pain is exacerbated by activity and alleviated by rest. Radicular symptoms may be present.

- **Multiple myeloma:** Typically, patients are older than 50 years of age. Back and bone pain may be the only presenting complaint. Anemia, neuropathy, hypercalcemia, and renal failure are also common.

- **Malingering:** This is defined as intentional faking of symptoms for secondary gain (eg, getting out of work).

Diagnostic Workup

The history and physical exam are often all that is required, as most patients with acute low back pain will improve within four weeks. Patients who require more extensive or urgent evaluation are those suspected of having pain caused by infection, cancer, abdominal aortic aneurysm, recurrent symptoms, or neurologic emergency (eg, cauda equina syndrome).

- **XR—L-spine:** Can show evidence of vertebral osteomyelitis, cancer, or fractures. Degenerative changes are expected in older patients and correlate poorly with clinical symptoms.

- **MRI—L-spine:** Provides the best anatomic detail and is the test of choice for suspected herniation, infection, or malignancy. Remember that asymptomatic disk herniation is common, so its presence does not necessarily correlate with clinical disease.

- **Rectal exam (including "saddle area" sensory exam):** To evaluate the prostate, rectal sphincter tone, and integrity of sacral nerve roots.

- **PSA:** Screening test for prostate cancer.

- **CBC, calcium, BUN/Cr:** To detect anemia, hypercalcemia, and renal failure, all of which may be clues to underlying multiple myeloma.

- **Serum and urine protein electrophoresis:** To detect a monoclonal paraprotein in myeloma. Both tests must be done because one could be negative.

Opening Scenario

John Matthews, a 25-year-old male, comes to the ED following a motor vehicle accident.

Vital Signs

BP: 123/88 mm Hg

Temp: 100°F (38°C)

RR: 22/minute

HR: 85/minute, regular

Examinee Tasks

1. Take a focused history.

2. Perform a focused physical exam (do not perform rectal, genitourinary, or female breast exam).

3. Explain your clinical impression and workup plan to the patient.

4. Write the patient note after leaving the room.

Checklist/SP Sheet

Patient Description

Patient is a 25 yo M.

Notes for the SP

- Exhibit pain in the left chest that worsens during inspiration and movement (ie, when you breathe in, hold your side and stop your breathing with a short gasp).
- Exhibit pain when your left chest is being palpated.
- Exhibit pain when your left upper abdomen is being palpated.
- Take fast, shallow breaths.
- Occasionally cough hard into a tissue.
- Moan occasionally and answer questions in short sentences.

Challenging Questions to Ask

"Do you think I am going to die?"

Sample Examinee Response

"Your condition raises concern and is obviously urgent. We will start by taking some images of your chest. Then, once we have a better idea of what is wrong, we can give you some medication to help you with your pain. If there is air or blood around your lungs, there is a procedure we can perform to release the pressure. We will be monitoring you very closely from this point on, and if you have any significant problems, we will be available to help."

Examinee Checklist

Building the Doctor-Patient Relationship

Entrance

☐ Examinee knocked on the door before entering.

☐ Examinee introduced self by name.

☐ Examinee identified his/her role or position.

☐ Examinee correctly used patient's name.

☐ Examinee made eye contact with the SP.

Reflective Listening

☐ Examinee asked an open-ended question and actively listened to the response.

☐ Examinee asked the SP to list his/her concerns and listened to the response without interrupting.

☐ Examinee summarized the SP's concerns, often using the SP's own words.

Information Gathering

☐ Examinee elicited data efficiently and accurately.

☑ Question	Patient Response
☐ Chief complaint	I'm having trouble breathing and have this excruciating pain (holds chest, left side).
☐ Onset	It started last night.
☐ Severity on a scale	It's some of the worst pain I've ever had. At least 8/10.
☐ Context	I was driving my car and was trying to answer my cell phone. When I looked up, I found that I had veered off the road. I immediately tried to slow down but hit a tree. I wasn't going very fast, and my car was basically okay. I was embarrassed, so I didn't call the police. I was wearing my seat belt and felt okay at first, so I didn't think I needed to come to the hospital.
☐ Alleviating factors	Nothing I do makes it better.
☐ Exacerbating factors	It gets even worse when I take a deep breath or try to move.
☐ Cough	I have been coughing for a couple of days, I guess.
☐ Sputum production	I have to use a tissue because I keep bringing up all this yellow junk.
☐ Fever/chills	I have been feeling a little warm and have noticed that my muscles ache, but I don't think I've had any shaking or chills.
☐ Other injuries	I have a few scratches on my arms from the car accident.
☐ Head trauma	No.
☐ Discharge from the ears, mouth, or nose (clear or bloody)	No.
☐ Loss of consciousness	No.
☐ Convulsions	No.

☑ Question	Patient Response
☐ Headache	No.
☐ Change in vision	No.
☐ Confusion, memory loss, or change in personality	No.
☐ Weakness or numbness in the extremities	No.
☐ Heart symptoms (palpitations)	No.
☐ Abdominal pain	Yes, I have sharp pain right here (points to the LUQ).
☐ Nausea/vomiting or stiff neck	No.
☐ Last meal/drink	I had breakfast this morning, about 5 hours ago. I didn't have any trouble keeping it down.
☐ Were you under the influence of alcohol or recreational drugs?	No.
☐ Pain on urination	No.
☐ Current medications	None.
☐ Past medical history	I had a sore throat, mild fever, and fatigue 2 weeks ago. My doctor told me I had infectious mononucleosis, but it is gone now.
☐ Past surgical history	None.
☐ Family history	My mother and father are both healthy.
☐ Occupation	I'm a banker.
☐ Alcohol use	Occasionally, on the weekends.
☐ Illicit drug use	No.
☐ Tobacco	No.
☐ Drug allergies	No.

Connecting with the Patient

☐ Examinee recognized the SP's emotions and responded with PEARLS.

Physical Examination

☐ Examinee washed his/her hands.

☐ Examinee asked permission to start the exam.

☐ Examinee used respectful draping.

☐ Examinee did not repeat painful maneuvers.

☑ Exam Component	Maneuver
☐ Head and neck exam	Inspection
☐ CV exam	Auscultation
☐ Pulmonary exam	Inspection, auscultation, palpation, percussion
☐ Abdominal exam	Inspection, auscultation, palpation (examined specifically for organomegaly such as splenomegaly)
☐ Neurologic exam	Mental status, cranial nerves, gross motor
☐ Skin exam	Inspection for abrasion, lacerations, bruising

Closure

☐ Examinee discussed initial diagnostic impressions.

☐ Examinee discussed initial management plans:

    ☐ Follow-up tests.

☐ Examinee asked if the SP had any other questions or concerns.

Sample Closure

Mr. Matthews, you should always seek medical treatment after an accident like this. We must now observe you closely until we can determine what is causing your pain. We are going to run a few tests and take some imaging studies of your chest. We will also give you something for your pain and will observe your breathing to make sure you are getting enough oxygen. Do you have any questions for me?

Patient Note

History

Physical Examination

Patient Note

Differential Diagnosis

Diagnosis #1

History Finding(s):   Physical Exam Finding(s):

Diagnosis #2

History Finding(s):   Physical Exam Finding(s):

Diagnosis #3

History Finding(s):   Physical Exam Finding(s):

Diagnostic Workup

Patient Note

History

HPI: *25 yo M c/o left chest pain and LUQ pain following an MVA. The patient struck a tree with his car at a slow speed. The chest pain is 8/10. It is exacerbated with movement or when he takes a deep breath, and nothing relieves it. He reports dyspnea and a productive cough with a low-grade fever but denies LOC, headache, change in mental status, or change in vision. No cardiovascular or neurologic symptoms. No nausea, vomiting, neck stiffness, or unusual fluid from the mouth or nose. No dysuria. His last meal was 5 hours ago. He denies being under the influence of alcohol or drugs.*

ROS: *As per HPI.*
Allergies: *NKDA.*
Medications: *None.*
PMH: *Infectious mononucleosis.*
PSH: *None.*
SH: *No smoking, occasional EtOH, no illicit drugs.*
FH: *Noncontributory.*

Physical Examination

Patient is in acute distress, dyspneic.

VS: *Temp 100°F, RR 22/minute.*
HEENT: *No JVD, no bruises, PERRLA, EOMI, no pharyngeal edema or exudates.*
Chest: *Two large bruises on left chest, left rib tenderness, decreased breath sounds over left lung field, right lung fields clear.*
Heart: *RRR; normal S1/S2; no murmurs, rubs, or gallops.*
Abdomen: *Soft, nondistended, ⊕ BS, LUQ tenderness, no rebound or guarding, no organomegaly.*
Skin: *No bruises or lacerations.*
Neuro: *Mental status: Alert and oriented × 3. Cranial nerves: 2–12 grossly intact. Motor: Strength 5/5 in all muscle groups. Sensation: Intact to pinprick and soft touch.*

Differential Diagnosis

Diagnosis #1: Pneumothorax	
History Finding(s):	*Physical Exam Finding(s):*
Left-sided chest pain following an MVA	Decreased breath sounds over left lung field
Pain is exacerbated by movement and deep breaths	RR 22/minute
Dyspnea	

Diagnosis #2: Hemothorax

History Finding(s):	Physical Exam Finding(s):
Left-sided chest pain following an MVA	Decreased breath sounds over left lung field
Dyspnea	RR 22/minute
Cough	

Diagnosis #3: Pneumonia

History Finding(s):	Physical Exam Finding(s):
Unilateral chest pain	Temperature 100°F
Productive cough	RR 22/minute
Low-grade fever	

Diagnostic Workup

CXR
Sputum and blood Gram stain and culture

CASE DISCUSSION

Patient Note Differential Diagnoses

The most important steps in any trauma are to assess the **ABCDEs**: **A**irway, **B**reathing, **C**irculation, **D**isability (neurologic), and **E**xposure. In this case, the exam is separated from the trauma by several hours and the patient is able to walk and talk, somewhat negating the urgency of a typical ED evaluation. At the same time, chest pain and dyspnea are serious symptoms that require swift evaluation and intervention.

- **Pneumothorax:** A pneumothorax forms when air collects between the pleural and visceral layers of the thorax. Physical findings include a unilateral loss of breath sounds with hyperresonance, shift of the trachea away from the injured side (in the case of tension pneumothorax), and JVD. Although no JVD is present, this patient's acute onset and distress suggest pneumothorax. CXR is the fastest diagnostic tool available.

- **Hemothorax:** This is defined by the presence of blood in the pleural space and is most commonly due to trauma. It presents with chest pain, shortness of breath, cough, decreased breath sounds on the involved side, and occasionally signs and symptoms of hypovolemic shock. The final diagnosis can be made by pleurocentesis or chest tube placement.

- **Pneumonia:** Most often community acquired and caused by *Streptococcus pneumoniae*, bacterial pneumonia can present with acute respiratory distress, fever, cough, pleuritic pain, and shaking chills. This patient has a productive cough, low-grade fever, and unilateral chest pain suggestive of pneumonia. However, traumatic causes should be ruled out first. Physical signs include tachypnea, crackles, egophony, and dullness to percussion. The CXR will show a lobar infiltrate, and sputum cultures may help identify the bacterial pathogen.

Additional Differential Diagnoses

- **Rib fracture:** Rib fractures are the most common chest injury and can result from almost any insult to the chest wall. A simple fracture could cause this patient's pain on inspiration and cough. Rib fractures can also lead to pneumothorax. They can be diagnosed with a CXR.

- **Splenic rupture:** Splenic injuries are always of great concern following a trauma because they can cause significant blood loss very quickly. If this patient was exposed to infectious mononucleosis, his chances of splenic injury or bleeding are greater. Given that this patient's pain is primarily left-sided in the chest area and LUQ, the spleen should be evaluated with an ultrasound exam followed by further imaging with an abdominal CT. On physical exam, it is important to evaluate for any signs or symptoms of organomegaly.

- **Pleuritis:** Inflammation of the pleural membrane can cause severe pain that increases with inspiration or movement. The physical exam is generally negative with the exception of the chest pain. This patient may have a simple viral pleuritis, but more emergent causes need to be ruled out first.

Diagnostic Workup

- **CXR:** On CXR, lobar consolidation may indicate pneumonia, hemothorax may cause linear consolidation, and tension pneumothorax will show mediastinal shift and tracheal deviation away from the pneumothorax. Rib fractures can also be diagnosed from the CXR if they are present.

- **Sputum and blood Gram stain and culture:** Used to screen sputum samples for the identification of bacterial pathogens such as *S pneumoniae*. Other stains, such as acid-fast stains and monoclonal antibodies, can identify tuberculosis and *Pneumocystis jiroveci* (formerly *P carinii*) and should be obtained if the history suggests that these are possibilities. A blood culture and Gram stain would also be useful given that the patient has a low-grade fever.

■ **Urine toxicology and blood alcohol level:** These tests should be considered for any driver following a motor vehicle accident. Even though this patient's car accident occurred a while ago, it is still necessary to evaluate his current situation.

■ **XR/CT—abdomen:** Although a CT scan may be a more effective means of assessing patients for internal abdominal injury, a FAST scan (focused assessment with sonography for trauma) can quickly assess for intra-abdominal bleeding, which may be advisable for this patient given his history of infectious mononucleosis. An AXR remains a quick way to rule out free air in the abdomen.

■ **Pulse oximetry:** Although not as sensitive as ABG analysis, pulse oximetry is a fast, noninvasive measure of oxygenation. Remember that a patient with long-standing lung disease such as COPD may have chronically suppressed oxygenation, which is necessary to maintain respiratory drive.

Opening Scenario

Tanya Parker, a 28-year-old female, comes to the clinic with a positive pregnancy test.

Vital Signs

BP: 120/70 mm Hg

Temp: 98.6°F (37°C)

RR: 14/minute

HR: 76/minute

Examinee Tasks

1. Take a focused history.

2. Perform a focused physical exam (do not perform rectal, genitourinary, or female breast exam).

3. Explain your clinical impression and workup plan to the patient.

4. Write the patient note after leaving the room.

Checklist/SP Sheet

Patient Description

Patient is a 28 yo F, married with no children.

Notes for the SP

If asked, tell the doctor that you feel tired all the time.

Challenging Questions to Ask

"We had not planned to have a baby so soon after marriage. What should I do, doctor?"

Sample Examinee Response

"I understand your anxiety about this unplanned pregnancy. I suggest that you discuss this with your husband. As your physician, I want to assure you that I am here to support and advise you in whatever decision you make. If you wish, I would be happy to discuss your options with both of you."

Examinee Checklist

Building the Doctor-Patient Relationship

Entrance

☐ Examinee knocked on the door before entering.

☐ Examinee introduced self by name.

☐ Examinee identified his/her role or position.

☐ Examinee correctly used patient's name.

☐ Examinee made eye contact with the SP.

Reflective Listening

☐ Examinee asked an open-ended question and actively listened to the response.

☐ Examinee asked the SP to list his/her concerns and listened to the response without interrupting.

☐ Examinee summarized the SP's concerns, often using the SP's own words.

Information Gathering

☐ Examinee elicited data efficiently and accurately.

☑ Question	Patient Response
☐ Chief complaint	Positive pregnancy test.
☐ Onset/duration	My periods have always been regular, but last month it was very light, and this month I haven't had one yet. So I checked a pregnancy test, and it was positive.
☐ Last menstrual period	Six weeks ago, and it was only light spotting.
☐ Menarche	At the age of 14.
☐ Menstrual history	My periods last 3–4 days and occur at the same time every month. Last month I had some spotting for only 1 or 2 days. Usually I have moderate flow and use 4–5 pads per day.
☐ Pain with periods	No.
☐ Spotting between periods	No.
☐ Contraception	My husband withdraws before ejaculation.
☐ Pregnancy/miscarriages	None.
☐ Sexual activity/partners	I am sexually active only with my husband.
☐ History of STDs	None.
☐ Nausea/vomiting	I do feel nauseated lately, but I have not been vomiting.
☐ Postcoital bleeding	No.
☐ Abdominal pain	No.
☐ Appetite changes	I don't feel like eating anything because of the nausea, especially with some smells of food.
☐ Weight changes	I haven't checked my weight recently, but I have been feeling bloated all the time.
☐ Fatigue	Yes. I'm really easily tired out by doing my daily activities.
☐ Breast discharge/tenderness	My breasts are a little fuller than before.
☐ Last Pap smear	Eight months ago, and it was normal.
☐ Fever	No.
☐ Bowel habits	Once a day.
☐ Urinary habits	I feel I have to use the bathroom frequently now. I have no burning or itching.
☐ Shortness of breath	No.

☑ Question	Patient Response
☐ Skin changes	I have not noticed anything.
☐ Exercise	I normally run 5 miles a day, but lately I've had to cut back because I feel so tired all the time.
☐ Current medications	Multivitamins.
☐ Past medical history	None.
☐ Past surgical history	My appendix was removed when I was 20.
☐ Family history	My father is a diabetic. My mom has thyroid and obesity problems.
☐ Occupation	Graduate student.
☐ Alcohol use	Occasionally 1 or 2 beers a week.
☐ Illicit drug use	None.
☐ Tobacco	None.
☐ Drug allergies	None.
☐ Planned pregnancy	No.
☐ Desired pregnancy	Unsure.
☐ Domestic abuse	No.

Connecting with the Patient

☐ Examinee recognized the SP's emotions and responded with PEARLS.

Physical Examination

☐ Examinee washed his/her hands.

☐ Examinee asked permission to start the exam.

☐ Examinee used respectful draping.

☐ Examinee did not repeat painful maneuvers.

☑ Exam Component	Maneuver
☐ HEENT exam	Inspection/palpation of thyroid
☐ CV exam	Auscultation
☐ Pulmonary exam	Auscultation
☐ Abdominal exam	Inspection, auscultation, palpation
☐ Skin exam	Inspected for pigmentation or pallor

Closure

☐ Examinee discussed initial diagnostic impressions.

☐ Examinee discussed initial management plans.

    ☐ Follow-up tests: Examinee mentioned the need for a pelvic/breast exam.

☐ Examinee asked if the SP had any other questions or concerns.

Sample Closure

Mrs. Parker, on the basis of my observations and what you have told me, it appears that you are pregnant. I will have to repeat a urine pregnancy test to confirm the diagnosis. Your last period may not have been a real menstrual period, as spotting can frequently occur in the first trimester. Unfortunately, natural methods of contraception such as pulling out before ejaculation are not very effective. We will also need to perform a pelvic ultrasound to estimate the age of the fetus and the expected date of delivery. If you are pregnant, we will check some more blood tests, a Pap smear, and some vaginal cultures that we routinely perform in every pregnancy. For now, I recommend stopping alcohol consumption and avoiding intense exercises and excess caffeine. I will be giving you some prenatal multivitamins to take orally, and we will schedule your future prenatal visits. I will be able to advise you further as soon as we receive these tests. Do you have any questions or concerns?

Patient Note

History

Physical Examination

Differential Diagnosis

Diagnosis #1

History Finding(s):   **Physical Exam Finding(s):**

Diagnosis #2

History Finding(s):   **Physical Exam Finding(s):**

Diagnosis #3

History Finding(s):   **Physical Exam Finding(s):**

Diagnostic Workup

Patient Note

History

HPI: *28 yo G0 presents with a positive pregnancy test. Her LMP was 6 weeks ago and was unusually scant. She reports bilateral breast engorgement, poor appetite, nausea with no vomiting, increased urinary frequency, and feeling bloated and fatigued. She is sexually active with her husband only, with coitus interruptus as the only method of contraception. This is an unplanned pregnancy, and she is unsure whether she will continue.*

OB/GYN: *G0, menarche at age 14, has regular periods 4–5/30. No history of STDs; last Pap smear was taken 8 months ago and was normal.*

ROS: *Denies abnormal bleeding, abdominal pain, fever, shortness of breath, or change in bowel habits.*
Allergies: *NKDA.*
Medications: *Multivitamins.*
PMH: *None.*
PSH: *Appendectomy at age 20.*
SH: *No smoking, 1–2 beers/week, no illicit drugs. Married graduate student; denies domestic violence.*
FH: *Father is a diabetic. Mother has thyroid problems and obesity.*

Physical Examination

Patient appears comfortable.

VS: *WNL.*
HEENT: *NC/AT, PERRLA, no icterus, no pallor, mouth and oropharynx normal.*
Neck: *No thyroid enlargement.*
Chest: *Clear breath sounds bilaterally.*
Heart: *RRR; normal S1/S2; no murmurs, rubs, or gallops.*
Abdomen: *Soft, nontender, nondistended, ⊕ BS, no evidence of guarding or hepatosplenomegaly.*

Differential Diagnosis

Diagnosis #1: Normal pregnancy	
History Finding(s):	**Physical Exam Finding(s):**
Amenorrhea for 6 weeks	
Positive pregnancy test	
Bilateral breast engorgement	
Nausea and weight gain	

Diagnosis #2: Ectopic pregnancy	
History Finding(s):	**Physical Exam Finding(s):**
Amenorrhea for 6 weeks	
Positive pregnancy test	

Diagnosis #3: Molar pregnancy

History Finding(s):	Physical Exam Finding(s):
Positive pregnancy test	
Nausea	

Diagnostic Workup

Urine hCG
U/S—pelvis
Breast/pelvic exams
Blood type, Rh, antibody screen

CASE DISCUSSION

Patient Note Differential Diagnoses

- **Normal pregnancy:** Any history of delayed periods or amenorrhea in a reproductive-age woman who is sexually active should prompt the diagnosis of pregnancy unless otherwise ruled out. This patient has symptoms of nausea, weight gain, and breast engorgement, all signs of early pregnancy.

- **Ectopic pregnancy:** Extrauterine implantation resulting in ectopic pregnancy should always be in the differential diagnosis of women with a positive pregnancy test until intrauterine pregnancy is identified.

- **Molar pregnancy:** Molar pregnancies are uncommon. Very high serum β-hCG levels, severe nausea and vomiting, new-onset hyperthyroidism, and a uterus that is larger than expected for gestational age should raise suspicion for molar pregnancy. The diagnosis is usually confirmed by pelvic ultrasound.

Diagnostic Workup

- **Urine hCG:** A urine hCG test can confirm pregnancy. Alternatively, a quantitative serum β-hCG can be ordered if an abnormal pregnancy (eg, abortion, ectopic pregnancy, molar pregnancy) is suspected.

- **U/S—pelvis:** It is important to confirm the location of the pregnancy (intrauterine vs. extrauterine) and the gestational age in patients with an uncertain LMP or irregular periods. This can also aid in the diagnosis of molar pregnancies, uterine fibroids, and adnexal masses.

- **Breast/pelvic exams:** Breast engorgement and galactorrhea are some of the physiologic changes that occur in pregnancy. A pelvic exam needs to be performed to evaluate the cervix (lesions, length, dilation, consistency), the uterus (size, fibroids), and the adnexa (masses) and to collect necessary specimens for cytology, cultures, and PCR studies.

- **Blood type, Rh, antibody screen:** To detect antibodies that could potentially cause hemolytic disease of the newborn. Rh(D)-negative women should receive anti-D immune globulin as indicated.

- **CBC:** To rule out anemia and to obtain a baseline for hemoglobin and platelets.

- **TSH:** Neurologic development may be adversely affected in children born to mothers with hypothyroidism, while maternal hyperthyroidism can lead to fetal and maternal complications.

- **RPR, rubella IgG, HBsAg, HIV antibody:** These infections can be transmitted perinatally, and early detection allows for measures that could decrease the possibility of transmission to the fetus. HIV screening should be discussed separately, and the patient's consent is required in some states. These are standard tests that every woman diagnosed with pregnancy should receive.

- **Pap smear:** To screen for cervical dysplasia and cervical cancer. However, since this patient had a normal Pap smear eight months ago, a repeat Pap smear is not necessarily indicated at this visit and could be postponed for another four months.

- **Cervical gonorrhea and chlamydia DNA testing:** Early diagnosis and treatment of these STDs can prevent serious neonatal infections.

- **UA, urine culture:** Pregnant women with untreated asymptomatic bacteriuria are at high risk of developing pyelonephritis. Therefore, all pregnant women need to be screened even if they do not complain of symptoms of a UTI.

CASE 6
DOORWAY INFORMATION

Opening Scenario

The mother of Louise Johnson, a 10-year-old female child, comes to the office because she is concerned that her daughter was recently diagnosed with diabetes.

Examinee Tasks

1. Take a focused history.

2. Explain your clinical impression and workup plan to the mother.

3. Write the patient note after leaving the room.

Checklist/SP Sheet

Patient Description

The patient's mother offers the history; her daughter is at school.

Notes for the SP

None.

Challenging Questions to Ask

- "Doctor, I have no history of diabetes in my family. Why is this happening to my daughter?"
- "Will my child ever be able to eat sweets again?"

Sample Examinee Response

"Your daughter probably had a genetic tendency to develop diabetes. Then certain unknown environmental factors led her to get full-blown diabetes. Your daughter may have either type 1 or type 2 diabetes. In type 1 diabetes, the immune system attacks the pancreas and destroys the cells that are responsible for making insulin. Since insulin regulates and maintains blood sugar, an insulin deficiency will lead to high levels of blood sugar. On the other hand, if your child is overweight and is not physically active, she may have type 2 diabetes, which is a combination of insulin deficiency and resistance to the action of insulin resulting from being overweight. In either case, it is not necessary to have a family history of diabetes. With regard to sweets being the cause of your daughter's diabetes, this is a myth. In fact, your daughter can still eat sweets, but in moderation. She will need to see a dietitian to develop healthy meal plans as well as to learn to recognize which foods contain carbohydrates and how much."

Examinee Checklist

Building the Doctor-Patient Relationship

Entrance

☐ Examinee knocked on the door before entering.

☐ Examinee introduced self by name.

☐ Examinee identified his/her role or position.

☐ Examinee correctly used patient's name.

☐ Examinee made eye contact with the SP.

Reflective Listening

☐ Examinee asked an open-ended question and actively listened to the response.

☐ Examinee asked the SP to list his/her concerns and listened to the response without interrupting.

☐ Examinee summarized the SP's concerns, often using the SP's own words.

Information Gathering

☐ Examinee elicited data efficiently and accurately.

☑ Question	Patient Response
☐ Chief complaint	My child was recently diagnosed with diabetes.
☐ Type of diabetes	I am not sure.
☐ Onset	A month ago.
☐ Presenting symptoms at the time of diagnosis	Excessive thirst and urination.
☐ Effect on child	She is concerned about the effect this will have on her normal activities, such as playing tennis and attending school.
☐ Depression	I'm not sure, but she seems more concerned than depressed.
☐ Irritability	No.
☐ Effect on parents	We were shocked.
☐ Medication	Insulin injections.
☐ Site of injection	In the tummy.
☐ Insulin injector	I do it when she is at home, but when she is away from me, she does the injections herself.
☐ Compliance with insulin	Yes.
☐ Schedule of insulin	Two types: one with meals and one at bedtime.
☐ Measuring glucose at home	Yes, before each meal and at bedtime.
☐ Ranges of blood glucose readings	Her blood sugar levels are normally in the low 100s in the morning and in the high 100s before meals.
☐ Recent level of glucose	Today her morning glucose was 96 in the fasting state.
☐ Hypoglycemia	Not really; the lowest blood glucose reading was 80 in the morning.
☐ Urination	Normal at present, but she had to go to the bathroom a lot, which is how she was first diagnosed.
☐ Abnormal thirst or extreme hunger	No, but she was excessively thirsty earlier.
☐ Weakness or fatigue	No.
☐ Vision problems (blurring of vision)	No.
☐ Weight changes	She has lost about 9 pounds within the past 3 months, but now her weight is stable.
☐ Patient's weight and height	She weighs 180 pounds and has been on the heavy side for a long time. She is 5 feet, 1 inch tall.

☑ Question	Patient Response
☐ Tingling or numbness in limbs	No.
☐ Infections of skin or gums	No.
☐ Itchy skin	No.
☐ Any specific diet	We are trying to give her a balanced diet with the help of the dietitian.
☐ Exercise and playful activities	Yes, she is active and plays tennis.
☐ When does she play?	Evenings.
☐ Loss of consciousness while playing	No.
☐ Last menstrual period	She has not yet started menstruating.
☐ Sleeping problems	No.
☐ Birth history	Normal.
☐ Child weight, height, and language development	She was always up to date with her development. She walked early, talked on time, and is doing well in school.
☐ Past medical history	None.
☐ Past surgical history	None.
☐ Drug allergies	No.

Connecting with the Patient

☐ Examinee recognized SP's emotions and responded with PEARLS.

Physical Examination

None.

Closure

☐ Examinee discussed initial diagnostic impressions.

☐ Examinee discussed initial management plans:

   ☐ Further examination.

   ☐ Follow-up tests.

☐ Examinee asked if the SP had any other questions or concerns.

Sample Closure

Mrs. Johnson, I can understand how you have felt since your daughter was diagnosed with diabetes. Diabetes may alter the dynamics of the entire family and affects everyone, so your life is going to be a little different now. We can manage this disease very well through a combination of insulin, a balanced diet, and regular exercise. First of all, you should understand the disease and know how to manage it. You will need to attend diabetes classes with your daughter. Second, everyone in your family, including your daughter, should learn to recognize signs of low glucose levels, such as confusion, disorientation, or fainting, and should know how to provide appropriate care. Your daughter should always carry a snack or juices as an "emergency kit." Her teachers and friends should also be aware of her disease. I hope you understood what we discussed today. Do you have any additional questions or concerns?

Patient Note

History

_____
_____
_____
_____
_____
_____
_____
_____
_____
_____
_____
_____
_____
_____
_____
_____
_____

Physical Examination

_____
_____
_____
_____
_____
_____
_____
_____
_____
_____
_____
_____
_____
_____
_____

Patient Note

Differential Diagnosis

Diagnosis #1

History Finding(s):   Physical Exam Finding(s):

Diagnosis #2

History Finding(s):   Physical Exam Finding(s):

Diagnosis #3

History Finding(s):   Physical Exam Finding(s):

Diagnostic Workup

Patient Note

History

HPI: *The source of the information is the patient's mother. The mother of a 10 yo F states that her child was diagnosed with DM 1 month ago, when she presented with excessive thirst and frequent urination. The parents were shocked after the diagnosis was made. The child seems concerned but not irritable or depressed. She is active, plays tennis, and is currently on a diet prescribed by a dietitian. She is on insulin injections and regularly monitors her blood glucose levels at home. Her compliance is good; she checks her blood glucose before each meal and at bedtime. Fasting glucose levels are usually 80 to the low 100s and in the high 100s before meals. She has not had any episodes of hypoglycemia. She has lost 9 lbs in the past 3 months, but her weight is stable now at about 180 lbs. She denies any weakness, fatigue, tingling over the limbs, visual symptoms, or rash/itch at the injection sites. She has not yet started menstruating.*

ROS: *Negative.*
Allergies: *NKDA.*
Medications: *Insulin.*
PMH: *None.*
PSH: *None.*
Birth history: *Normal.*
Developmental history: *Normal.*
FH: *No family history of diabetes.*

Physical Examination

None.

Differential Diagnosis

Diagnosis #1: Type 1 diabetes mellitus	
History Finding(s):	**Physical Exam Finding(s):**
Polyuria, polydipsia	
Recent weight loss	
Hyperglycemia	

Diagnosis #2: Type 2 diabetes mellitus	
History Finding(s):	**Physical Exam Finding(s):**
Polyuria, polydipsia	
Obesity	
Hyperglycemia	

Diagnosis #3: Secondary causes of diabetes (eg, Cushing's syndrome)

History Finding(s):	Physical Exam Finding(s):
Obesity	

Diagnostic Workup

Insulin and C-peptide levels
Islet cell antibodies
HbA_{1c}
Electrolytes, glucose
UA and urine microalbumin
24-hour urine free cortisol

CASE DISCUSSION

Patient Note Differential Diagnoses

- **Diabetes mellitus (DM):** Although most cases of DM in the pediatric population are type 1, the increasing prevalence of obesity and physical inactivity in the urban population has led to a growing incidence of type 2 DM among children. In every suspected case of DM, it is mandatory to rule out other causes.

- **Secondary causes of diabetes (hyperglycemia):** DM can be secondary to other factors or medical conditions, such as drugs (eg, thiazide diuretics, glucocorticoids), Cushing's syndrome, pancreatitis, cystic fibrosis, hemochromatosis, and acromegaly.

Diagnostic Workup

- **Insulin and C-peptide levels:** When combined, can be a useful tool in identifying type 1 DM.

- **Islet cell antibodies:** This finding will support the diagnosis of type 1 DM.

- **HbA$_{1c}$:** Used to diagnose DM and to monitor treatment. HbA$_{1c}$ estimates blood glucose control during the preceding 2–3 months. Elevated levels suggest existing DM as well as lack of control of blood glucose levels within the past 2–3 months.

- **Electrolytes, glucose:** To assess for hypernatremia, which may be seen in DM, as well as for glycemic control in conjunction with HbA$_{1c}$. A random glucose test $\geq$ 200 mg/dL can help make the diagnosis of DM.

- **UA, urine microalbumin:** To screen for diabetic nephropathy.

- **24-hour urine free cortisol:** To rule out coexisting Cushing's syndrome.

CASE 7
DOORWAY INFORMATION

Opening Scenario

Richard Green, a 74-year-old male, comes to the ED complaining of pain in his right arm.

Vital Signs

BP: 135/85 mm Hg

Temp: 98.0°F (36.7°C)

RR: 12/minute

HR: 76/minute, regular

Examinee Tasks

1. Take a focused history.

2. Perform a focused physical exam (do not perform rectal, genitourinary, or female breast exam).

3. Explain your clinical impression and workup plan to the patient.

4. Write the patient note after leaving the room.

Checklist/SP Sheet

Patient Description

Patient is a 74 yo M.

Notes for the SP

- Sit up on the bed.
- Hold your right arm close to your body with your left hand and keep it externally rotated and slightly abducted.
- Show pain when the examinee tries to move your right shoulder in any direction.
- Do not allow the examinee to bring your shoulder to its full range of motion in flexion, extension, abduction, or external rotation.

Challenging Questions to Ask

"Doctor, do you think I will be able to move my arm again like before?"

Sample Examinee Response

"I hope so, but first we need to find out exactly what is causing your problem."

Examinee Checklist

Building the Doctor-Patient Relationship

Entrance

☐ Examinee knocked on the door before entering.

☐ Examinee introduced self by name.

☐ Examinee identified his/her role or position.

☐ Examinee correctly used patient's name.

☐ Examinee made eye contact with the SP.

Reflective Listening

☐ Examinee asked an open-ended question and actively listened to the response.

☐ Examinee asked the SP to list his/her concerns and listened to the response without interrupting.

☐ Examinee summarized the SP's concerns, often using the SP's own words.

Information Gathering

☐ Examinee elicited data efficiently and accurately.

☑ Question	Patient Response
☐ Chief complaint	Pain in the right arm.
☐ Onset	Three days ago.
☐ Precipitating events	I was playing with my grandchildren in the garden when I tripped and fell.
☐ Description of the fall	I tripped over a toy on the ground and fell on my hand. My arm was outstretched.
☐ Loss of consciousness	No.
☐ Location	The upper and middle parts of the arm.
☐ Weakness/paralysis	None.
☐ Numbness/loss of sensation	None.
☐ Progression of pain	I didn't feel any pain at the time, and then the pain started gradually. It is stable now, but it is still there.
☐ Pain anywhere else	No.
☐ Seen by a doctor since then	No.
☐ Any treatments	I used a sling and took some Tylenol, but the pain didn't get that much better.
☐ Alleviating factors	Not moving my arm and Tylenol.
☐ Exacerbating factors	Moving my arm.
☐ Reason for not seeking medical attention	Well, it wasn't that bad, and I thought it would get better on its own (looks anxious). Also, my son didn't have time to bring me to the hospital; he was busy.
☐ Living conditions	I live with my son. He is married and has 3 children. Life has been hard on him lately. He lost his job and is looking for a new one.
☐ Social history	I am a widower. My wife died 3 years ago, and since then I have lived with my son.
☐ Bad treatment in his son's house	No (looks anxious). They are all nice.
☐ Do you feel safe at home?	Yes (looks anxious).

☑ Question	Patient Response
☐ Current medications	Tylenol, albuterol inhaler.
☐ Allergies	Yes, I am allergic to aspirin.
☐ Nature of reaction to aspirin	I get an itchy rash all over my body.
☐ Past medical history	Asthma.
☐ Past surgical history	They removed part of my prostate 2 years ago. It was very difficult for me to urinate, but that has gotten much better. They said there was no evidence of cancer.
☐ Occupation	Retired schoolteacher.
☐ Alcohol use	No.
☐ Tobacco	No.
☐ Exercise	Every day I walk for 20 minutes to the grocery store and back.

Connecting with the Patient

☐ Examinee recognized the SP's emotions and responded with PEARLS.

Physical Examination

☐ Examinee washed his/her hands.

☐ Examinee asked permission to start the exam.

☐ Examinee used respectful draping.

☐ Examinee did not repeat painful maneuvers.

☑ Exam Component	Maneuver
☐ Head and neck exam	Checked for bruises, neck movements
☐ CV exam	Auscultation
☐ Pulmonary exam	Auscultation
☐ Exam of the arms	Compared both arms in terms of strength, range of motion (shoulder, elbow, wrist), joint stability, sensation, DTRs, pulses

Closure

☐ Examinee discussed initial diagnostic impressions.

☐ Examinee discussed initial management plans:

    ☐ Follow-up tests.

    ☐ Alternative living options such as assisted living.

    ☐ Social work assistance.

☐ Examinee offered a statement of support: "Your safety is my primary concern, and I am here for help and support when you need it."

☐ Examinee asked if the SP had any other questions or concerns.

Sample Closure

Mr. Green, you may have a fractured bone, a simple sprain, or a dislocation of the shoulder joint. We will need to obtain an x-ray of your shoulder and arm to make a diagnosis, and more precise imaging studies such as an MRI may be necessary as well. Your safety is my primary concern, and I am here to offer you help and support whenever you need it. Sometimes living with a family can be stressful for the whole household. Have you ever considered moving to an assisted-living community or to an apartment complex for seniors? If you are interested, I can arrange a meeting with our social worker, who can assess your social situation and help you find the resources you need. Do you have any questions for me?

Patient Note

History

Physical Examination

Patient Note

Differential Diagnosis

Diagnosis #1

History Finding(s):   **Physical Exam Finding(s):**

Diagnosis #2

History Finding(s):   **Physical Exam Finding(s):**

Diagnosis #3

History Finding(s):   **Physical Exam Finding(s):**

Diagnostic Workup

Patient Note

History

HPI: *74 yo M c/o right arm pain for the past 3 days. The pain started after he fell on his outstretched right arm and persisted despite his use of Tylenol and a sling at home. No loss of consciousness before or after the fall. No paralysis or loss of sensation. The pain is in the upper and middle part of the arm, increases with any movement of the arm, and is alleviated by rest. When asked why he delayed seeking medical assistance, the patient looked anxious and stated that his son didn't have time to take him to the hospital.*

ROS: *Negative except as above.*

Allergies: *Aspirin (rash).*

Medications: *Tylenol, albuterol inhaler.*

PMH: *Asthma, probable BPH s/p prostate surgery.*

PSH: *As above.*

SH: *No smoking, no EtOH. Widower for the past 3 years; lives with his son, who recently lost his job. Walks 20 minutes every morning.*

Physical Examination

Patient is in no acute distress.

VS: *WNL.*

HEENT: *Normocephalic, atraumatic, no bruises.*

Neck: *Supple, full range of motion in all directions, no bruises.*

Chest: *Clear breath sounds bilaterally.*

Heart: *RRR; normal S1/S2; no murmurs, rubs, or gallops.*

Extremities: *Right arm held closely against chest wall. Nonlocalized tenderness over middle and upper right arm and right shoulder; pain and restricted range of motion on flexion, extension, abduction, and external rotation of right shoulder. Right elbow and wrist are normal. Pulses normal and symmetric in brachial and radial arteries. Unable to assess muscle strength due to pain. DTRs intact and symmetric. Sensation intact to pinprick and soft touch.*

Differential Diagnosis

Diagnosis #1: Humeral fracture	
History Finding(s):	**Physical Exam Finding(s):**
Pain following recent fall on outstretched arm	Tenderness over upper and middle right arm
Pain increases with arm movement	Restricted range of motion

Patient Note

Diagnosis #2: Shoulder dislocation

History Finding(s):	Physical Exam Finding(s):
Pain following recent fall on outstretched arm	Right arm externally rotated and slightly abducted
Pain increases with arm movement	Pain and restricted range of motion on shoulder exam

Diagnosis #3: Osteoporosis

History Finding(s):	Physical Exam Finding(s):
Advanced age	

Diagnostic Workup

XR—right shoulder and arm
MRI—shoulder
Bone density scan (DEXA)

CASE DISCUSSION

Patient Note Differential Diagnoses

- **Humeral fracture:** Most commonly occurs in elderly persons, usually after a fall. The axillary nerve can be injured in a proximal humerus fracture, causing sensory loss along the lateral aspect of the deltoid region. The radial nerve can be injured in a fracture of the midshaft/distal third of the humerus, causing wrist drop.

- **Shoulder dislocation:** The glenohumeral joint is the most commonly dislocated joint in the human body. It most often dislocates anteriorly and inferiorly and usually results from a fall on an outstretched arm with forceful abduction, extension, and external rotation of the shoulder. On exam, the patient's arm is typically externally rotated and slightly abducted. Movement is avoided owing to pain.

- **Osteoporosis:** Suspect underlying osteoporosis in elderly patients (especially women) presenting with fractures following minimal trauma. The most common sites of osteoporotic fractures are the thoracic and lumbar vertebral bodies, the neck of the femur, and the distal radius.

Additional Differential Diagnoses

- **Elder abuse:** The history contains red flags (bruises, anxious behavior) that may point to elder abuse. The American Medical Association has defined elder abuse as "an act or omission which results in harm or threatened harm to the health or welfare of an elderly person." The diagnosis of elder abuse is not readily made because often both the abuser and the victim deny abuse. Thus, diagnosis is often inferential, and supporting evidence must be sought.

- **Rotator cuff tear:** Patients usually present with nonspecific pain localized to the shoulder, but pain is often referred down the proximal lateral arm owing to shared innervation. There may be an inability to abduct or flex the shoulder. Patients may also demonstrate significant weakness in internal or external rotation strength.

Diagnostic Workup

- **XR—right shoulder and arm:** AP and lateral views that include the joints above and below the injury can show fracture or dislocation. An axillary view is useful to help diagnose proximal humeral fracture or dislocation.

- **MRI—shoulder:** Required to diagnose rotator cuff tears, labral disease, and other disorders.

- **Bone density scan (DEXA):** To diagnose and quantify osteoporosis.

CASE 8
DOORWAY INFORMATION

Opening Scenario

Raymond Stern, a 56-year-old male, comes to the clinic for diabetes follow-up.

Vital Signs

BP: 139/85 mm Hg

Temp: 98.0°F (36.7°C)

RR: 15/minute

HR: 75/minute, regular

Examinee Tasks

1. Take a focused history.

2. Perform a focused physical exam (do not perform rectal, genitourinary, or female breast exam).

3. Explain your clinical impression and workup plan to the patient.

4. Write the patient note after leaving the room.

Checklist/SP Sheet

Patient Description

Patient is a 56 yo M.

Notes for the SP

- Pretend that you have a loss of sharp and dull sensations, vibration sense, and position sense in both feet (stocking distribution).
- Pretend to have a normal knee jerk and absent ankle reflex.

Challenging Questions to Ask

"Will I lose my feet, doctor?"

Sample Examinee Response

"Amputation is a last resort in patients with diabetes who develop an infection in their feet, and fortunately we are not at that point. The nerve damage to your feet is uncomfortable, but it will not lead to amputation as long as you take the proper measures to protect your feet from injury. If we continue to keep your blood sugar and cholesterol well controlled, we should be able to avoid amputation. We'll discuss more on how to do this later in the visit."

Examinee Checklist

Building the Doctor-Patient Relationship

Entrance

☐ Examinee knocked on the door before entering.

☐ Examinee introduced self by name.

☐ Examinee identified his/her role or position.

☐ Examinee correctly used patient's name.

☐ Examinee made eye contact with the SP.

Reflective Listening

☐ Examinee asked an open-ended question and actively listened to the response.

☐ Examinee asked the SP to list his/her concerns and listened to the response without interrupting.

☐ Examinee summarized the SP's concerns, often using the SP's own words.

Information Gathering

☐ Examinee elicited data efficiently and accurately.

☑ Question	Patient Response
☐ Chief complaint	I am here for a diabetes checkup. The last time I saw my doctor was 6 months ago.
☐ Onset	I have had diabetes mellitus for the past 25 years.
☐ Treatment	NPH insulin, 20 units in the morning and 15 units in the evening.
☐ Compliance with medications	I never miss any doses.
☐ Last blood sugar reading	Three days ago, and it was 135.
☐ Blood sugar monitoring	I have a blood sugar monitor at home, and I check my blood sugar twice a week. It usually ranges between 120 and 145.
☐ Last HbA$_{1c}$	The last was 6 months ago, and it was 7.
☐ Last time eyes were checked	One year ago, and there were no signs of diabetic eye disease.
☐ How he is feeling today	Good.
☐ Medication side effects	No.
☐ Heart symptoms (chest pain, palpitations)	Sometimes I feel my heart racing, and I start sweating.
☐ Description of these symptoms	It happens rarely if I miss a meal. I feel better after drinking orange juice.
☐ Pulmonary complaints (shortness of breath, cough)	No.
☐ Neurologic complaints (headaches, dizziness, weakness, numbness)	I have tingling and numbness in my feet all the time, especially at night, and it's gotten worse over the past 2 months.
☐ Polyuria, dysuria, hematuria	No.
☐ Abdominal complaints (pain, dyspepsia, nausea)	No.
☐ Change in bowel habits	No.
☐ Visual problems (blurred vision)	No.
☐ Foot infection	No.
☐ Marital or work problems	No, my wife is great, and I am very happy in my job.

☑ Question	Patient Response
☐ Feelings of anxiety or stress	No.
☐ Weight changes	No.
☐ Appetite changes	No.
☐ Hypertension	No.
☐ History of hypercholesterolemia	Yes, it was diagnosed 2 years ago.
☐ Previous heart problems	I had a heart attack last year.
☐ History of TIA or stroke	No.
☐ Current medications	Insulin, lovastatin, aspirin, atenolol.
☐ Past medical history	Heart attack last year; high cholesterol for 2 years.
☐ Past surgical history	None.
☐ Family history	My father died at age 60 of a stroke. My mother is healthy.
☐ Occupation	Clerk.
☐ Diet	I eat everything that my wife cooks—meat, vegetables, etc. I don't follow any special diet.
☐ Exercise	No.
☐ Alcohol use	Yes, whiskey on the weekends.
☐ CAGE questions	No (to all 4).
☐ Illicit drug use	No.
☐ Tobacco	No.
☐ Social history	I am married and live with my wife.
☐ Sexual activity	I am not doing my job the way I used to, but my wife understands and is supportive. They told me it is the diabetes. Is it?
☐ Type of sexual problem	I can't get it up, doc. I don't even wake up with erections anymore.
☐ Libido	Good.
☐ Duration	One or two years ago.
☐ Feelings of depression	No.
☐ Drug allergies	No.

Connecting with the Patient

☐ Examinee recognized the SP's emotions and responded with PEARLS.

Physical Examination

☐ Examinee washed his/her hands.

☐ Examinee asked permission to start the exam.

☐ Examinee used respectful draping.

☐ Examinee did not repeat painful maneuvers.

☑ Exam Component	Maneuver
☐ Eye exam	Funduscopic exam
☐ Neck exam	Carotid auscultation
☐ CV exam	Palpation, auscultation
☐ Pulmonary exam	Auscultation
☐ Abdominal exam	Auscultation, palpation, percussion
☐ Extremities	Inspected feet, peripheral pulses
☐ Neurologic exam	DTRs, Babinski's sign, sensation and strength in lower extremities

Closure

☐ Examinee discussed initial diagnostic impressions.

☐ Examinee discussed initial management plans:

    ☐ Follow-up tests.

    ☐ Lifestyle modification (diet, exercise).

☐ Examinee asked if the SP had any other questions or concerns.

Sample Closure

Mr. Stern, the palpitations and sweating you have experienced are most likely due to episodes of low blood sugar, which may have resulted from a higher-than-normal dose of insulin or from skipping or delaying meals. The numbness you describe in your feet is probably related to the effect of diabetes on your nervous system; better control of your blood sugar may help improve this problem. Many factors, including diabetes, can cause the erection difficulties you describe. I will need to perform an examination of your genital area and run some blood tests, and at some point we may also need to conduct some more complex tests to identify the cause of your problems. Do you have any questions for me?

Patient Note

History

Physical Examination

Patient Note

Differential Diagnosis

Diagnosis #1

History Finding(s):   Physical Exam Finding(s):

Diagnosis #2

History Finding(s):   Physical Exam Finding(s):

Diagnosis #3

History Finding(s):   Physical Exam Finding(s):

Diagnostic Workup

Patient Note

History

HPI: *56 yo M presents for diabetes follow-up.*

- *25-year history of DM, treated with insulin.*
- *Compliant with medications.*
- *Monitors blood glucose twice a week, readings between 120 and 145 mg/dL.*
- *Last HbA$_{1c}$ 6 months ago was 7%.*
- *Occasional episodes of palpitations and diaphoresis, occurring after missing meals and resolving with drinking orange juice.*
- *Tingling and numbness in feet all the time, especially at night, worse over past 2 months.*
- *Loss of erections × 2 years; absence of early-morning erections.*
- *No weight or appetite changes.*
- *No special diet.*

ROS: *Negative except as above.*

Allergies: *NKDA.*

Medications: *Lovastatin, NPH insulin, aspirin, atenolol.*

PMH: *Hypercholesterolemia diagnosed 2 years ago; MI 1 year ago.*

PSH: *None.*

SH: *No smoking, drinks whiskey on weekends (CAGE 0/4), no illicit drugs. Works as a clerk. He is married and lives with his wife.*

FH: *Father died of a stroke at age 60.*

Physical Examination

Patient is in no distress.

VS: *WNL.*

HEENT: *PERRLA, no funduscopic abnormalities.*

Neck: *No carotid bruits, no JVD.*

Chest: *Clear breath sounds bilaterally.*

Heart: *Apical impulse not displaced; RRR; normal S1/S2; no murmurs, rubs, or gallops.*

Abdomen: *Soft, nondistended, nontender, ⊕ BS, no bruits, no organomegaly.*

Extremities: *No edema, no skin breakdown, 2+ dorsalis pedis pulses.*

Neuro: *Motor: Strength 5/5 in bilateral lower extremities. DTRs: Symmetric 2+ knee jerks, absent ankle jerks and ⊖ Babinski bilaterally. Sensation: Decreased pinprick; soft touch, vibratory, and position sense in bilateral lower extremities.*

Patient Note

Differential Diagnosis

Diagnosis #1: Insulin-induced hypoglycemia

History Finding(s)	Physical Exam Finding(s)
Episodes of palpitations and diaphoresis that resolve with drinking orange juice	
Tight glycemic control	

Diagnosis #2: Diabetic peripheral neuropathy

History Finding(s)	Physical Exam Finding(s)
History of diabetes mellitus	Absent ankle jerk
Constant numbness and tingling in feet	

Diagnosis #3: Organic erectile dysfunction

History Finding(s)	Physical Exam Finding(s)
Loss of erection for 2 years with absence of early-morning erection	
History of diabetes mellitus	
History of alcohol use	
Taking lovastatin and atenolol	

Diagnostic Workup

Genital exam
Serum glucose, HbA_{1c}
UA, urine microalbumin, BUN/Cr
Doppler U/S—penis
Nerve conduction studies

CASE DISCUSSION

Patient Note Differential Diagnoses

- **Insulin-induced hypoglycemia:** The patient's history suggests episodes of hypoglycemia. Typical signs and symptoms of hypoglycemia include sweating, tachycardia, palpitations, tremor, anxiety, weakness, confusion, and seizures. Maintaining tight glycemic control may occasionally result in hypoglycemia, and patients should be educated about how to recognize and treat this complication.

- **Diabetic peripheral neuropathy:** Involvement of the peripheral nervous system in diabetes may lead to symmetric sensory or mixed polyneuropathy (among other patterns of neuropathy). Burning foot paresthesias that worsen at night and loss of ankle reflexes, as seen in this case, are classic.

- **Erectile dysfunction (ED):** In diabetics, ED is usually related to vascular disease, autonomic neuropathy, or medications taken for associated conditions (eg, antihypertensives). In general, impotence unaccompanied by loss of libido with absence of early-morning erections suggests organic ED of either a vascular or a neurologic origin. Alcohol also causes an autonomic neuropathy and may contribute to ED, as can medications such as statins and β-blockers.

Additional Differential Diagnoses

The differential for nondiabetic peripheral neuropathy includes hereditary, toxic, metabolic, infectious, inflammatory, and paraneoplastic disorders. No specific cause is determined in up to 50% of cases. The history and exam guide us to some of the common causes discussed below.

- **Alcoholic peripheral neuropathy:** This causes a distal sensorimotor polyneuropathy marked by painful leg paresthesias and is directly attributable to alcohol or to associated nutritional deficiencies (eg, thiamine and vitamin B_{12}).

- **Multiple myeloma:** Myeloma or other paraproteinemias must be ruled out in a patient with peripheral neuropathy.

- **Renal failure:** Uremia may cause a sensory peripheral neuropathy that may affect diabetic patients.

- **Hypothyroidism:** Peripheral neuropathy and other neurologic symptoms may be associated with hypothyroidism.

- **Vasculitides:** Polyarteritis nodosa, rheumatoid arthritis, and other vasculitides may cause peripheral neuropathy and can be detected by monitoring ESR, ANCA, RF, and anti–cyclic citrullinated peptide (anti-CCP) antibody.

Diagnostic Workup

- **Genital exam:** To rule out Peyronie's disease (eg, penile scarring or plaque formation).
- **Serum glucose, HbA$_{1c}$:** To assess glycemic control.
- **UA, urine microalbumin, BUN/Cr:** To screen for diabetic nephropathy.
- **Doppler U/S—penis:** A helpful noninvasive test to measure penile blood flow.
- **Nerve conduction studies:** To confirm that symptoms arise from a peripheral nerve origin and to indicate an axonal vs. demyelinating mechanism.

- **CBC, serum calcium, ESR, serum protein electrophoresis:** To detect paraproteinemias (eg, multiple myeloma); anemia is often an associated finding. Other findings include elevated blood calcium levels and an elevated ESR.

- **Other studies:** In select cases, other studies used to evaluate peripheral neuropathy include ESR, BUN/Cr, TSH, liver enzymes, RF, ANA, ANCA, anti-CCP antibody, hepatitis B and C serologies, RPR, HIV antibody, urine heavy metal screen, CSF examination, CXR, and cutaneous nerve biopsy (eg, to diagnose amyloidosis).

Opening Scenario

Julia Melton, a 25-year-old female, comes to the ED after being assaulted.

Vital Signs

BP: 120/85 mm Hg

Temp: 98.0°F (36.7°C)

RR: 17/minute

HR: 90/minute, regular

Examinee Tasks

1. Take a focused history.

2. Perform a focused physical exam (do not perform rectal, genitourinary, or female breast exam).

3. Explain your clinical impression and workup plan to the patient.

4. Write the patient note after leaving the room.

Checklist/SP Sheet

Patient Description

Patient is a 25 yo F.

Notes for the SP

- Look depressed and tearful.
- Start weeping when asked about physical and/or sexual assaults.
- Pretend to have right chest pain with deep inspiration, cough, and palpation.

Challenging Questions to Ask

"This is all my fault, doctor. Do you think my friends will ever accept me again?"

Sample Examinee Response

"I am so sorry for what happened to you; it is horrific and must be very difficult for you to handle. However, it is not your fault by any means. Whoever did this to you should be held accountable."

Examinee Checklist

Building the Doctor-Patient Relationship

Entrance

☐ Examinee knocked on the door before entering.

☐ Examinee introduced self by name.

☐ Examinee identified his/her role or position.

☐ Examinee correctly used patient's name.

☐ Examinee made eye contact with the SP.

Reflective Listening

☐ Examinee asked an open-ended question and actively listened to the response.

☐ Examinee asked the SP to list his/her concerns and listened to the response without interrupting.

☐ Examinee summarized the SP's concerns, often using the SP's own words.

Information Gathering

☐ Examinee elicited data efficiently and accurately.

☑ Question	Patient Response
☐ Chief complaint	I was attacked by 2 men.
☐ Onset	About 3 hours ago. I came to the ED right away.
☐ Incident location	It happened outside the bar that I usually go to.
☐ Did you recognize the assailants?	I have seen them in the bar but never talked to them.
☐ Did you report the incident?	No.
☐ Description of the assault	I was walking toward my car, and then all of a sudden I was pulled into a storage room. I started screaming, but the men started to slap me and beat me up with their fists.
☐ Assault objects	They used their fists and their bodies to hold me down. I couldn't move at all even though I tried to struggle against them.
☐ Sexual assault	Yes.
☐ Did they use condoms?	No.
☐ Did ejaculation occur?	I don't know.
☐ Type of intercourse (oral, vaginal, anal)	Vaginal.
☐ Foreign objects used	None.
☐ Last menstrual period	Three weeks ago.
☐ Contraceptives	I'm not on the pill or anything.
☐ Pain	Yes, I feel sore all over, especially on the right side of my chest.
☐ Location of the worst pain	The right chest.
☐ Radiation	No.
☐ Severity on a scale	About 8/10.
☐ Alleviating factors	It improves when I sit still.
☐ Exacerbating factors	It gets worse whenever I move or take a deep breath.
☐ Bleeding or bruises	No.
☐ Loss of consciousness	No.
☐ Headache	No.

☑ Question	Patient Response
☐ Change in vision	No.
☐ Dizziness	No.
☐ Weakness	No, I am just tired.
☐ Numbness	No.
☐ Shortness of breath	Yes, I feel that I can't get enough air.
☐ Palpitations	Yes.
☐ Blood in stool/urine	No, but I haven't gone to the bathroom since the incident.
☐ Vaginal bleeding	No.
☐ Nausea/vomiting	No.
☐ Abdominal pain	Yes, it hurts everywhere.
☐ Joint pain	My wrists hurt where they were holding me down.
☐ Current medications	None.
☐ Past medical history	None.
☐ Past surgical history	None.
☐ Family history	None.
☐ Occupation	Student.
☐ Alcohol use	Occasionally.
☐ Illicit drug use	Never.
☐ Tobacco	No.
☐ Drug allergies	No.

Connecting with the Patient

☐ Examinee recognized the SP's emotions and responded with PEARLS.

Physical Examination

☐ Examinee washed his/her hands.

☐ Examinee asked permission to start the exam.

☐ Examinee used respectful draping.

☐ Examinee did not repeat painful maneuvers.

☑ Exam Component	Maneuver
☐ Head and neck exam	Inspection, palpation
☐ Mouth exam	Inspection
☐ CV exam	Auscultation
☐ Pulmonary exam	Inspection, auscultation, palpation, percussion
☐ Abdominal exam	Inspection, auscultation, palpation
☐ Neurologic exam	Mental status, cranial nerves, gross motor
☐ Musculoskeletal exam	Inspection, palpation

Closure

☐ Examinee discussed initial diagnostic impressions.

☐ Examinee discussed initial management plans:

    ☐ Follow-up tests: Examinee mentioned the need for a pelvic exam.

☐ Examinee asked if the SP had any other questions or concerns.

Sample Closure

Ms. Melton, I am really sorry for what happened to you. I want to emphasize that it is not your fault, and you should not feel guilty about it. I recommend that you report the incident to the police. In the meantime, I will need to do a pelvic examination to make sure you have no injuries in the genital area. In addition, I will need to collect some specimens and swabs from your body and genital area so that they can be used as evidence if you choose to file charges, and also to look for STDs. We will run some blood tests for potential STDs and will order a pregnancy test and some x-rays. If your pregnancy test is negative, we will offer you some options for emergency contraception. It would also be prudent to give you some antibiotics to protect you from infections. Finally, I can have our social worker come talk to you and provide you with phone numbers for support groups and other resources. Do you have any questions for me?

Patient Note

History

Physical Examination

Patient Note

Differential Diagnosis

Diagnosis #1

History Finding(s):   **Physical Exam Finding(s):**

Diagnosis #2

History Finding(s):   **Physical Exam Finding(s):**

Diagnosis #3

History Finding(s):   **Physical Exam Finding(s):**

Diagnostic Workup

Patient Note

History

HPI: *25 yo F comes to the ED after being sexually and physically assaulted. The event happened about 3 hours ago as she was leaving a bar. She was beaten and raped by 2 unknown men. They had vaginal intercourse with her without using condoms, and she is unsure if ejaculation occurred. Her LMP was 3 weeks ago. She does not use any form of contraception. She also c/o shortness of breath, palpitations, and right chest pain that is nonradiating. The chest pain is exacerbated by movement and deep breaths and is relieved by sitting still. No nausea or vomiting. No dizziness or headache. No weakness or numbness in her extremities; no vaginal, rectal, or urinary bleeding.*

ROS: *Negative except as above.*
Allergies: *NKDA.*
Medications: *None.*
PMH: *None.*
PSH: *None.*
SH: *No smoking, occasional EtOH, no illicit drugs.*
FH: *Noncontributory.*

Physical Examination

Patient is anxious and in acute distress.

VS: *WNL.*
HEENT: *No JVD, PERRLA, EOMI.*
Chest: *Clear breath sounds bilaterally; tenderness on palpation of right chest wall.*
Heart: *Normal S1/S2; no murmurs, rubs, or gallops.*
Abdomen: *Soft, nontender, nondistended, ⊕ BS, no rebound or organomegaly.*
Neuro: *Mental status: Alert and oriented × 3. Cranial nerves: 2–12 grossly intact. Motor: Strength 5/5 in all muscle groups.*

Differential Diagnosis

Diagnosis #1: Rib fracture	
History Finding(s)	**Physical Exam Finding(s)**
Physical assault	Tenderness on palpation of right chest wall
Right chest pain	
Pain is exacerbated by movement and deep breaths	

Diagnosis #2: STD	
History Finding(s)	**Physical Exam Finding(s)**
Sexual assault by 2 men	
No condom use	

Diagnosis #3: Pregnancy

History Finding(s)	Physical Exam Finding(s)
Unprotected vaginal intercourse with possible ejaculation	
No OCP use	
Last menstrual period 3 weeks ago	

Diagnostic Workup

Pelvic exam
XR—skeletal survey
CXR
Urine hCG
Wet mount, KOH prep, cervical culture, gonorrhea and chlamydia tests
HIV antibody, VDRL, HBV antigen

CASE DISCUSSION

Patient Note Differential Diagnoses

- **Rib fracture:** This can result from any insult to the chest wall. A simple fracture can cause pain on inspiration and cough.

- **STDs:** Sexual assault victims may acquire a variety of pathogens during the incident, including trichomoniasis, chlamydia, gonorrhea, HIV, and hepatitis B.

- **Pregnancy:** All sexual assault victims should be evaluated for possible existing pregnancy and should be offered emergency contraception.

Additional Differential Diagnoses

- **Pneumothorax/hemothorax:** Defined as the presence of air or blood in the pleural space between the visceral and parietal pleurae. Physical findings include unilateral loss of breath sounds with hyperresonance, shifting of the trachea away from the injured side, and JVD. Because this patient suffered physical trauma, she may have a traumatic pneumothorax. A CXR is a fast and easy tool with which to evaluate patients for a pneumothorax.

- **Muscle rupture:** Chest pain in trauma victims may be musculoskeletal in origin.

Diagnostic Workup

- **Pelvic exam:** To evaluate for any possible physical injury of the genital or anal area and to collect specimens for medical and forensic purposes.

- **XR—skeletal survey:** To detect possible bone or rib fractures.

- **CXR:** To detect rib fractures, pneumothorax, and pleural effusions.

- **Urine hCG:** To rule out pregnancy.

- **Wet mount, KOH prep, cervical culture, gonorrhea and chlamydia tests:** The vaginal discharge is examined microscopically to evaluate for infection. The presence of epithelial cells covered with bacteria (clue cells) suggests bacterial vaginosis, and the presence of hyphae and spores points to candidal infection. Motile organisms are seen in trichomonal infection. A "fishy" odor after the addition of KOH to the discharge is indicative of bacterial vaginosis. If sperm are detected in the victim, testing of sperm DNA may aid in the identification of the assailants.

- **HIV antibody, VDRL, HBV antigen:** To rule out HIV, syphilis, and hepatitis B infection.

- **Evidence collection using rape kit:** Rape kits are available to facilitate and guide the evidence collection process. Tissue swabs should be collected from the victim as soon as possible to assist in evidence collection. Careful consideration should be given to maintaining a set chain of custody of the evidence collected.

Opening Scenario

Riva George, a 35-year-old female, comes to the hospital complaining of pain in her right calf.

Vital Signs

BP: 130/70 mm Hg

Temp: 99.9°F (37.7°C)

RR: 13/minute

HR: 88/minute

Examinee Tasks

1. Take a focused history.

2. Perform a focused physical exam (do not perform rectal, genitourinary, or female breast exam).

3. Explain your clinical impression and workup plan to the patient.

4. Write the patient note after leaving the room.

Checklist/SP Sheet

Patient Description

Patient is a 35 yo F, married with two children.

Notes for the SP

- Exhibit pain in your calf when the doctor dorsiflexes your right ankle.
- Place a bandage on your right leg to cover the cuts that you got after a fall.

Challenging Questions to Ask

"My father had a clot in his leg. What do you think I should do to make sure I don't get one too?"

Sample Examinee Response

"There are several measures you can take that may prevent you from having a clot. Above all, you should avoid immobilization for long periods of time—for example, while sitting at your computer desk or on long-distance plane trips. Try to move in place and perhaps take a short walk. If you are on oral contraceptive pills, I strongly recommend that you stop taking them, as they are known to precipitate clotting. Studies have also shown that obesity increases your risk of having a clot, so I suggest that you exercise regularly and manage your diet."

Examinee Checklist

Building the Doctor-Patient Relationship

Entrance

☐ Examinee knocked on the door before entering.

☐ Examinee introduced self by name.

☐ Examinee identified his/her role or position.

☐ Examinee correctly used patient's name.

☐ Examinee made eye contact with the SP.

Reflective Listening

☐ Examinee asked an open-ended question and actively listened to the response.

☐ Examinee asked the SP to list his/her concerns and listened to the response without interrupting.

☐ Examinee summarized the SP's concerns, often using the SP's own words.

Information Gathering

☐ Examinee elicited data efficiently and accurately.

☑ Question	Patient Response
☐ Chief complaint	Pain in my right calf muscle.
☐ Onset	The pain started a few days ago and has gotten worse.
☐ Frequency	It is present all the time.
☐ Progression	The pain was mild in the beginning, but now it hurts even when I take just a single step.
☐ Severity on a scale	8/10.
☐ Radiation	No.
☐ Quality	Pressure, spasms.
☐ Alleviating factors	Pain medication (ibuprofen). It also helps if I prop up my leg with a pillow.
☐ Exacerbating factors	Walking and extending my knee.
☐ Swelling	At the end of the day, my legs feel heavy and pit on pressure.
☐ Injury	Yes, I fell down and scratched my right leg (points to bandage).
☐ Redness	Yes.
☐ Warmth	My right leg feels warmer than my left.
☐ Varicose veins	No.
☐ Shortness of breath	No.
☐ Chest pain	No.
☐ Recent immobilization	I travel frequently as part of my consulting business, and a week ago I took a 15-hour flight to meet an important client.
☐ Fever	I have felt warm recently but haven't measured my temperature.
☐ Last menstrual period	Two weeks ago.
☐ Contraceptives	I have been taking oral contraceptives for 2 years.
☐ Frequency of menstrual periods	Regular. My periods last 3 days, and I use 3–4 pads. They are not accompanied by pain.

☑ Question	Patient Response
☐ Obstetric history	I have had 2 kids, both with a normal delivery.
☐ Last Pap smear	One year ago; it was normal.
☐ Weight changes	I gained 50 pounds after having my last child 3 years ago.
☐ Past medical history	None.
☐ Past surgical history	None.
☐ Family history	My dad had a clot in his leg.
☐ Occupation	Executive consultant.
☐ Alcohol use	No.
☐ Illicit drug use	No.
☐ Tobacco	No.
☐ Sexual activity	With my husband.
☐ Drug allergies/herbal medication	No.

Connecting with the Patient

☐ Examinee recognized the SP's emotions and responded with PEARLS.

Physical Examination

☐ Examinee washed his/her hands.

☐ Examinee asked permission to start the exam.

☐ Examinee used respectful draping.

☐ Examinee did not repeat painful maneuvers.

☑ Exam Component	Maneuver
☐ CV/pulmonary exam	Inspection, auscultation, palpation; compared pulses (femoral, popliteal, dorsalis pedis) on both sides
☐ Joint exam	Inspection, palpation, range of motion (knee, ankle, hip joint on both sides)
☐ Extremities	Inspection, palpation; checked for Homans' sign
☐ Neurologic exam	Sensory and motor reflexes (knee, ankle)

Closure

☐ Examinee discussed initial diagnostic impressions.

☐ Examinee discussed initial management plans:

    ☐ Follow-up tests.

☐ Examinee asked if the SP had any other questions or concerns.

Sample Closure

Mrs. George, on the basis of your history and my physical examination, I believe it is possible that you had a blood clot. However, we will also look for other possible causes of your symptoms, such as an infection or a ruptured cyst. We will be running a few blood tests as well as some imaging studies that should help us make a final diagnosis. If your test results show a clot, we will start you on blood thinners to prevent further complications, such as the possibility of a clot traveling to your lungs. Do you have any questions for me?

Patient Note

History

_____
_____
_____
_____
_____
_____
_____
_____
_____
_____
_____
_____
_____
_____
_____
_____
_____

Physical Examination

_____
_____
_____
_____
_____
_____
_____
_____
_____
_____
_____
_____
_____
_____

Patient Note

Differential Diagnosis

Diagnosis #1

History Finding(s):   Physical Exam Finding(s):

Diagnosis #2

History Finding(s):   Physical Exam Finding(s):

Diagnosis #3

History Finding(s):   Physical Exam Finding(s):

Diagnostic Workup

Patient Note

History

HPI: *35 yo F c/o right calf pain of a few days' duration. The pain is constant, 8/10 in intensity, not radiating, aggravated on walking and extending the knee, and associated with swelling, redness, and warmth. It is alleviated on elevation of the foot and with ibuprofen. The patient took a 15-hour flight 1 week ago. She has a history of weight gain postpartum and cuts to the right leg secondary to a fall. She has 2 children, both normal deliveries. LMP was 2 weeks ago. The patient says she has gained 50 lbs in the past 3 years. She has been on OCPs for 2 years. No history of chest pain or shortness of breath.*

ROS: *Negative except as above.*

Allergies: *NKDA.*

Medications: *OCPs, ibuprofen.*

PMH: *None.*

PSH: *None.*

SH: *No smoking, no EtOH, no illicit drugs.*

FH: *Father had DVT. No history of sudden deaths in the family.*

Physical Examination

Patient is in severe pain.

VS: *WNL except for low-grade fever.*

Chest: *Clear breath sounds bilaterally; no rales or rhonchi.*

Heart: *RRR; normal S1/S2; no murmurs, rubs, or gallops.*

Abdomen: *Soft, nontender, nondistended, ⊕ BS.*

Extremities: *Inspection: Right calf appears red and swollen compared to left; contours of the muscles appear normal; no ulcers or pigmentation. Palpation: Right leg is warmer compared to left; pitting pedal edema ⊕ on right side; multiple healing cuts covered with bandage on right leg; dorsalis pedis pulse felt and equal on both sides; mobility normal at ankle joint, knee, and hip joint; ⊕ Homans' sign on right side.*

Neuro: *Mental status: Alert and oriented. DTRs: Symmetric 2+. Motor/sensation: Normal. Cranial nerves: 2–12 intact. Gait: Normal.*

Differential Diagnosis

Diagnosis #1: Deep venous thrombosis	
History Finding(s)	**Physical Exam Finding(s)**
Recent 15-hour airplane flight	Homans' sign
Weight gain of 50 lbs over past 3 years	Pitting edema
Taking OCPs for 2 years	Swollen, tender, red, warm right calf
Father with DVT (possible familial thrombophilia)	

Diagnosis #2: Cellulitis

History Finding(s)	Physical Exam Finding(s)
Cuts to right leg secondary to fall	Swollen, tender, red, warm right calf
Low-grade fever	Temperature 99.9°F

Diagnosis #3: Rupture of Baker's cyst

History Finding(s)	Physical Exam Finding(s)
Spasmodic pain in right calf	Swollen, tender, warm right calf

Diagnostic Workup

Doppler U/S—legs
D-dimer
Hypercoagulability testing
CBC with differential
Wound and blood cultures

CASE DISCUSSION

Patient Note Differential Diagnoses

- **Deep venous thrombosis (DVT):** DVT is common in the lower limbs and may arise under conditions of stasis, hypercoagulability, and venous endothelial injury. Conditions that result in prolonged immobilization (eg, postsurgery, trauma, sedentary jobs, extended airplane or automobile travel) are predisposing factors. Other risk factors include advancing age, pregnancy, synthetic estrogens, prior DVT, obesity, malignancy, and thrombophilia. DVT may produce pain and edema of the affected limb or may be asymptomatic. A positive Homans' sign (pain on dorsiflexion of the ankle) is suggestive of DVT but not diagnostic.

- **Cellulitis:** Trauma can lead to cellulitis of the skin and subcutaneous tissue or to myositis of the calf muscle. All the classic signs of inflammation associated with fever (calor, dolor, rubor, tumor) may point to this diagnosis. Regional lymph node enlargement and tenderness are commonly seen. Myositis ossificans may occur as a complication of this disorder, causing hardening of the muscle and pain on contraction. Radiographs may show ossification in the muscle.

- **Rupture of Baker's cyst:** Baker's cysts (also known as popliteal cysts) are seen in the popliteal fossa. Arthritis or a cartilage tear of the knee joint may cause excess synovial fluid to be accumulated, forming a cyst. A ruptured Baker's cyst may mimic a DVT. Ruptures can present with tightness and swelling behind the knee, pain on knee extension, and stiffness of the calf muscle.

Additional Differential Diagnoses

- **Hematoma:** Injuries can cause bleeding intramuscularly (in which no bruising occurs) or intermuscularly (in which bruising is usually present). Patients present with pain, swelling, and restricted movement. The condition may lead to posterior compartment syndrome.

- **Rupture of the gastrocnemius muscle:** This presents with sudden pain associated with rupture at the musculotendinous junction of the gastrocnemius muscle, halfway between the knee and the heel. There may be bruising and pain on standing on the tips of the toes. Patients also present with pain on dorsiflexion of the ankle against resistance.

- **Spasm/sprain:** Undue strain may cause physical tearing of muscles or tendons, inducing spasm and pain. Ligaments can be ruptured or torn as a result of overstretching or injuries.

Diagnostic Workup

- **Doppler U/S—legs:** An initial diagnostic test that is noninvasive and can visualize clots in the veins of the leg.

- **D-dimer:** A cross-linked fibrin degradation product that may be increased in DVT. It is usually indicated in cases with a low to intermediate probability of thromboembolism. The negative predictive value of this test is sufficiently high to rule out DVT.

- **Hypercoagulability testing:** Several autoantibodies are implicated in thrombophilic states. Proteins C and S deficiency, partial antithrombin deficiency, prothrombin gene mutations, factor V Leiden, hyperhomocysteinemia, antiphospholipid antibody syndrome, and paroxysmal nocturnal hemoglobinuria may all lead to increased coagulability. Hypercoagulability testing should be done on patients with no predisposing factors, recurrent DVT, or a family history of DVT.

- **CBC with differential:** To detect infections such as cellulitis.

- **Wound and blood cultures:** To work up an infectious etiology of cellulitis.

- **CPK and myoglobin:** Both can be elevated in muscle injury (myositis).

- **CT/MRI:** CT venography is used to diagnose DVT in conjunction with contrast-enhanced spiral CT to rule out pulmonary embolism. MRI is noninvasive and can detect acute, symptomatic proximal DVTs as well as muscle or tendon rupture.

CASE 11
DOORWAY INFORMATION

Opening Scenario

Oliver Jefferson, a 62-year-old male, comes to the office complaining of hoarseness.

Vital Signs

BP: 115/75 mm Hg

Temp: 99.9°F (37.7°C)

RR: 16/minute

HR: 74/minute, regular

Examinee Tasks

1. Take a focused history.

2. Perform a focused physical exam (do not perform rectal, genitourinary, or female breast exam).

3. Explain your clinical impression and workup plan to the patient.

4. Write the patient note after leaving the room.

Checklist/SP Sheet

Patient Description

Patient is a 62 yo M, married with 4 children.

Notes for the SP

Speak slowly and in a hoarse voice.

Challenging Questions to Ask

"Am I going to get my voice back?"

Sample Examinee Response

"I see that you are very concerned about your voice, and I am concerned too. I am not yet sure what has caused your hoarseness. We will need to do some tests to find out what the problem is and decide on your treatment."

Examinee Checklist

Building the Doctor-Patient Relationship

Entrance

☐ Examinee knocked on the door before entering.

☐ Examinee introduced self by name.

☐ Examinee identified his/her role or position.

☐ Examinee correctly used patient's name.

☐ Examinee made eye contact with the SP.

Reflective Listening

☐ Examinee asked an open-ended question and actively listened to the response.

☐ Examinee asked the SP to list his/her concerns and listened to the response without interrupting.

☐ Examinee summarized the SP's concerns, often using the SP's own words.

Information Gathering

☐ Examinee elicited data efficiently and accurately.

☑ Question	Patient Response
☐ Chief complaint	Hoarseness.
☐ Onset	Three months ago.
☐ Suddenly or gradually	It started gradually.
☐ Constant or intermittent	It is all the time.
☐ Progression	It is getting worse.
☐ Similar episodes in the past	No.
☐ Pain during speaking	No.
☐ Voice overuse recently	I was a teacher for 20 years, but now I am retired.
☐ Exposure to cold weather or dust	No.
☐ Recent upper respiratory infection (eg, sore throat, runny nose)	I had the flu 4 weeks ago.
☐ Alleviating factors	Nothing.
☐ Exacerbating factors	Nothing.
☐ Heartburn	Yes, I have heartburn all the time, but I don't take any medication for it.
☐ History of stroke or TIA	No.
☐ Weight changes	I have lost 10 pounds over the past 3 months.
☐ Appetite changes	I have a poor appetite.
☐ Swollen glands or lymph nodes	Yes, I feel like there's a lump in my throat.
☐ Fever, night sweats	I feel hot, but I didn't measure my temperature, and I don't have chills or night sweats.
☐ Fatigue	Yes, I don't have the same energy as before.
☐ GI symptoms (eg, nausea/vomiting, constipation)	No.
☐ Cardiac symptoms (eg, palpitations)	No.
☐ Pulmonary symptoms (eg, shortness of breath, hemoptysis, cough)	No.
☐ Past medical history	High cholesterol, but I don't take any medication for it.
☐ Past surgical history	None.
☐ Diet	The usual. No change in my diet. Just eating less.

☑ Question	Patient Response
☐ Current medications	None.
☐ Family history	My mother had thyroid disease and my father had lung cancer.
☐ Occupation	Retired teacher.
☐ Alcohol use	Three glasses of wine every day.
☐ CAGE questions	No (to all 4).
☐ Tobacco	Yes, I have been smoking a pack a day for the past 30 years.
☐ Illicit drug use	None.
☐ Drug allergies	None.

Connecting with the Patient

☐ Examinee recognized the SP's emotions and responded with PEARLS.

Physical Examination

☐ Examinee washed his/her hands.

☐ Examinee asked permission to start the exam.

☐ Examinee used respectful draping.

☐ Examinee did not repeat painful maneuvers.

☑ Exam Component	Maneuver
☐ HEENT	Inspected conjunctivae, mouth and throat, lymph nodes; examined thyroid gland
☐ CV exam	Auscultation
☐ Pulmonary exam	Auscultation
☐ Abdominal exam	Auscultation, palpation, percussion
☐ Extremities	Inspection, DTRs

Closure

☐ Examinee discussed initial diagnostic impressions.

☐ Examinee discussed initial management plans:

    ☐ Follow-up tests.

☐ Examinee asked if the SP had any other questions or concerns.

Sample Closure

Mr. Jefferson, there are a few things that could be causing your hoarseness, such as an infection or a benign or cancerous growth. To find out, I need to do a laryngoscopy, which is a procedure to view the inside of your throat, and a CT scan of your neck. These tests will likely reveal the underlying problem. Since cigarette smoking is dangerous to your health, I advise you to quit smoking; we have many ways to help you if you are interested. I also recommend that you stop drinking, as alcohol and smoking are associated with laryngeal cancer. Do you have any questions for me?

Patient Note

History

Physical Examination

Patient Note

Differential Diagnosis

Diagnosis #1

History Finding(s):	Physical Exam Finding(s):

Diagnosis #2

History Finding(s):	Physical Exam Finding(s):

Diagnosis #3

History Finding(s):	Physical Exam Finding(s):

Diagnostic Workup

History

HPI: *62 yo M c/o hoarseness × 3 months.*

- *Painless, gradually getting worse.*
- *Mild fever, fatigue, and "lump in my throat."*
- *Poor appetite; lost 10 lbs in 3 months.*
- *History of flu 4 weeks ago.*

ROS: *Negative except as above in addition to heartburn.*
Allergies: *None.*
Medications: *None.*
PMH: *High cholesterol.*
PSH: *None.*
SH: *Drinks 3 glasses of wine/day/30 years; smoked 30 packs/year; CAGE (0/4). History of voice overuse (worked as a teacher for 20 years).*
FH: *Mother with hypothyroidism, father with lung cancer.*

Physical Examination

Patient is in no acute distress.

VS: *WNL except for low-grade fever.*
HEENT: *Nose, mouth, and pharynx WNL.*
Neck: *Right anterior cervical chain with lymphadenopathy. No lymphadenopathy on the left.*
Chest: *Nontender, bilateral clear BS.*
Heart: *PMI not displaced, regular rhythm, no murmurs or rubs.*
Abdomen: *⊕ BS, nondistended, no organomegaly.*
Extremities: *DTRs are equal.*

Differential Diagnosis

Diagnosis #1: Laryngeal cancer	
History Findings(s):	**Physical Exam Finding(s)**
Cervical lymphadenopathy	Temperature 99.9°F
Worsening hoarseness over past 3 months	
Weight loss, decreased appetite, and low-grade fever	
History of cigarette smoking and alcohol use	
Advanced age	

Diagnosis #2: Laryngitis	
History Finding(s)	**Physical Exam Finding(s)**
History of flu 4 weeks ago	Temperature 99.9°F
Low-grade fever	
GERD	
History of cigarette smoking	

Diagnosis #3: Vocal cord polyp/nodule	
History Finding(s)	**Physical Exam Finding(s)**
Vocal overuse from teaching for 20 years	

Diagnostic Workup

Laryngoscopy
ESR
CT—chest and neck
U/S—neck

CASE DISCUSSION

Patient Note Differential Diagnoses

- **Laryngeal cancer:** This is the most likely diagnosis given the patient's constitutional symptoms (low-grade fever, weight loss, fatigue, poor appetite) and long history of smoking and drinking.

- **Laryngitis:** This is a common condition of the larynx and can be acute or chronic. The acute form is most likely viral and is self-limited. Common causes of the chronic form are cigarette smoke, polluted air, and GERD. This patient has a long history of untreated GERD, so it could be a sign of chronic laryngitis.

- **Vocal cord polyps/nodules:** Benign vocal fold lesions are sometimes related to overuse of the voice and can be easily identified by means of laryngoscopy. However, this diagnosis does not explain the constitutional symptoms that the patient describes.

Additional Differential Diagnoses

- **Hypothyroidism:** Hoarseness is one of the manifestations of hypothyroidism. Hypothyroidism can explain some of the patient's complaints, such as loss of appetite and fatigue, but does not explain all his symptoms.

- **Mitral valve stenosis (MVS):** Hoarseness in MVS is due to enlargement of the left atrium and compression of the recurrent laryngeal nerve. MVS is more common in women and usually presents with a history of rheumatic fever. Other symptoms include palpitations and easy fatigue. The physical exam findings include diastolic murmur and tachycardia.

- **Gastroesophageal reflux disease (GERD):** Longstanding acid reflux can cause chronic irritation and inflammation of the vocal cords, leading to hoarseness.

Diagnostic Workup

- **Laryngoscopy:** The gold standard for evaluating the larynx; allows direct visualization of the vocal cords. It also allows biopsy of suspicious lesions for pathologic evaluation.

- **ESR:** Will be increased in infectious and malignant causes.

- **CT—chest and neck:** Can identify the location and extent of most laryngeal lesions.

- **U/S—neck:** To identify the presence of lymphadenopathy.

- **Esophageal pH monitoring:** To diagnose GERD as a cause of laryngitis.

- **CBC:** Anemia can be associated with hypothyroidism, and an elevated WBC count is common in infections.

- **TSH:** To diagnose thyroid disease.

- **Cardiac echocardiography:** Essential in diagnosing cardiac valvular diseases.

CASE 12
DOORWAY INFORMATION

Opening Scenario

Carol Holland, a 67-year-old female, comes to the office complaining of neck pain.

Vital Signs

BP: 115/75 mm Hg

Temp: 98.0°F (36.7°C)

RR: 16/minute

HR: 74/minute, regular

Examinee Tasks

1. Take a focused history.

2. Perform a focused physical exam (do not perform rectal, genitourinary, or female breast exam).

3. Explain your clinical impression and workup plan to the patient.

4. Write the patient note after leaving the room.

Checklist/SP Sheet

Patient Description

Patient is a 67 yo F who lives with her husband.

Notes for the SP

- Sit still with your back slightly hunched and head straight ahead; avoid turning your neck, and instead just move your eyes to make eye contact with the examinee.
- Show pain when moving your neck and when the examinee palpates your neck.
- Pretend to have numbness in the back of your left forearm.

Challenging Questions to Ask

"I'm supposed to visit my sister in Florida in 3 days. Will I still be able to go?"

Sample Examinee Response

"Before I am comfortable with you traveling, I want to make sure you don't have a serious injury, like a broken bone or a nerve compression in your spine. I would like to see the results of some tests first to make sure you'll be safe."

Examinee Checklist

Building the Doctor-Patient Relationship

Entrance

☐ Examinee knocked on the door before entering.

☐ Examinee introduced self by name.

☐ Examinee identified his/her role or position.

☐ Examinee correctly used patient's name.

☐ Examinee made eye contact with the SP.

Reflective Listening

☐ Examinee asked an open-ended question and actively listened to the response.

☐ Examinee asked the SP to list his/her concerns and listened to the response without interrupting.

☐ Examinee summarized the SP's concerns, often using the SP's own words.

Information Gathering

☐ Examinee elicited data efficiently and accurately.

☑ Question	Patient Response
☐ Chief complaint	Pain in my neck.
☐ Onset	Two days ago.
☐ Associated/precipitating events	Someone called my name and I turned my head to the left to look. Since then it hurts to move.
☐ Progression	It has stayed the same.
☐ Severity on a scale	2/10 at rest, 8/10 with motion.
☐ Location	The whole neck, but worse on the left.
☐ Radiation	It radiates down my left arm.
☐ Quality	Sharp.
☐ Alleviating factors	Holding my head still.
☐ Exacerbating factors	Turning my head in either direction.
☐ Weakness/numbness	No weakness, but my left arm tingles.
☐ Recent trauma	No.
☐ Recent heavy lifting	No.
☐ History of neck pain/trauma	I have thrown my neck out before, but not like this.
☐ Trouble breathing	No.
☐ Fever, night sweats, weight loss	I've lost about 10 pounds in the past 6 months, and my appetite has decreased.
☐ Headaches, dizziness, photophobia, nausea, vomiting	No.
☐ Past medical history	None.
☐ Past surgical history	None.
☐ Health maintenance	I am up to date on mammograms and had a normal colonoscopy last year. I was found to have osteopenia at my last osteoporosis screening.
☐ Current medications	I take calcium and vitamin D supplements.

☑ Question	Patient Response
☐ Family history	My mother had osteoporosis, and my father had a heart attack at 68.
☐ Occupation	Retired magazine editor.
☐ Travel history, sick contact	No.
☐ Alcohol use	Just a glass of wine with dinner on weekends.
☐ Illicit drug use	Never.
☐ Tobacco	Never.
☐ Drug allergies	None.

Connecting with the Patient

☐ Examinee recognized the SP's emotions and responded with PEARLS.

Physical Examination

☐ Examinee washed his/her hands.

☐ Examinee asked permission to start the exam.

☐ Examinee used respectful draping.

☐ Examinee did not repeat painful maneuvers.

☑ Exam Component	Maneuver
☐ Neck exam	Inspection, palpation, stiffness, range of motion, Lhermitte's sign, Spurling's test
☐ Extremities	Inspection, palpation of peripheral pulses, range of motion
☐ Neurologic exam	Motor, DTRs, sensory exam, Kernig's and Brudzinski's signs

Closure

☐ Examinee discussed initial diagnostic impressions.

☐ Examinee discussed initial management plans:

    ☐ Follow-up tests.

☐ Examinee asked if the SP had any other questions or concerns.

Sample Closure

Mrs. Holland, given your symptoms, I am concerned that you may have a pinched nerve in your neck. Since you have a history of low bone density, I want to make sure your symptoms weren't caused by a fracture. And although it's unlikely, certain cancers may spread to the neck and spine and cause similar symptoms. I want to run some tests to rule out this possibility. I would like to start by getting an x-ray of your neck. Do you have any other questions for me?

Patient Note

History

Physical Examination

Differential Diagnosis

Diagnosis #1

History Finding(s):	Physical Exam Finding(s):

Diagnosis #2

History Finding(s):	Physical Exam Finding(s):

Diagnosis #3

History Finding(s):	Physical Exam Finding(s):

Diagnostic Workup

Patient Note

History

HPI: *67 yo F with 2 days of neck pain and left upper extremity numbness.*

- *Started after quick rotation to the left.*
- *Sharp pain 2/10 at rest, 8/10 with motion.*
- *Associated left arm numbness. Denies weakness.*
- *10-lb weight loss in past 6 months attributed to poor appetite.*
- *No recent trauma or heavy lifting.*
- *No dyspnea, fevers, night sweats.*
- *Screenings up to date.*

ROS: *Negative except as above.*
Allergies: *NKDA.*
Medications: *Calcium and vitamin D supplements.*
PMH: *Osteopenia on last DEXA.*
PSH: *None.*
SH: *Social alcohol use, no tobacco or drugs. Retired magazine editor.*
FH: *Mother with osteoporosis, father with MI at 68.*

Physical Examination

Patient sitting rigid and still, avoiding moving neck.

VS: *WNL.*
Neck: *No scars or deformities, limited ROM 2/2 pain. Tenderness to palpation on cervical spinous processes.* ⊖ *Lhermitte and Spurling tests.*
Extremities: *No scars or deformities, brachial and radial pulses full. Full range of motion.*
Neuro: *Motor: Strength 5/5 throughout upper extremities. DTRs: 2+ symmetric,* ⊖ *Babinski bilaterally. Sensation: Loss of pinprick sensation noted on dorsum of left hand and posterior left arm and forearm; all other sensation normal.*

Differential Diagnosis

Diagnosis #1: Disk herniation	
History Finding(s)	**Physical Exam Finding(s)**
Neck pain that increases with movement	Loss of pinprick sensation noted on dorsum of left hand and posterior left arm and forearm
Radiculopathy (left arm numbness)	

Diagnosis #2: Cervical fracture

History Finding(s)	Physical Exam Finding(s)
Rapid rotation of neck preceded pain	
Pain increases with movement	
Osteopenia on last DEXA	

Diagnosis #3: Neck muscle strain

History Finding(s)	Physical Exam Finding(s)
Rapid rotation of neck preceded pain	

Diagnostic Workup

XR—C-spine
MRI—C-spine
Nerve conduction studies

CASE DISCUSSION

Patient Note Differential Diagnoses

- **Disk herniation:** As with other areas of the spine, pain at the site of compression with the addition of signs of nerve compression suggests radiculopathy caused by disk herniation.

- **Cervical fracture:** Cervical fractures are dangerous, acute findings that can compromise innervation to the diaphragm if they interrupt the phrenic nerve. The exam would presumably show tenderness to palpation, but it is critical to include this in the differential given the patient's history of osteopenia.

- **Neck muscle strain:** Many people experience neck strains caused by quick turning of the head. The patient's radiculopathy suggests that this is more than a simple strain.

Additional Differential Diagnoses

- **Osteoarthritis:** Degenerative disease of the spine could cause the findings seen by the same routes as herniation and fracture—compression of the nerves.

- **Cervical spondylosis:** A spondylosis would be caused by the same channels as degenerative disk disease.

- **Metastatic cancer:** Breast and lung cancers, among others, can metastasize to the bone and cause cord compression. A possible spinal lesion in conjunction with weight loss in an older woman should raise concern for metastatic disease.

- **Multiple myeloma:** Although a rarer malignancy, multiple myeloma is a cause of spinal lesions in both men and women. Associated findings may include symptoms of anemia, renal failure, and hypercalcemia in addition to the constitutional symptoms typically found in malignancy.

Diagnostic Workup

- **XR—C-spine:** The first test to order for pain that raises concern for fracture or radiculopathy. Check for space narrowing or fractures.

- **MRI—C-spine:** MRI is indicated for patients who have neck pain with neurologic signs or symptoms regardless of plain film findings. MRI is the most sensitive method with which to diagnose disk, spine, and spinal cord pathology. Because of its high sensitivity, MRI may detect clinically insignificant abnormalities.

- **Nerve conduction studies:** Nerve stimulation will determine if the patient's loss of sensation is due to a conduction issue in the peripheral nerve. Although they are specific, nerve conduction studies are not necessarily sensitive for cervical pathology.

- **CBC, calcium, BUN/Cr:** To detect anemia, hypercalcemia, and renal failure, all of which may be clues to underlying multiple myeloma.

- **Serum and urine protein electrophoresis:** To detect a monoclonal paraprotein in myeloma.

Opening Scenario

Sharon Smith, a 48-year-old female, comes to the clinic complaining of abdominal pain.

Vital Signs

BP: 135/70 mm Hg

Temp: 98.5°F (36.9°C)

RR: 16/minute

HR: 76/minute, regular

Examinee Tasks

1. Take a focused history.

2. Perform a focused physical exam (do not perform rectal, genitourinary, or female breast exam).

3. Explain your clinical impression and workup plan to the patient.

4. Write the patient note after leaving the room.

Checklist/SP Sheet

Patient Description

Patient is a 48 yo F, married with 4 children.

Notes for the SP

- Sit up on the bed.
- Show pain on palpation of the right upper abdomen that is exacerbated during inspiration.
- Exhibit epigastric tenderness on palpation.
- If ultrasound is mentioned by the examinee, ask, "What does 'ultrasound' mean?"

Challenging Questions to Ask

"My father had pancreatic cancer. Could I have it too?"

Sample Examinee Response

"It's highly unlikely, as your symptoms are very unusual for pancreatic cancer. Regardless, some routine blood and x-ray tests should help us exclude that as a possibility."

Examinee Checklist

Building the Doctor-Patient Relationship

Entrance

☐ Examinee knocked on the door before entering.

☐ Examinee introduced self by name.

☐ Examinee identified his/her role or position.

☐ Examinee correctly used patient's name.

☐ Examinee made eye contact with the SP.

Reflective Listening

☐ Examinee asked an open-ended question and actively listened to the response.

☐ Examinee asked the SP to list his/her concerns and listened to the response without interrupting.

☐ Examinee summarized the SP's concerns, often using the SP's own words.

Information Gathering

☐ Examinee elicited data efficiently and accurately.

☑ Question	Patient Response
☐ Chief complaint	Abdominal pain.
☐ Onset	Two weeks ago.
☐ Constant/intermittent	Well, I don't have the pain all the time. It comes and goes.
☐ Frequency	At least once every day.
☐ Progression	It is getting worse.
☐ Severity on a scale	When I have the pain, it is 7/10, and then it can go down to 0.
☐ Location	It is here (points to the epigastrium).
☐ Radiation	No.
☐ Quality	Burning.
☐ Alleviating factors	Food, antacids, and milk.
☐ Exacerbating factors	Heavy meals and hunger.
☐ Types of food that exacerbate pain	Heavy, fatty meals, like pizza.
☐ Relationship of food to pain	Well, usually the pain will decrease or stop completely when I eat, but it comes back after 2–3 hours.
☐ Previous episodes of similar pain	No.
☐ Nausea/vomiting	Sometimes I feel nauseated when I am in pain. Yesterday I vomited for the first time.
☐ Description of vomitus	It was a sour, yellowish fluid.
☐ Blood in vomitus	No.
☐ Diarrhea/constipation	No.
☐ Weight changes	No.
☐ Appetite changes	No.
☐ Change in stool color	No.
☐ Current medications	Maalox, ibuprofen (2 pills 2–3 times a day if asked).
☐ Past medical history	I had a urinary tract infection 1 year ago, treated with amoxicillin, and arthritis in both knees, for which I take ibuprofen.

☑ Question	Patient Response
☐ Past surgical history	I had 2 C-sections.
☐ Family history	My father died at 55 of pancreatic cancer. My mother is alive and healthy.
☐ Occupation	Housewife.
☐ Alcohol use	No.
☐ Illicit drug use	No.
☐ Tobacco	No.
☐ Sexual activity	With my husband (laughs).
☐ Drug allergies	No.

Connecting with the Patient

☐ Examinee recognized the SP's emotions and responded with PEARLS.

Physical Examination

☐ Examinee washed his/her hands.

☐ Examinee asked permission to start the exam.

☐ Examinee used respectful draping.

☐ Examinee did not repeat painful maneuvers.

☑ Exam Component	Maneuver
☐ CV exam	Auscultation
☐ Pulmonary exam	Auscultation
☐ Abdominal exam	Inspection, auscultation, palpation (including Murphy's sign), percussion

Closure

☐ Examinee discussed initial diagnostic impressions.

☐ Examinee discussed initial management plans:

    ☐ Follow-up tests: Examinee mentioned the need for a rectal exam.

☐ Examinee asked if the SP had any other questions or concerns.

Sample Closure

Mrs. Smith, there are a number of disorders that can cause pain similar to what you have described. Pain of this type is most commonly due to an ulcer, an abdominal infection, or a gallstone. We will have to run some tests to confirm the diagnosis and to rule out more serious illness. These tests will include a rectal exam, an ultrasound of your abdomen, blood tests, and possibly an upper endoscopy, which examines your stomach by means of a tiny camera passed through your mouth. Once we have made the diagnosis, we will be able to treat your condition and help alleviate your pain. Do you have any questions for me?

USMLE STEP 2 CS **Patient Note**

History

Physical Examination

PRACTICE CASES

Patient Note

Differential Diagnosis

Diagnosis #1

History Finding(s):   **Physical Exam Finding(s):**

Diagnosis #2

History Finding(s):   **Physical Exam Finding(s):**

Diagnosis #3

History Finding(s):   **Physical Exam Finding(s):**

Diagnostic Workup

History

HPI: *48 yo F c/o intermittent, burning, nonradiating epigastric pain that started for the first time 2 weeks ago. The pain occurs at least once a day, usually 2–3 hours after meals. It is exacerbated by hunger and heavy, fatty foods and is alleviated by milk, antacids, and other food. It reaches 7/10 in severity and then diminishes to 0/10. It is sometimes accompanied by nausea. The patient vomited once yesterday: a sour, yellowish, nonbloody fluid. No diarrhea or constipation. No changes in weight or appetite. No changes in the color of the stool.*

ROS: *Negative except as above.*

Allergies: *NKDA.*

Medications: *Maalox, ibuprofen.*

PMH: *Arthritis in the knees, treated with ibuprofen. UTI last year, treated with amoxicillin.*

PSH: *2 C-sections.*

SH: *No smoking, no EtOH, no illicit drugs. Sexually active with husband only.*

FH: *Father died of pancreatic cancer at age 55.*

Physical Examination

Patient is in no acute distress.

VS: *WNL.*

Chest: *No tenderness, clear breath sounds bilaterally.*

Heart: *RRR; normal S1/S2; no murmurs, rubs, or gallops.*

Abdomen: *Soft, nondistended, C-section scar, epigastric tenderness without rebound, ⊕ Murphy's sign, ⊕ BS, no hepatosplenomegaly.*

Differential Diagnosis

Diagnosis #1: Cholecystitis	
History Finding(s):	**Physical Exam Finding(s):**
Pain is exacerbated by heavy, fatty foods	Epigastric tenderness
Associated with nausea and vomiting	Positive Murphy's sign
Female gender, age in 40s	

Diagnosis #2: Peptic ulcer disease	
History Finding(s):	**Physical Exam Finding(s):**
History of NSAID use	Epigastric tenderness
Epigastric pain 2–3 hours after meals	
Pain is exacerbated by hunger and fatty foods and is relieved by antacids	

Diagnosis #3: Gastritis

History Finding(s):	Physical Exam Finding(s):
History of NSAID use	Epigastric tenderness
Epigastric pain associated with food	
Nausea and vomiting	

Diagnostic Workup

Rectal exam, stool for occult blood
U/S—abdomen
Upper endoscopy
H pylori antibody testing

CASE DISCUSSION

Patient Note Differential Diagnoses

Although the causes of abdominal pain are many, this presentation should prompt you to ponder the common etiologies:

- **Cholecystitis:** Several features suggest this diagnosis, including pain following fatty meals, nausea and vomiting, and the patient's age and gender ("female and forty"). However, the pain in acute cholecystitis is usually unremitting and is not alleviated by milk or antacids. The patient's intermittent pain may be due to "biliary colic," representing transient obstruction of the cystic duct, usually due to gallstones. The positive Murphy's sign is sensitive for cholecystitis, and the location of the pain is classically the RUQ.

- **Peptic ulcer disease:** The history of NSAID use and burning epigastric pain alleviated by antacids and food are consistent with this diagnosis (although the clinical history cannot accurately distinguish duodenal from gastric ulcers). In addition, the abdominal exam reveals epigastric pain, the classic location for pain related to peptic ulcers. Although the positive Murphy's sign is more suggestive of cholecystitis, the maneuver itself could easily cause discomfort in any patient with upper abdominal pain because of the deep palpation that is required to perform it.

- **Gastritis:** Gastritis is a common cause of epigastric pain, nausea, and vomiting in patients taking NSAIDs, but the pain associated with gastritis is typically milder than that of peptic ulcer disease. Although epigastric pain more likely signals the presence of an ulcer, true differentiation would best be made on upper endoscopy.

Additional Differential Diagnoses

- **Functional or nonulcer dyspepsia:** This is the most common cause of chronic dyspepsia. After thorough evaluation, no obvious organic etiology is discovered.

- **Perforated ulcer:** These patients appear toxic and have severe diffuse abdominal pain with rebound tenderness and involuntary guarding.

- **Gastric cancer:** Although this patient does not have early satiety, anorexia, weight loss, or a left supraclavicular mass (Virchow's node), it should be noted that signs and symptoms are minimal until late in the course of this rare disease.

- **Other etiologies:** Less likely possibilities include pancreatitis, atypical GERD, choledocholithiasis, mesenteric ischemia, and extra-abdominal causes.

Diagnostic Workup

- **Rectal exam, stool for occult blood:** May document occult blood loss due to peptic ulcer, gastritis, cancer, or other causes.

- **U/S—abdomen:** A quick, inexpensive imaging technique with which to examine a patient with suspected acute cholecystitis (it may show stones, pericholecystic fluid, a thickened gallbladder wall, and a sonographic Murphy's sign).

- **Upper endoscopy:** Peptic ulcer, gastritis, and gastric cancer have lesions that can be visualized (biopsy is required for gastric cancer diagnosis and is sometimes necessary for the diagnosis of H pylori).

- **Noninvasive *H pylori* testing:** Serologic tests for antibodies to *H pylori* are adequate for diagnosis but not to document cure, as antibody levels often remain detectable after treatment (indicating exposure, not necessarily active infection). The urease breath test is a useful means of confirming *H pylori* eradication in peptic ulcer disease.

- **AST/ALT/bilirubin/alkaline phosphatase, lipase:** To look for evidence of hepatocellular injury, biliary obstruction, or pancreatitis.

- **HIDA (hepatobiliary) scan:** Uses scintigraphy with technetium-99m DISIDA (a bilirubin analog) to diagnose acute and chronic cholecystitis. HIDA can reveal obstruction of the cystic duct and is usually ordered if ultrasound fails to establish a diagnosis.

CASE 14
DOORWAY INFORMATION

Opening Scenario

Kelly Clark, a 35-year-old female, comes to the ED complaining of headache.

Vital Signs

BP: 135/80 mm Hg

Temp: 98.6°F (37°C)

RR: 16/minute

HR: 76/minute, regular

Examinee Tasks

1. Take a focused history.
2. Perform a focused physical exam (do not perform rectal, genitourinary, or female breast exam).
3. Explain your clinical impression and workup plan to the patient.
4. Write the patient note after leaving the room.

Checklist/SP Sheet

Patient Description

Patient is a 35 yo F, married with 3 children.

Notes for the SP

Hold the right side of your head during the encounter and look as if you are in severe pain.

Challenging Questions to Ask

"Do you have anything that will make me feel better? Please, doctor, I am in pain."

Sample Examinee Response

"Yes, we have many options for medicines to relieve your pain, but first I need to learn as much as I can about your pain so that I can recommend the best medicine."

Examinee Checklist

Building the Doctor-Patient Relationship

Entrance

☐ Examinee knocked on the door before entering.

☐ Examinee introduced self by name.

☐ Examinee identified his/her role or position.

☐ Examinee correctly used patient's name.

☐ Examinee made eye contact with the SP.

Reflective Listening

☐ Examinee asked an open-ended question and actively listened to the response.

☐ Examinee asked the SP to list his/her concerns and listened to the response without interrupting.

☐ Examinee summarized the SP's concerns, often using the SP's own words.

Information Gathering

☐ Examinee elicited data efficiently and accurately.

☑ Question	Patient Response
☐ Chief complaint	Headache.
☐ Onset	Two weeks ago.
☐ Constant/intermittent	Well, I don't have the pain all the time. It comes and goes.
☐ Frequency	At least once a day.
☐ Progression	It is getting worse (2–3 times a day).
☐ Severity on a scale	When I have the pain, it is 9/10 and prevents me from working.
☐ Location	It is here (points to the right side of the head).
☐ Duration	One or two hours.
☐ Radiation (changes its location)	No.
☐ Quality	Sharp and pounding.
☐ Aura (warning that the headache is about to come)	No.
☐ Timing (the same time every day/morning/evening)	The headache may come at any time. I'm having one now.
☐ Relationship with menses	No.
☐ Alleviating factors	Resting in a quiet, dark room; sleep, aspirin.
☐ Exacerbating factors	Stress, light, and noise.
☐ Nausea/vomiting	Sometimes I feel nauseated when I am in pain. Yesterday I vomited for the first time.
☐ Headache wakes you up from sleep	No.
☐ Visual changes/tears/red eye	No.
☐ Weakness/numbness	No.
☐ Speech difficulties	No.
☐ Runny nose during the attack	No.
☐ Similar episodes before	Yes, in college I had a similar headache that was accompanied by nausea.
☐ Weight/appetite changes	No.
☐ Joint pain/fatigue	Occasional aches and pains treated with ibuprofen.

☑ Question	Patient Response
☐ Stress	Yes, I am working on a new project that I have to finish this month. Last month was a disaster. I worked hard on my designs, but they were rejected, and I have to start all over again.
☐ Head trauma	No.
☐ Last menstrual period	Two weeks ago.
☐ Current medications	Ibuprofen.
☐ Past medical history	An episode of sinusitis 4 months ago, treated with amoxicillin (but the pain was different from what I have now).
☐ Past surgical history	Tubal ligation 8 years ago.
☐ Family history	My father died at age 65 of a brain tumor. My mother is alive and has migraines.
☐ Occupation	Engineer.
☐ Alcohol use	No.
☐ Illicit drug use	No.
☐ Tobacco use	No.
☐ Social history	I live with my husband and 3 children.
☐ Sexual activity	With my husband.
☐ Use of OCPs	No, I had a tubal ligation after my third child 8 years ago.
☐ Drug allergies	No.

Connecting with the Patient

☐ Examinee recognized the SP's emotions and responded with PEARLS.

Physical Examination

☐ Examinee washed his/her hands.

☐ Examinee asked permission to start the exam.

☐ Examinee used respectful draping.

☐ Examinee did not repeat painful maneuvers.

☑ Exam Component	Maneuver
☐ HEENT	Palpation (head, facial sinuses, temporomandibular joints), funduscopic exam; inspected nose, mouth, teeth, and throat
☐ Neck exam	Inspection, palpation
☐ CV exam	Auscultation
☐ Pulmonary exam	Auscultation
☐ Neurologic exam	Cranial nerves, muscle strength, DTRs

Closure

☐ Examinee discussed initial diagnostic impressions.

☐ Examinee discussed initial management plans:

    ☐ Follow-up tests.

☐ Examinee asked if the SP had any other questions or concerns.

Sample Closure

Mrs. Clark, it sounds as if your symptoms are due to a migraine headache, so the first thing I will do is prescribe some medications that will alleviate your pain. To ensure that there isn't something else going on, however, I would like to get a CT scan of your head to rule out a mass or vascular problem as the cause of your headache. A blood test may also show if you have problems other than migraine. Do you have any questions for me?

USMLE STEP 2 CS **Patient Note**

History

Physical Examination

Patient Note

Differential Diagnosis

Diagnosis #1

History Finding(s):	Physical Exam Finding(s):

Diagnosis #2

History Finding(s):	Physical Exam Finding(s):

Diagnosis #3

History Finding(s):	Physical Exam Finding(s):

Diagnostic Workup

History

HPI: *35 yo F c/o daily headaches for 2 weeks. These headaches occur 2–3 times a day and last for 1–2 hours. The pain is sharp and pounding. The pain is located on the right hemisphere of the head, with no radiation or preceding aura. The pain reaches 9/10 in severity and prevents the patient from continuing her activities. Headaches are exacerbated by stress, light, and noise and are alleviated by resting in a dark room, sleeping, and taking aspirin. The pain is sometimes accompanied by nausea and vomiting. No changes in weight or appetite.*

ROS: *Occasional aches and pains.*

Allergies: *NKDA.*

Medications: *Ibuprofen, aspirin.*

PMH: *Headaches at age 20, accompanied by nausea. One episode of sinusitis 4 months ago, treated with amoxicillin.*

PSH: *Tubal ligation 8 years ago.*

SH: *No smoking, no EtOH, no illicit drugs. Patient is an engineer, lives with husband and 3 children, and is sexually active with husband only.*

FH: *Father died of a brain tumor at age 65. Mother has migraines.*

Physical Examination

Patient is in severe pain.

VS: *WNL.*

HEENT: *NC/AT, nontender to palpation, PERRLA, EOMI, no papilledema, no nasal congestion, no pharyngeal erythema or exudates, dentition good.*

Neck: *Supple, no lymphadenopathy.*

Chest: *Clear breath sounds bilaterally.*

Heart: *RRR; normal S1/S2; no murmurs, rubs, or gallops.*

Neuro: *Mental status: Alert and oriented × 3, good concentration. Cranial nerves: 2–12 grossly intact. Motor: Strength 5/5 throughout. DTRs: 2+ intact, symmetric.*

Differential Diagnosis

Diagnosis #1: Migraine	
History Finding(s):	**Physical Exam Finding(s):**
Unilateral, sharp headaches	Severe pain with lack of neurologic findings
Associated with nausea and vomiting	
Photophobia	

Diagnosis #2: Tension headache

History Finding(s):	Physical Exam Finding(s):
Chronic headaches	Severe pain with lack of neurologic findings
Associated with stress at work	
Improve with sleep	

Diagnosis #3: Intracranial mass lesion

History Finding(s):	Physical Exam Finding(s):
Headaches associated with nausea and vomiting	
Family history of brain tumor	

Diagnostic Workup

CBC
CT—head or MRI—brain
LP
CT—sinus

CASE DISCUSSION

Patient Note Differential Diagnoses

Headaches without neurologic findings on exam are common and have routine causes, but less common pathology should still be considered:

- **Migraine:** Despite lacking an aura, the patient's presentation is classic for this diagnosis. Migraines are more common in women and typically appear as a unilateral headache. They are often associated with aura, nausea, vomiting, and photophobia. A positive family history makes the diagnosis even more likely.

- **Tension headache:** This is often associated with stress but is usually bilateral and squeezing. It lasts from hours to days and worsens as the day progresses. Tension headaches are often associated with stress and sleep deprivation.

- **Intracranial mass lesion:** One-third of patients with brain tumors present with a primary complaint of headache. Headache is nonspecific and may mimic features of migraine. Certain brain tumors may have a familial basis. The patient's lack of weight loss or neurologic findings on exam casts doubt on but does not rule out this diagnosis.

Additional Differential Diagnoses

- **Depression:** Headaches may be worse on arising in the morning and are associated with other symptoms of depression. The patient also reports stress and rejection at work.

- **Pseudotumor cerebri:** In pseudotumor cerebri, headaches may be focal but are usually accompanied by diplopia and other visual symptoms. The physical exam should reveal papilledema but may be normal during the first few days after the onset of illness.

- **Cluster headache:** This involves unilateral periorbital pain, often accompanied by ipsilateral nasal congestion, rhinorrhea, lacrimation, redness of the eye, and/or Horner's syndrome. Episodes of daily pain occur in clusters and often awaken patients at night. However, this rarely occurs in women (a similar entity seen in women is termed *chronic paroxysmal hemicrania*).

- **Sinusitis:** This is a rare cause of headache. Although the patient had a sinus infection several months ago, there are no signs or symptoms of sinus or respiratory infection in this case.

Diagnostic Workup

- **CBC:** To look for leukocytosis, a nonspecific sign of infection or inflammation. Mild normocytic anemia and thrombocytosis may also be seen in temporal arteritis.

- **CT—head or MRI—brain:** Headache syndromes are largely clinical diagnoses. Neuroimaging is generally reserved for patients with acute severe headache, chronic unexplained headache, or abnormalities on neurologic exam. MRI provides greater anatomic detail, but CT is preferred to rule out acute bleeds.

- **LP:** To look for elevated opening pressure in pseudotumor. CSF is otherwise normal. RBCs and xanthochromia can be seen in subarachnoid hemorrhage (perform if suspicion is high despite a negative CT scan).

- **CT—sinus:** To look for sinusitis.

CASE 15
DOORWAY INFORMATION

Opening Scenario

Patricia Garrison, a 36-year-old female, comes to the office complaining of not having menstrual periods recently.

Vital Signs

BP: 120/85 mm Hg

Temp: 98.0°F (36.7°C)

RR: 13/minute

HR: 65/minute, regular

Examinee Tasks

1. Take a focused history.
2. Perform a focused physical exam (do not perform rectal, genitourinary, or female breast exam).
3. Explain your clinical impression and workup plan to the patient.
4. Write the patient note after leaving the room.

Checklist/SP Sheet

Patient Description

Patient is a 36 yo F.

Notes for the SP

None.

Challenging Questions to Ask

"Am I going through menopause?"

Sample Examinee Response

"I doubt it. It would be extremely unusual at your age. I need to learn more by asking you about other symptoms and doing an exam. Then we can discuss possible reasons you are not having periods."

Examinee Checklist

Building the Doctor-Patient Relationship

Entrance

☐ Examinee knocked on the door before entering.

☐ Examinee introduced self by name.

☐ Examinee identified his/her role or position.

☐ Examine correctly used patient's name.

☐ Examinee made eye contact with the SP.

Reflective Listening

☐ Examinee asked an open-ended question and actively listened to the response.

☐ Examinee asked the SP to list his/her concerns and listened to the response without interrupting.

☐ Examinee summarized the SP's concerns, often using the SP's own words.

Information Gathering

☐ Examinee elicited data efficiently and accurately.

☑ Question	Patient Response
☐ Chief complaint	I haven't had a period in 3 months.
☐ Menstrual history	I used to have regular periods every month lasting for 4–5 days, but over the past year I started having them less frequently—every 5–6 weeks, lasting for 7 days.
☐ Pads/tampons changed a day	It was 2–3 a day, but the blood flow is becoming less, and I use only 1 a day now.
☐ Age at menarche	Age 14.
☐ Weight changes	I have gained 15 pounds over the past year.
☐ Cold intolerance	No.
☐ Skin/hair changes	Actually, I recently noticed some hair on my chin that I have been plucking.
☐ Voice change	No.
☐ Change in bowel habits	No.
☐ Appetite changes	I have a good appetite.
☐ Fad diet or diet pills	No, I've been a vegetarian for 10 years.
☐ Fatigue	No.
☐ Depression/anxiety/stress	No.
☐ Hot flashes	No.
☐ Vaginal dryness/itching	No.
☐ Sleeping problems (falling asleep, staying asleep, early waking, snoring)	No.
☐ Urinary frequency	No.
☐ Nipple discharge	Yes, just last week I noticed some milky discharge from my left breast.
☐ Visual changes	No.
☐ Headache	No.
☐ Abdominal pain	No.
☐ Sexual activity	Once a week on average with my husband.
☐ Contraceptives	The same pills for 8 years.
☐ Pregnancies	I have 1 child; he is 10 years old.

☑ Question	Patient Response
☐ Problems during pregnancy/delivery	No, it was a normal delivery, and my child is healthy.
☐ Miscarriages/abortions	No.
☐ Last Pap smear	Ten months ago. It was normal.
☐ History of abnormal Pap smears	No.
☐ Current medications	None.
☐ Past medical history	None.
☐ Past surgical history	None.
☐ Family history	My father and mother are healthy; my mother began menopause at age 55.
☐ Occupation	Nurse.
☐ Alcohol use	None.
☐ Illicit drug use	Never.
☐ Tobacco	No.
☐ Exercise	I run 2 miles 3 times a week.
☐ Drug allergies	No.

Connecting with the Patient

☐ Examinee recognized the SP's emotions and responded with PEARLS.

Physical Examination

☐ Examinee washed his/her hands.

☐ Examinee asked permission to start the exam.

☐ Examinee used respectful draping.

☐ Examinee did not repeat painful maneuvers.

☑ Exam Component	Maneuver
☐ Neck exam	Examined thyroid gland
☐ CV exam	Auscultation
☐ Pulmonary exam	Auscultation
☐ Extremities	Inspection
☐ Neurologic exam	Visual fields, extraocular movements, checked DTRs

Closure

☐ Examinee discussed initial diagnostic impressions.

☐ Examinee discussed initial management plans:

    ☐ Follow-up tests: Examinee mentioned the need for pelvic and breast exams.

☐ Examinee asked if the SP had any other questions or concerns.

Sample Closure

Mrs. Garrison, there are a few reasons you may not be having regular periods. The first thing we need to do is determine whether you are pregnant. We can do that with a simple urine test. The other thing we need to do is conduct breast and pelvic exams, especially since you have had some nipple discharge, and look for any signs of menopause. Menopause is highly unlikely at your age, but on rare occasions it may occur. A blood test to measure your hormone levels will also help us determine if you are menopausal or have a hormonal imbalance. This will give us a good start in figuring out why you haven't had your period, and we will go from there. Do you have any questions for me?

Patient Note

History

Physical Examination

Differential Diagnosis

Diagnosis #1

History Finding(s):   **Physical Exam Finding(s):**

Diagnosis #2

History Finding(s):   **Physical Exam Finding(s):**

Diagnosis #3

History Finding(s):   **Physical Exam Finding(s):**

Diagnostic Workup

History

HPI: *36 yo F c/o amenorrhea for 3 months. She recently noticed some milky discharge from her left breast as well as abnormal facial hair but denies visual changes or headache. She also describes oligomenorrhea, hypomenorrhea, and a 15-lb weight gain over the past year but denies dry skin, cold intolerance, voice change, constipation, depression, fatigue, or sleep problems. She also denies hot flashes and vaginal dryness or itching.*

OB/GYN: *Menarche at age 14. For the past year, menses have cycled every 5–6 weeks and lasted for 7 days, with decreased blood flow. Before that, menses cycled every 4 weeks. G1P1; 1 uncomplicated vaginal delivery 10 years ago. Last Pap smear 10 months ago; no history of abnormal Pap smears. Sexually active with husband once a week on average; uses OCPs for contraception.*

ROS: *Negative except as above.*

Allergies: *NKDA.*

Medications: *None.*

PMH/PSH: *None.*

SH: *Denies tobacco, alcohol, or illicit drug use. Exercises regularly. Vegetarian; hasn't changed her diet recently.*

FH: *Mother had menopause at age 55.*

Physical Examination

Patient is in no acute distress.

VS: *WNL.*

HEENT: *EOMI without diplopia or lid lag; visual fields full to confrontation.*

Neck: *No thyromegaly.*

Chest: *Clear breath sounds bilaterally.*

Heart: *RRR; normal S1/S2; no murmurs, rubs, or gallops.*

Abdomen: *Soft, nontender, nondistended, ⊕ BS, no hepatosplenomegaly.*

Extremities: *No edema, no tremor.*

Neuro: *See HEENT. Normal DTRs in lower extremities bilaterally.*

Differential Diagnosis

Diagnosis #1: Pregnancy	
History Finding(s):	**Physical Exam Finding(s):**
Change in menstrual cycles	
Regular sexual activity	
Previous successful pregnancy	

Patient Note

Diagnosis #2: Hyperprolactinemia	
History Finding(s):	**Physical Exam Finding(s):**
Galactorrhea	
Oligomenorrhea	

Diagnosis #3: Polycystic ovary syndrome	
History Finding(s):	**Physical Exam Finding(s):**
Weight gain	
Hirsutism	
Oligomenorrhea	

Diagnostic Workup

Urine hCG
Pelvic and breast exams
Prolactin, TSH
LH/FSH

CASE DISCUSSION

Patient Note Differential Diagnoses

- **Pregnancy:** Although this patient's symptoms suggest a hormonal cause of oligomenorrhea, any change in the menstrual cycle warrants consideration of pregnancy. Pregnancy is the most common cause of secondary amenorrhea in women of childbearing age and should be ruled out during the initial evaluation. Menstruation may not necessarily cease completely during pregnancy.

- **Hyperprolactinemia:** This causes menstrual cycle disturbances, galactorrhea, and infertility. It may result from a variety of conditions, including pregnancy, pituitary lesions, hypothyroidism, renal failure, and cirrhosis, or it can be a side effect of medications. Roughly 70% of women with secondary amenorrhea and galactorrhea will have hyperprolactinemia.

- **Polycystic ovary syndrome (PCOS):** This manifests variably as hirsutism, obesity, virilization, infertility, and glucose intolerance. About one-half of patients have amenorrhea (due to chronic anovulation). The patient's oligomenorrhea and hirsutism in the context of recent weight gain suggest this diagnosis.

Additional Differential Diagnoses

- **Thyroid disease:** Both hyper- and hypothyroidism can cause menstrual irregularities, although amenorrhea is more commonly due to hypothyroidism. Except for galactorrhea and weight gain, the patient does not have other signs or symptoms of thyroid disease.

- **Premature ovarian failure:** This refers to primary hypogonadism that occurs before age 40. Causes include autoimmunity against the ovary, pelvic radiation therapy, chemotherapy, surgical bilateral oophorectomy, and familial factors. The patient's lack of menopausal symptoms (eg, fatigue, insomnia, headache, diminished libido, depression, and hot flashes) makes this diagnosis unlikely.

- **Asherman's syndrome:** This describes amenorrhea due to endometrial scarring, which can occur following uterine infections. The vaginal estrogen effect is normal.

Diagnostic Workup

- **Urine hCG:** To rule out pregnancy.

- **Pelvic and breast exams:** Required to check for genital virilization (ie, clitoromegaly), uterine or adnexal enlargement, and estrogen effects (via inspection of vaginal mucosa) and to elicit breast discharge.

- **Prolactin, TSH:** To screen for hyperprolactinemia and thyroid disease. FT_4 is also useful if hyperthyroidism (or central hypothyroidism) is suspected.

- **LH/FSH:** PCOS is a clinical diagnosis; an increased LH/FSH ratio is often seen but is neither necessary nor sufficient to make the diagnosis. Physiologically, increased levels of estrone (derived from obesity) are believed to suppress pituitary FSH, leading to a relative increase in LH. Constant LH stimulation of the ovary then results in anovulation (and often amenorrhea). An elevated FSH (> 40 mIU/mL) is diagnostic for premature ovarian failure.

- **Electrolytes, BUN/Cr, glucose, AST/ALT/bilirubin/alkaline phosphatase:** To check renal and hepatic function and to screen for evidence of hypercortisolism (eg, high sodium and low potassium).

- **Testosterone, DHEAS:** To screen for hyperandrogenism when amenorrhea is accompanied by hirsutism and virilization. Mild elevations are often due to PCOS, but high levels may be due to ovarian or adrenal tumors.

- **MRI—brain:** Required to evaluate the pituitary region in patients suspected of having amenorrhea due to a mass effect (eg, prolactinoma).

- **Hysteroscopy:** To look for endometrial adhesions that are diagnostic for Asherman's syndrome.

Opening Scenario

Stephanie McCall, a 28-year-old female, comes to the office complaining of pain during sex.

Vital Signs

BP: 120/85 mm Hg

Temp: 98.0°F (36.7°C)

RR: 13/minute

HR: 65/minute, regular

Examinee Tasks

1. Take a focused history.

2. Perform a focused physical exam (do not perform rectal, genitourinary, or female breast exam).

3. Explain your clinical impression and workup plan to the patient.

4. Write the patient note after leaving the room.

Checklist/SP Sheet

Patient Description

Patient is a 28 yo F.

Notes for the SP

None.

Challenging Questions to Ask

When asked about vaginal discharge, ask, "Do you think I have a sexually transmitted disease?"

Sample Examinee Response

"There are many causes of vaginal discharge, only some of which are due to sexually transmitted infections. I will try to look for clues by asking you more questions and examining you, and we will definitely send a sample of the discharge to the lab to check for infection."

Examinee Checklist

Building the Doctor-Patient Relationship

Entrance

☐ Examinee knocked on the door before entering.

☐ Examinee introduced self by name.

☐ Examinee identified his/her role or position.

☐ Examinee correctly used patient's name.

☐ Examinee made eye contact with the SP.

Reflective Listening

☐ Examinee asked an open-ended question and actively listened to the response.

☐ Examinee asked the SP to list his/her concerns and listened to the response without interrupting.

☐ Examinee summarized the SP's concerns, often using the SP's own words.

Information Gathering

☐ Examinee elicited data efficiently and accurately.

☑ Question	Patient Response
☐ Chief complaint	I have been experiencing pain during sex.
☐ Onset	Three months ago.
☐ Describe pain	Aching and burning.
☐ Timing	It happens every time I try to have sex.
☐ Location	In the vaginal area. It starts on the outside, and I feel it on the inside with deep thrusting.
☐ Vaginal discharge	Yes, recently.
☐ Color/amount/smell	White, small amount every day (I don't have to wear a pad); it smells like fish.
☐ Itching	Yes, a little bit.
☐ Douching	No.
☐ Last menstrual period	Two weeks ago.
☐ Frequency of menstrual periods	Regular, every month; lasts for 3 days.
☐ Pads/tampons changed a day	Three.
☐ Painful periods	Yes, they have started to be painful over the past year.
☐ Postcoital or intermenstrual bleeding	No.
☐ Sexual partner	I have had the same boyfriend for the past year; before that, I had a relationship with my ex-boyfriend for 5 years.
☐ Contraception	I am using the patch.
☐ Sexual desire	Good.
☐ Conflicts with partner	No, we are pretty close.
☐ Feeling safe at home	Yes, I have my own apartment.
☐ History of physical, sexual, or emotional abuse	I don't usually talk about it, but I was raped in college, and that was when I contracted gonorrhea.
☐ History of vaginal infections or STDs	I had gonorrhea 10 years ago in college.
☐ Last Pap smear	Six months ago; it was normal.
☐ History of abnormal Pap smears	No.
☐ Depression/anxiety	No.
☐ Hot flashes	No.

☑ Question	Patient Response
☐ Vaginal dryness during intercourse	No.
☐ Sleeping problems	No.
☐ Urinary frequency/pain with urination	No.
☐ Pregnancies	I have never been pregnant.
☐ Current medications	None.
☐ Past medical history	None.
☐ Past surgical history	None.
☐ Family history	Both parents are healthy.
☐ Occupation	Editor for a fashion magazine.
☐ Alcohol use	A couple of beers on the weekends; sometimes a glass of wine on a romantic dinner.
☐ CAGE questions	No (to all 4).
☐ Illicit drug use	Marijuana in college, but I don't use anything now.
☐ Tobacco	No.
☐ Exercise	I swim and run 3 times a week.
☐ Drug allergies	No.

Connecting with the Patient

☐ Examinee recognized the SP's emotions and responded with PEARLS.

Physical Examination

☐ Examinee washed his/her hands.

☐ Examinee asked permission to start the exam.

☐ Examinee used respectful draping.

☐ Examinee did not repeat painful maneuvers.

☑ Exam Component	Maneuver
☐ CV exam	Auscultation
☐ Pulmonary exam	Auscultation
☐ Abdominal exam	Auscultation, palpation, percussion

Closure

☐ Examinee discussed initial diagnostic impressions.

☐ Examinee discussed initial management plans:

   ☐ Follow-up tests: Examinee mentioned the need for a pelvic exam.

☐ Examinee asked if the SP had any other questions or concerns.

Sample Closure

Ms. McCall, your most likely diagnosis is an infection in the vagina or cervix. However, there are other, less common causes of your problem. I can't make a diagnosis until I do a pelvic exam and take a look at what I find under a microscope. I will also take a cervical swab and send it for gonorrhea and chlamydia testing. Do you have any questions for me?

Patient Note

History

Physical Examination

Patient Note

Differential Diagnosis

Diagnosis #1

History Finding(s):   **Physical Exam Finding(s):**

Diagnosis #2

History Finding(s):   **Physical Exam Finding(s):**

Diagnosis #3

History Finding(s):   **Physical Exam Finding(s):**

Diagnostic Workup

Patient Note

History

HPI: *28 yo F c/o pain during intercourse for 3 months, located both superficially and with deep thrusting. She also noticed a scant white vaginal discharge with a fishy odor, accompanied by mild vaginal pruritus. She denies postcoital or intermenstrual vaginal bleeding. She is sexually active with her boyfriend (only) for the past year, and her sexual desire is normal. She feels safe at home and denies any conflicts with her partner. She also denies vaginal dryness, hot flashes, hirsutism, depression, fatigue, sleep problems, dysuria, and urinary frequency.*

OB/GYN: *G0P0. Last menstrual period 2 weeks ago; has regular menses but started to be painful over the past year. No history of abnormal Pap smears; most recent was 6 months ago. Uses patch for contraception.*

ROS: *Negative except as above.*

Allergies: *NKDA.*

Medications: *None.*

PMH: *History of rape 10 years ago; subsequently contracted gonorrhea.*

PSH: *None.*

SH: *No tobacco. Drinks a couple of beers on the weekends, occasional wine, CAGE 0/4; used marijuana in college. Exercises regularly.*

FH: *Noncontributory.*

Physical Examination

Patient is in no acute distress.

VS: *WNL.*

Chest: *Clear breath sounds bilaterally.*

Heart: *RRR; normal S1/S2; no murmurs, rubs, or gallops.*

Differential Diagnosis

Diagnosis #1: Vulvovaginitis	
History Finding(s):	**Physical Exam Finding(s):**
White vaginal discharge	
Fishy odor of discharge	
Vaginal pruritus	

Diagnosis #2: Cervicitis	
History Finding(s):	**Physical Exam Finding(s):**
White vaginal discharge	
Dyspareunia	
Sexual activity without barrier contraception	

Diagnosis #3: Endometriosis

History Finding(s):	Physical Exam Finding(s):
Dysmenorrhea	
Dyspareunia	

Diagnostic Workup

Pelvic exam
Wet mount, KOH prep, "whiff test"
Cervical cultures (chlamydia and gonorrhea DNA probes)
Laparoscopy

CASE DISCUSSION

Patient Note Differential Diagnoses

- **Vulvovaginitis:** This describes infection or inflammation of the vagina. Etiologies include pathogens (eg, *Gardnerella*), allergic or contact reactions, and friction from intercourse. The presence of a vaginal discharge accompanied by a fishy odor and pruritus makes this the most likely diagnosis.

- **Cervicitis:** The presence of vaginal discharge and pain with deep thrusting suggests infection or inflammation of the cervix. Although the patient is in a monogamous relationship, she does not use barrier contraception and could still contract an STD if her partner were to acquire one.

- **Endometriosis:** This describes abnormal ectopic endometrial tissue, which can cause inflammation and scarring in the lower pelvis. Endometriosis may account for the patient's dysmenorrhea over the past year and, if so, could also cause dyspareunia with deep thrusting.

Additional Differential Diagnoses

- **Pelvic inflammatory disease (PID):** The patient's history of gonorrhea infection (if it caused PID) also puts her at risk for pelvic scarring and subsequent dyspareunia (due to impaired mobility of the pelvic organs).

- **Vulvodynia:** This is the leading cause of dyspareunia in premenopausal women but is not well understood. Pain may be constant or intermittent, focal or diffuse, and superficial or deep. Physical findings are often absent, making it a diagnosis of exclusion. However, vulvar erythema can be seen in a subset of vulvodynia termed *vulvar vestibulitis*.

- **Domestic violence:** Physicians must screen for this in any woman presenting with dyspareunia. Serial screening is required, as victims may not disclose this history initially.

- **Pelvic tumor:** This could account for the patient's pain with deep thrusting and possibly for her history of dysmenorrhea. However, pelvic tumors are not associated with vaginal discharge and pruritus.

- **Vaginismus:** This describes severe involuntary spasm of muscles around the introitus and often results from fear, pain, or sexual or psychological trauma. The muscle contractions generally preclude penetration. Although this patient was raped in the past, she does not describe the muscle contractions characteristic of vaginismus.

Diagnostic Workup

- **Pelvic exam:** To localize and reproduce the pain or discomfort and to determine if any pathology is present. A complete exam includes external genital inspection and palpation, a speculum exam, and bimanual and rectal exams.

- **Wet mount, KOH prep, "whiff test":** The vaginal discharge is examined microscopically. The presence of epithelial cells covered with bacteria (clue cells) suggests bacterial vaginosis, and the presence of hyphae and spores indicates candidal infection. Motile organisms are seen in trichomonal infection. A "fishy" odor following exposure of the discharge to a drop of potassium hydroxide is characteristic of bacterial vaginosis.

- **Cervical cultures:** To diagnose chlamydia, gonorrhea, and occasionally HSV infection (the latter is characterized by the presence of vesicles or ulcers on the cervix).

- **Laparoscopy:** The gold standard for confirming a clinical diagnosis of endometriosis or scarring of the pelvic organs from prior infections or surgeries.

- **U/S—pelvis:** Can be used to assess the size and positioning of pelvic organs and to help rule out masses or other pathology.

Opening Scenario

Paul Stout, a 75-year-old male, comes to the office complaining of hearing loss.

Vital Signs

BP: 132/68 mm Hg

Temp: 98.4°F (36.9°C)

RR: 18/minute

HR: 84/minute, regular

Examinee Tasks

1. Take a focused history.

2. Perform a focused physical exam (do not perform rectal, genitourinary, or female breast exam).

3. Explain your clinical impression and workup plan to the patient.

4. Write the patient note after leaving the room.

Checklist/SP Sheet

Patient Description

Patient is a 75 yo M.

Notes for the SP

- Ask the examinee to speak up if he or she did not speak in a loud and clear manner.

- Pretend that you have difficulty hearing in both ears.

- On physical exam, demonstrate that you have no lateralization on the Weber test (ie, show that your hearing is equal in both ears).

- Pretend that you cannot hear when spoken to from behind.

Challenging Questions to Ask

"Do you think I am going deaf?"

Sample Examinee Response

"Your symptoms and the results of my exam show that you have some kind of hearing deficit. We need to perform more tests to figure out the cause of the problem, whether it is going to get worse, and whether we can halt its progression or improve your hearing. In the meantime, I would like you to stop taking aspirin."

Examinee Checklist

Building the Doctor-Patient Relationship

Entrance

☐ Examinee knocked on the door before entering.

☐ Examinee introduced self by name.

☐ Examinee identified his/her role or position.

☐ Examinee correctly used patient's name.

☐ Examinee made eye contact with the SP.

Reflective Listening

☐ Examinee asked an open-ended question and actively listened to the response.

☐ Examinee asked the SP to list his/her concerns and listened to the response without interrupting.

☐ Examinee summarized the SP's concerns, often using the SP's own words.

Information Gathering

☐ Examinee elicited data efficiently and accurately.

☑ Question	Patient Response
☐ Chief complaint	I can't hear as well as I used to.
☐ Description	My wife has told me that I can't hear well, and lately I have noticed that I have been reading lips.
☐ Onset	This has been going on for a year.
☐ Progression	It has been getting worse.
☐ Location	It seems like I'm having trouble with both ears, but I'm not sure.
☐ Is hearing lost for all sounds or for anything specific?	Nothing specific.
☐ Do words sound jumbled or distorted?	Yes, especially in crowded places or when I watch television.
☐ Can you locate the source of sound?	Yes.
☐ Do you have any problems understanding speech?	No.
☐ Treatments tried	I saw my doctor a month ago, and he cleaned out some wax from my ears. That seemed to help for a while, but now it's just as bad as it was before.
☐ Did that help you?	No.
☐ Ear pain	No.
☐ Ear discharge	No.
☐ Sensation of room spinning around you	No.
☐ Feeling of imbalance	No.
☐ Recent infections	I had a urinary infection about a year ago. My doctor gave me an antibiotic, but I don't remember its name.
☐ Ringing in the ears	Sometimes, in both ears.
☐ Trauma to the ears	No.
☐ Exposure to loud noises	Yes. I was in the army, and it was always loud.
☐ Headaches	Rarely.
☐ Insertion of foreign body	No.

☑ Question	Patient Response
☐ Nausea/vomiting	No.
☐ Neurologic problems, loss of sensation, muscle weakness, numbness or tingling anywhere in the body	No.
☐ Current medications	Hydrochlorothiazide. For the past 25 years, I have also taken aspirin daily to protect my heart.
☐ Past medical history	Hypertension. I take my blood pressure every day, and it's well controlled.
☐ Past surgical history	None.
☐ Family history of hearing loss	No.
☐ Occupation	Retired military veteran.
☐ Alcohol use	Never.
☐ Illicit drug use	Never.
☐ Tobacco	Never.
☐ Sexual activity	Only with my wife.
☐ Drug allergies	I develop a rash when I take penicillin.

Connecting with the Patient

☐ Examinee recognized the SP's emotions and responded with PEARLS.

Physical Examination

☐ Examinee washed his/her hands.

☐ Examinee asked permission to start the exam.

☐ Examinee used respectful draping.

☐ Examinee did not repeat painful maneuvers.

☑ Exam Component	Maneuver
☐ HEENT exam	Tested hearing by speaking with back turned; inspected sinuses, nose, mouth, and throat; funduscopic exam and otoscopy; assessed hearing with Rinne and Weber tests and whisper test
☐ CV/pulmonary exam	Auscultation
☐ Neurologic exam	Cranial nerves, sensation, motor, reflexes, cerebellar—finger to nose, heel to shin

Closure

☐ Examinee discussed initial diagnostic impressions.

☐ Examinee discussed initial management plans:

   ☐ Follow-up tests.

☐ Examinee asked if the SP had any other questions or concerns.

Sample Closure

Mr. Stout, I know that you are concerned about your problem. I can confirm that you do have some hearing loss. I would like to run several tests, including some blood tests. I would also like you to stop taking aspirin, because this may be contributing to your hearing loss. I will refer you to an audiometrist, who will assess you for a hearing aid. Do you have any questions for me?

Patient Note

History

Physical Examination

Patient Note

Differential Diagnosis

Diagnosis #1	
History Finding(s):	**Physical Exam Finding(s):**

Diagnosis #2	
History Finding(s):	**Physical Exam Finding(s):**

Diagnosis #3	
History Finding(s):	**Physical Exam Finding(s):**

Diagnostic Workup

Patient Note

History

HPI: *75 yo M c/o bilateral hearing loss for all sounds that started 1 year ago and is progressively worsening. He had cerumen removal 1 month ago with moderate improvement. He reports occasional tinnitus and rare headaches. He notes that words sound jumbled in crowded places or when he is watching TV. He denies inserting any foreign body into the ear canal. No ear pain, no ear discharge, no vertigo, no loss of balance. No history of trauma to the ears; no difficulty comprehending or locating the source of sounds.*

ROS: *Negative.*
Allergies: *Penicillin, causes rash.*
Medications: *HCTZ, aspirin (for 25 years).*
PMH: *Hypertension. UTI 1 year ago, treated with antibiotics.*
PSH: *None.*
SH: *No smoking, no EtOH, no illicit drugs. Retired veteran. Sexually active with wife only.*
FH: *No history of hearing loss.*

Physical Examination

Patient is in no acute distress.

VS: *WNL.*

HEENT: *NC/AT, PERRLA, EOMI, no nystagmus, no papilledema, no cerumen. TMs with light reflex, no stigmata of infection, no redness to ear canal, no tenderness of auricle or periauricle, no lymphadenopathy, oropharynx normal. Weber test without lateralization; ⊕ Rinne test (revealed air conduction > bone conduction).*

Chest: *Clear breath sounds bilaterally.*

Heart: *RRR; S1/S2; no murmurs, rubs, or gallops.*

Neuro: *Cranial nerves: 2–12 grossly intact except for decreased hearing. Motor: Strength 5/5 throughout. DTRs: 2+ throughout. Sensation: Intact. Gait: Normal; no past pointing and ⊖ heel to shin.*

Differential Diagnosis

Diagnosis #1: Presbycusis	
History Finding(s):	**Physical Exam Finding(s):**
Bilateral, progressive hearing loss	Positive Rinne test
Advanced age	Lack of lateralization on Weber test
Hypertension	

Diagnosis #2: Cochlear nerve damage	
History Finding(s):	**Physical Exam Finding(s):**
Prior exposure to loud noise	Positive Rinne test
Bilateral hearing loss	Lack of lateralization on Weber test

Patient Note

Diagnosis #3: Otosclerosis

History Finding(s):	*Physical Exam Finding(s):*
Bilateral, progressive hearing loss	Lack of lateralization on Weber test
Advanced age	

Diagnostic Workup

Audiometry
Tympanography
Brain stem auditory evoked potentials

CASE DISCUSSION

Patient Note Differential Diagnoses

- **Presbycusis:** This is a process of the inner ear in which bone loss is greater than air loss, leading to a gradual loss of hearing. It is typically bilateral. Presbycusis is a common diagnosis as people age and can be detected by performing the Rinne test. Chronic hypertension can lead to vascular changes that reduce blood flow to the cochlea and can contribute to the development of presbycusis, as can other conditions that affect the vasculature, such as diabetes and smoking. This patient should be referred to an audiologist who works in conjunction with an ENT specialist. He will likely need a hearing aid.

- **Cochlear nerve damage:** The cochlear nerve can become damaged as a result of loud noise. This patient is a military veteran and admits to a history of exposure to loud noises. Cochlear nerve damage would present in a manner similar to presbycusis. As with presbycusis, patients with suspected damage should be referred to an audiologist working in conjunction with an ENT specialist. Such patients will likely need hearing aids as well.

- **Otosclerosis:** This is a disease of the elderly that presents as gradual hearing loss resulting from abnormal temporal bone growth. It is a conductive hearing loss, so air loss exceeds bone loss. Otosclerosis is usually bilateral, but in a minority of patients the disease can be unilateral or can affect one side more than the other.

Additional Differential Diagnoses

- **Ménière's disease:** This condition usually presents with hearing loss, tinnitus, and episodic vertigo. It is caused by endolymphatic disruption in the inner ear. Causes include head trauma and syphilis. It can be unilateral or bilateral.

- **Ototoxicity:** Hearing loss caused by antibiotics will become more pronounced and may even continue to worsen for a time after the drug is discontinued. Any sensorineural hearing loss associated with these drugs is permanent. Aspirin can also cause hearing loss, but such loss is reversible with discontinuation of the drug. While workup is pending in this patient, aspirin should be withheld.

- **Acoustic neuroma:** It is unlikely that the patient has an intracranial lesion such as a brain tumor in the absence of any other signs. However, this diagnosis should be considered if evidence of focal neurologic deficits is found.

Diagnostic Workup

- **Audiometry:** To assess hearing function and deafness to specific frequencies.
- **Tympanography:** A graphic display that represents the conduction of sound in the middle ear. It may help distinguish middle ear from inner ear dysfunction.
- **Brain stem auditory evoked potentials:** Used to diagnose auditory neuropathy.
- **CT—head:** Used to rule out any intracranial process, tumor, bleed, or CVA. An MRI of the brain would be better for an acoustic neuroma or a schwannoma.
- **VDRL/RPR:** To rule out syphilis associated with Ménière's disease.

Opening Scenario

The mother of David Whitestone, a 5-day-old male child, calls the office complaining that her child has yellow skin and eyes.

Examinee Tasks

1. Take a focused history.

2. Explain your clinical impression and workup plan to the mother.

3. Write the patient note after leaving the room.

Checklist/SP Sheet

Patient Description

The patient's mother offers the history.

Notes for the SP

Show concern about your child's health, but add that you do not want to come to the office unless you have to because you do not have transportation.

Challenging Questions to Ask

"Can this jaundice hurt my baby? Why is he like this?"

Sample Examinee Response

"Newborns often develop a mild case of natural jaundice after birth. This type of physiologic jaundice will resolve and rarely poses a threat to the baby. However, if your newborn has a more severe type of jaundice, his yellow pigment levels, known as bilirubin levels, may rise too high and cause damage to his brain. To determine the severity of your child's illness, I must examine him in the office and obtain some blood tests. After seeing him, I should be able to give you a more accurate assessment of his condition."

Examinee Checklist

Building the Doctor-Patient Relationship

Entrance

☐ Examinee introduced self by name.

☐ Examinee identified his/her role or position.

☐ Examinee correctly used patient's name and identified caller and relationship of caller to patient.

Reflective Listening

☐ Examinee asked an open-ended question and actively listened to the response.

☐ Examinee asked the SP to list his/her concerns and listened to the response without interrupting.

☐ Examinee summarized the SP's concerns, often using the SP's own words.

Information Gathering

☐ Examinee elicited data efficiently and accurately.

☑ Question	Patient Response
☐ Chief complaint	My baby has yellow skin and eyes.
☐ Onset	I noticed it yesterday.
☐ Progression	It is not getting worse, but I'm still concerned.
☐ Parts of body involved	It is mainly visible on his face and hands.
☐ Age of child	Five days old.
☐ Vomiting	None.
☐ Abdominal distention	No.
☐ Frequency of bowel movements	He has 2–3 bowel movements a day.
☐ Color of stool	Brown.
☐ Blood in stool	No.
☐ Urinary frequency	Every 3–4 hours.
☐ Number of wet diapers	About 7–8 diapers per day.
☐ Breast-feeding and frequency	Started soon after birth. Every 4–5 hours.
☐ Sucking well	Yes.
☐ Activities and cry	Yes, he is playful and active. He cries occasionally.
☐ Awake and responsive	Yes.
☐ Recent URI	No.
☐ Fever	No.
☐ Breathing fast	No.
☐ Dry mouth	No.
☐ Shaking (seizures)	No.
☐ Your own blood group and the blood groups of your husband and baby	I'm B Rh positive and my husband is A Rh positive. My baby is also B Rh positive.
☐ Ill contacts	Not to my knowledge.
☐ Other pregnancies and miscarriages	I have a 3-year-old daughter and have had no miscarriages. She is healthy.
☐ Birth history	It was an uncomplicated vaginal delivery.
☐ Complications during pregnancy	Yes, I had a positive culture for some bacteria and received antibiotics before delivery.
☐ Delivery at term or premature	At term.
☐ Smoking, alcohol, or recreational drugs during pregnancy	No.
☐ First bowel movement of baby	Soon after delivery.

☑ Question	Patient Response
☐ Discharge from hospital	Uneventful.
☐ Current medications	None.
☐ Past medical history	None.
☐ Past surgical history	None.
☐ Family history	My daughter also had jaundice after the first week of birth. She was admitted to the hospital.
☐ Drug allergies	None. He hasn't taken any medications.

Connecting with the Patient

☐ Examinee recognized the SP's emotions and responded with PEARLS.

Physical Examination

None.

Closure

☐ Examinee discussed initial diagnostic impressions.

☐ Examinee discussed initial management plans:

   ☐ Follow-up tests.

☐ Examinee asked if the SP had any other questions or concerns.

Sample Closure

Mrs. Whitestone, given the information you have provided, I'm considering the possibility of physiologic or natural jaundice. This condition usually peaks on day 4 or 5 after birth and then gradually disappears within 1–2 weeks. However, breast-feeding, some other pathologic conditions, and certain birth defects can also cause jaundice in infants, and these need to be ruled out. I suggest that you bring your child to the medical center for further evaluation. I hope you understood what we discussed today. Do you have any concerns or questions?

Patient Note

History

Physical Examination

Patient Note

Differential Diagnosis

Diagnosis #1

History Finding(s):   Physical Exam Finding(s):

Diagnosis #2

History Finding(s):   Physical Exam Finding(s):

Diagnosis #3

History Finding(s):   Physical Exam Finding(s):

Diagnostic Workup

Patient Note

History

HPI: *The source of information is the patient's mother. The mother of a 5-day-old M c/o her child having yellow discoloration of the eyes and skin for 2 days. It has not worsened. The child is awake, responsive, playful, and active. He is breast-fed. His stomach is soft and he has 2–3 daily bowel movements. The color of his stools is brown. She denies any h/o recent fever, vomiting, seizure, URI, or breathlessness. There is no noticeable dryness of the mouth. He is wetting 7–8 diapers per day every 3–4 hours. He was delivered vaginally at full term. The mother did receive antibiotics for a positive culture before delivery. The blood group of both mother and neonate is B positive, while that of the father is A positive.*

ROS: *Negative.*

Allergies: *NKDA.*

Medications: *None.*

PMH: *None.*

PSH: *None.*

FH: *His elder sister was hospitalized after the first week of birth for jaundice.*

Physical Examination

None.

Differential Diagnosis

Diagnosis #1: Physiologic jaundice	
History Finding(s):	**Physical Exam Finding(s):**
Infant in first week of life	
No changes in feeding, urination, or bowel movements	

Diagnosis #2: ABO or Rh incompatibility	
History Finding(s):	**Physical Exam Finding(s):**
Infant in first week of life	
Mother and father with different ABO types	

Diagnosis #3: Neonatal sepsis	
History Finding(s):	**Physical Exam Finding(s):**
History of maternal infection	

Diagnostic Workup

Total and indirect bilirubin
Blood typing
Direct Coombs test
CRP

CASE DISCUSSION

Patient Note Differential Diagnoses

Neonatal jaundice can be divided into causes that predominate in the first week of life (early onset) and those that appear thereafter (late onset). The patient's age (five days) makes early-onset causes more likely.

- **Physiologic jaundice:** A condition that peaks between the third and seventh days of life. Underlying causes include accelerated destruction of erythrocytes, decreased excretory capacity, and decreased activity of the bilirubin-conjugating enzymes in hepatic cells. It is most commonly seen in preterm infants.

- **ABO or Rh incompatibility:** Although both the mother and father are Rh positive, the fact that they have different blood types puts the neonate at risk for ABO incompatibility. The hemolysis that results from blood group incompatibility may also cause clinically significant jaundice in neonates within the first week of life.

- **Neonatal sepsis:** Jaundice may be a manifestation of early-onset neonatal sepsis. A history of maternal infections, particularly with group B streptococcus, may be a clue to this diagnosis. However, neonatal sepsis typically manifests with other signs of infection, such as lethargy, vomiting, poor feeding, fever, hypothermia, and/or abnormally colored urine. Additionally, intrauterine infections (commonly referred to as TORCH—toxoplasmosis, rubella, CMV, HSV, and others) could present with neonatal jaundice within the first week of life. These infants may exhibit other findings that may help reach the correct diagnosis, such as small size for gestational age, rash, microcephaly, cataracts, microphthalmia, and/or hepatosplenomegaly.

Additional Differential Diagnoses:

Early-onset neonatal jaundice (within the first week of life):

- **Cephalohematoma:** As this scalp hemorrhage reabsorbs, it can also serve as a source of increased bilirubin production. There is no mention of cephalohematoma in this presentation.

- **Breast-feeding jaundice:** This is a condition that results from poor breast-feeding, which in turn results in slow bowel movements and insufficient removal of bilirubin. This child's mother reports good feeding as well as frequent bowel movements.

- **Polycythemia:** This condition may also lead to abnormally elevated levels of bilirubin resulting from increased total RBC mass.

- **Familial neonatal hyperbilirubinemia:** Look for a positive history of a sibling who had neonatal jaundice requiring phototherapy. The patient's sister had jaundice after birth, making this differential a possibility.

Late-onset neonatal jaundice (after the first week of life):

- **Breast milk jaundice:** This condition results from insufficient mechanisms in the neonatal digestive tract to adequately excrete bilirubin. In contrast to breast-feeding jaundice, neonates with this condition typically feed well and therefore increase their bilirubin loads.

- **Biliary atresia:** This condition would also present with jaundice but is considerably rarer than the others listed here. Labs show a direct hyperbilirubinemia, and an abdominal ultrasound may be diagnostic.

- **Metabolic disorders:** These include hypothyroidism, galactosemia, and hereditary hemolytic disorders such as spherocytosis or G6PD deficiency.

Diagnostic Workup

- **Total and indirect bilirubin:** The first step in determining the severity and type of jaundice. Phototherapy is usually indicated and is maintained on the basis of bilirubin measurements (eg, phototherapy should be initiated when total serum bilirubin levels exceed 15 mg/dL in an otherwise well two-day-old term infant).

- **Blood typing and direct Coombs testing:** To evaluate for jaundice stemming from blood group incompatibility. All infants who are born to mothers with type O blood should routinely receive direct Coombs testing to check for maternal-fetal incompatibility. Such children should also be closely followed for evidence of jaundice from hemolysis.

- **CRP:** To monitor for signs of infection.

- **CBC:** To evaluate the status of blood parameters such as hematocrit and hemoglobin due to suspected underlying hemolysis. Differential counts may provide additional clues about infections causing neonatal sepsis, although these can be more subtle in infants than in adults, since the neonatal immune system is immature.

- **Serology for CMV, toxoplasmosis, and rubella; RPR for syphilis; and urine culture for CMV:** In suspected intrauterine (TORCH) infections.

Opening Scenario

The mother of Josh White, a 7-month-old male child, comes to the office complaining that her child has a fever.

Examinee Tasks

1. Take a focused history.

2. Explain your clinical impression and workup plan to the mother.

3. Write the patient note after leaving the room.

Checklist/SP Sheet

Patient Description

The patient's mother offers the history; she is a fair historian.

Notes for the SP

Show concern regarding your child's situation.

Challenging Questions to Ask

- "Is my baby going to be okay?"
- "Do I need to bring my baby to the hospital?"

Sample Examinee Response

"I understand you are concerned and want answers, but I will need to examine your child first. Although I suspect that he has a viral infection, I need to make sure he does not have anything more serious that might require a trip to the hospital."

Examinee Checklist

Building the Doctor-Patient Relationship

Entrance

☐ Examinee knocked on the door before entering.

☐ Examinee introduced self by name.

☐ Examinee identified his/her role or position.

☐ Examinee correctly used patient's name.

☐ Examinee made eye contact with the SP.

Reflective Listening

☐ Examinee asked an open-ended question and actively listened to the response.

☐ Examinee asked the SP to list his/her concerns and listened to the response without interrupting.

☐ Examinee summarized the SP's concerns, often using the SP's own words.

Information Gathering

☐ Examinee elicited data efficiently and accurately.

☑ Question	Patient Response
☐ Chief complaint	My child has a fever.
☐ Onset	Yesterday.
☐ Temperature	I measured it on his forehead, and it was 101.
☐ Runny nose	Yes.
☐ Ear pulling/ear discharge	No.
☐ Cough	No.
☐ Shortness of breath	I think so; he is breathing quickly.
☐ Difficulty breathing	I have not noticed any belly breathing or flaring of his nostrils.
☐ Difficulty swallowing	I don't know, but he hasn't eaten anything since yesterday and is refusing to drink from his bottle or my breast.
☐ Rash	No.
☐ Nausea/vomiting	No.
☐ Change in bowel habits or in stool color or consistency	No.
☐ Change in urinary habits, urine smell, or color (change in normal number of wet diapers)	No.
☐ Shaking (seizures)	No.
☐ How has the baby looked (lethargic, irritated, playful, etc.)?	He has looked tired and irritated since yesterday.
☐ Appetite changes	He is not eating anything at all.
☐ Ill contacts	His 3-year-old brother had an upper respiratory tract infection a week ago, but he is fine now.
☐ Day care center	Yes.
☐ Ill contacts in day care center	I don't know.
☐ Vaccinations	Up to date.
☐ Last checkup	Two weeks ago, and everything was perfect with him.
☐ Birth history	It was a 40-week vaginal delivery with no complications.
☐ Child weight, height, and language development	Normal.
☐ Eating habits	I am breast-feeding him, and I give him all the vitamins that his pediatrician prescribes. He has refused my breast since yesterday. He also gets baby food 3 times a day.
☐ Sleeping habits	Last night he did not sleep well and cried when I laid him down.

☑ Question	Patient Response
☐ Current medications	Tylenol.
☐ Past medical history	Jaundice in the first week of life.
☐ Past surgical history	None.
☐ Drug allergies	No.

Connecting with the Patient

☐ Examinee recognized the SP's emotions and responded with PEARLS.

Physical Examination

None.

Closure

☐ Examinee discussed initial diagnostic impressions.

☐ Examinee discussed initial management plans:

    ☐ Follow-up tests.

☐ Examinee asked if the SP had any other questions or concerns.

Sample Closure

Mrs. White, your child's fever may be due to a simple upper respiratory tract infection, or it may be attributable to an ear infection caused by a virus or certain types of bacteria. I would like to examine him so that I can better determine the cause of his fever and exclude more serious causes, such as meningitis. In addition to a detailed physical exam, your baby may need some blood tests, a urinalysis, and possibly a chest x-ray. Do you have any questions for me?

Patient Note

History

Physical Examination

Patient Note

Differential Diagnosis

Diagnosis #1

History Finding(s):	Physical Exam Finding(s):

Diagnosis #2

History Finding(s):	Physical Exam Finding(s):

Diagnosis #3

History Finding(s):	Physical Exam Finding(s):

Diagnostic Workup

Patient Note

History

HPI: *History obtained from mother. The patient is a 7-month-old M with fever × 1 day. Temperature recorded by forehead thermometer at home reached 101°F yesterday. The child has been tired, irritated, and breathing rapidly for the past day. The mother denies any abdominal retractions or nasal flaring. The mother also notes rhinorrhea and refusal of breast and baby food. The child has a history of sick contact with his 3 yo brother, who had a URI 1 week ago that has since resolved. He attends day care. No cough, ear pulling, ear discharge, or rash.*

ROS: *Negative except as above.*

Allergies: *NKDA.*

Medications: *Tylenol.*

PMH: *Jaundice in the first week of life.*

PSH: *None.*

Birth history: *40-week vaginal delivery with no complications.*

Dietary history: *Breast-feeding and supplemental vitamins.*

Immunization history: *UTD.*

Developmental history: *Last checkup was 2 weeks ago and showed normal weight, height, and developmental milestones.*

Physical Examination

None.

Differential Diagnosis

Diagnosis #1: Viral URI	
History Finding(s):	**Physical Exam Finding(s):**
Fever (101°F)	
Rhinorrhea	
Sibling with URI	
Day care attendance	
Increased breathing rate	

Diagnosis #2: Pneumonia	
History Finding(s):	**Physical Exam Finding(s):**
Fever (101°F)	
Day care attendance	
Sibling with URI	
Increased breathing rate	

Diagnosis #3: Otitis media	
History Finding(s):	**Physical Exam Finding(s):**
Fever (101°F)	
Irritability	
Day care attendance	

Diagnostic Workup

CBC with differential
Blood culture
UA and urine culture
CXR
Respiratory viral panel
Pneumatic otoscopy

CASE DISCUSSION

Patient Note Differential Diagnoses

- **Viral URI:** Clues suggesting this diagnosis as the source of fever include rhinorrhea and recent exposure to a sibling with a URI. URIs are usually viral, self-limited, and benign, but lower respiratory tract infection must first be ruled out in light of the child's apparent dyspnea and tachypnea.

- **Pneumonia:** Fever, rhinorrhea, tachypnea, and dyspnea support this diagnosis even though cough is not present. The physical exam may reveal retractions, nasal flaring, grunting, dullness on chest percussion, and rales.

- **Otitis media:** Otalgia and ear drainage in an ill, febrile child can suggest a diagnosis of acute otitis media but are often not present (as in this case). The physical exam is important and may reveal a hyperemic, bulging tympanic membrane (TM), loss of TM landmarks, and decreased TM mobility on pneumatic otoscopy.

Additional Differential Diagnoses

- **Meningitis:** Findings are often subtle and nonspecific and may be limited to fever, irritability, and poor feeding, as seen in this case. The physical exam may reveal a bulging fontanelle. Meningeal signs may not be obvious in infants (nuchal rigidity and focal neurologic signs are more commonly seen in older children).

- **UTI:** Infants with a UTI may not have symptoms referable to the urinary tract. Infants who do may have dribbling or colic before and during voiding. Patients with high fever and CVA tenderness are presumed to have pyelonephritis until proven otherwise.

- **Gastroenteritis:** This patient has fever but no GI symptoms. Viral gastroenteritis typically causes vomiting and/or watery diarrhea, whereas bacterial infection may cause fever, tenesmus, bloody diarrhea, and severe abdominal pain.

- **Occult bacteremia:** This is an important consideration for children with high fever (> 102°F/38.9°C) and no obvious source. However, occult bacteremia has significantly declined among children with fever without a localizing source who have received universal infant immunizations in the United States, including conjugate vaccines against *Streptococcus pneumoniae* and *Haemophilus influenzae* type b. On the other hand, a relatively high proportion of unimmunized or incompletely immunized children with no identifiable fever source will have a positive blood culture that can progress to sepsis if left untreated. An extensive workup (see below) is not necessarily indicated in this case, as fever is < 102°F and the child is appropriately immunized.

Diagnostic Workup

- **CBC with differential, blood culture, UA, and urine culture:** The workup for sepsis or occult bacteremia in children with unexplained high fever. Notably, a WBC count > 15,000/μL suggests occult bacteremia. Occult UTI is a prominent cause of fever without a localizing source, especially in fully immunized children, and must be investigated.

- **CXR:** To diagnose pneumonia.

- **Respiratory viral panel (rapid antigen or PCR tests):** Used to diagnose common viral causes of respiratory tract infection that may present as fever with no localizing source.

- **Pneumatic otoscopy:** Key to look for the TM erythema and decreased mobility seen in otitis media.

- **Tympanometry:** Useful in infants older than six months of age; confirms abnormal TM mobility in otitis media. Not routinely used in primary pediatric care settings.

- **LP—CSF analysis:** Should be performed if there is any concern for meningitis. CSF analysis includes cell count and differential, glucose, protein, Gram stain, culture, PCR for specific viruses, and occasionally latex agglutination for common bacterial antigens.

- **CT—head:** Used mainly to rule out brain abscess or hemorrhage.

- **Bronchoscopy:** Rarely used in the initial workup for fever without a localizing source. A diagnostic aid in cases of severe or refractory pneumonia.

- **Serum antibody titers:** To identify causative viruses in pediatric infections (not commonly used).

Opening Scenario

Eric Glenn, a 26-year-old male, comes to the office complaining of cough.

Vital Signs

BP: 120/80 mm Hg

Temp: 99.9°F (37.7°C)

RR: 15/minute

HR: 75/minute, regular

Examinee Tasks

1. Take a focused history.

2. Perform a focused physical exam (do not perform rectal, genitourinary, or female breast exam).

3. Explain your clinical impression and workup plan to the patient.

4. Write the patient note after leaving the room.

Checklist/SP Sheet

Patient Description

Patient is a 26 yo M.

Notes for the SP

- Cough as the examinee enters the room.

- Continue coughing every 3–4 minutes during the encounter.

- Chest auscultation: When asked to take a breath, pretend to inhale while the examinee is listening to your right chest by moving your shoulders up, but do not actually breathe in.

- Chest palpation: When the examinee palpates your right chest and asks you to say "99," turn your face to the right side, and say it in a coarse, deep voice.

- If asked about sputum, ask the examinee, "What does 'sputum' mean?"

- During the encounter, pretend to have a severe attack of coughing. Note whether the examinee offers you a glass of water or a tissue.

Challenging Questions to Ask

"Do I need antibiotics to get better?"

Sample Examinee Response

"Possibly. Antibiotics don't help with bronchitis because this condition is primarily caused by viruses that are not sensitive to antibiotics. However, if I find that you have bacterial pneumonia, antibiotics will be needed."

Examinee Checklist

Building the Doctor-Patient Relationship

Entrance

☐ Examinee knocked on the door before entering.

☐ Examinee introduced self by name.

☐ Examinee identified his/her role or position.

☐ Examinee correctly used patient's name.

☐ Examinee made eye contact with the SP.

Reflective Listening

☐ Examinee asked an open-ended question and actively listened to the response.

☐ Examinee asked the SP to list his/her concerns and listened to the response without interrupting.

☐ Examinee summarized the SP's concerns, often using the SP's own words.

Information Gathering

☐ Examinee elicited data efficiently and accurately.

☐ Examinee offered the SP a glass of water or a tissue during the severe bout of coughing.

☑ Question	Patient Response
☐ Chief complaint	Cough.
☐ Onset	One week ago.
☐ Preceding symptoms/events	I had a runny nose, fever, and sore throat 2 weeks ago for a week, but everything is better now.
☐ Fever/chills	I think I had a mild fever, but I didn't take my temperature; no chills.
☐ Sputum production	Small amounts of white mucus.
☐ Blood in sputum	No.
☐ Chest pain	Yes, I feel a sharp pain when I cough or take a deep breath.
☐ Location	Right chest.
☐ Quality	It feels like a knife. I can't take a deep breath.
☐ Alleviating/exacerbating factors	It increases when I take a deep breath and when I cough. I feel better when I sleep on my right side.
☐ Radiation of pain	No.
☐ Severity on a scale	8/10.
☐ Night sweats	No.
☐ Exposure to TB	None.
☐ Pet, animal exposure	None.
☐ Recent travel	None.
☐ Last PPD	Never had it.

☑ Question	Patient Response
☐ Associated symptoms (shortness of breath, wheezing, abdominal pain, nausea/vomiting, diarrhea/constipation)	None.
☐ Weight/appetite changes	No.
☐ Current medications	Tylenol.
☐ Past medical history	I had gonorrhea 2 years ago and was treated with antibiotics.
☐ Past surgical history	None.
☐ Family history	My father and mother are alive and in good health.
☐ Occupation	Pizza delivery person.
☐ Alcohol use	I drink a lot on the weekends. I never count.
☐ CAGE questions	No (to all 4).
☐ Illicit drug use	Never.
☐ Tobacco	Yes, I smoke a pack a day. I started when I was 15 years old.
☐ Sexual activity	Well, I've had many girlfriends. Every Saturday night, I pick up a new girl from the nightclub.
☐ Use of condoms	Nope, I don't enjoy it with a condom.
☐ Drug allergies	No.

Connecting with the Patient

☐ Examinee recognized the SP's emotions and responded with PEARLS.

Physical Examination

☐ Examinee washed his/her hands.

☐ Examinee asked permission to start the exam.

☐ Examinee used respectful draping.

☐ Examinee did not repeat painful maneuvers.

☑ Exam Component	Maneuver
☐ Head and neck exam	Examined mouth, throat, lymph nodes
☐ CV exam	Auscultation, palpation
☐ Pulmonary exam	Auscultation, palpation, percussion
☐ Extremities	Inspection

Closure

☐ Examinee discussed initial diagnostic impressions.

☐ Examinee discussed initial management plans:

  ☐ Follow-up tests.

  ☐ Safe sex practices.

  ☐ HIV testing (and discussed consent).

☐ Examinee asked if the SP had any other questions or concerns.

Sample Closure

Mr. Glenn, your cough is most likely due to an infection that can be either bacterial or viral. The chest pain you are experiencing is probably due to irritation of your lung membranes by an infection. Some of these infections can be more common with HIV, and given your sexual history, I recommend that we test for it. Another reason for your cough may be acid reflux, more commonly known as heartburn. We are going to test your blood and sputum and will obtain a chest x-ray to help us make a definitive diagnosis. We may also need to obtain a PPD to test for tuberculosis if your cough is persistent. In the meantime, I strongly recommend that you use condoms during intercourse to prevent STDs such as HIV as well as to prevent unwanted pregnancies. Do you have any questions for me?

Patient Note

History

Physical Examination

Patient Note

Differential Diagnosis

Diagnosis #1

History Finding(s):   Physical Exam Finding(s):

Diagnosis #2

History Finding(s):   Physical Exam Finding(s):

Diagnosis #3

History Finding(s):   Physical Exam Finding(s):

Diagnostic Workup

Patient Note

History

HPI: *26 yo M c/o cough × 1 week.*

- *2 weeks ago: fever, rhinorrhea, sore throat.*
- *Persistent productive cough with small amount of white mucus but no hemoptysis.*
- *Sharp, stabbing 8/10 pain in right chest, exacerbated by cough and deep inspiration.*
- *Mild fever.*
- *Denies chills, night sweats, SOB, or wheezing.*
- *No recent travel.*
- *No TB exposure.*
- *No weight or appetite changes.*

ROS: *Negative except as above.*

Allergies: *NKDA.*

Medications: *Tylenol.*

PMH: *Gonorrhea 2 years ago, treated with antibiotics.*

SH: *1 PPD since age 15; drinks heavily on weekends. CAGE 0/4. Unprotected sex with multiple female partners.*

FH: *Noncontributory.*

Physical Examination

Patient is in no acute distress.

VS: *WNL except for low-grade fever.*

HEENT: *Nose, mouth, and pharynx WNL.*

Neck: *No JVD, no lymphadenopathy.*

Chest: *Increase in tactile fremitus and decrease in breath sounds on the right side. No rhonchi, rales, or wheezing.*

Heart: *Apical impulse not displaced; RRR; normal S1/S2; no murmurs, rubs, or gallops.*

Extremities: *No cyanosis or edema.*

Differential Diagnosis

Diagnosis #1: Pneumonia	
History Finding(s):	**Physical Exam Finding(s):**
Persistent cough	Increased tactile fremitus
Low-grade fever	Decreased breath sounds on the right
	Temperature 99.9°F

Diagnosis #2: URI-associated cough (postinfectious cough)	
History Finding(s):	**Physical Exam Finding(s):**
Recent URI	Temperature 99.9°F
Low-grade fever	
Persistent cough	

Diagnosis #3: Acute bronchitis	
History Finding(s):	**Physical Exam Finding(s):**
Low-grade fever	Increased tactile fremitus
Persistent cough	Temperature 99.9°F
White sputum production	

Diagnostic Workup

CXR
CBC with differential
Sputum Gram stain and culture

CASE DISCUSSION

Patient Note Differential Diagnoses

This young man's acute productive cough and pleuritic pain are likely caused by a viral respiratory infection or pneumonia. Rarely, severe coughing can lead to a rib fracture, which in turn can cause severe pleuritis.

- **Pneumonia:** Pleuritic pain may signal lower respiratory tract infection. This diagnosis is often confirmed by characteristic chest exam findings, which may be difficult to elicit in an otherwise healthy patient. In this patient, increased tactile fremitus suggests airspace consolidation, but there are no bronchial breath sounds or rales to help suggest a focal pneumonia. The absence of dyspnea also argues against this diagnosis.

- **URI-associated cough:** Acute cough frequently follows URI ("postinfectious") and commonly persists for 1–2 weeks (or up to 6–8 weeks in patients with underlying asthma). Causes range from rhinosinusitis to acute bronchitis.

- **Acute bronchitis:** Cough can also accompany acute URI. The acute onset of this patient's symptoms points to an acute, not chronic, bronchitis.

Additional Differential Diagnoses

- **Pleurodynia:** An uncommon acute illness usually caused by one of the coxsackieviruses. It occurs in summer and early fall and presents with acute, severe paroxysmal pain of the thorax or abdomen that worsens with cough or breathing. Most patients recover within three days to one week.

- **Other etiologies:** Other causes of acute cough include aspiration (for which alcoholic, elderly, and neurologically impaired patients are at risk), pulmonary embolism (extremely rare in a young patient with no risk factors), and pulmonary edema (signs and symptoms of heart failure would be present). Given the patient's history, he should be screened for HIV infection. Notably, there is no evidence of immunosuppression on exam (eg, no thrush), and in *Pneumocystis jiroveci* pneumonia, cough is usually nonproductive and accompanied by dyspnea.

Diagnostic Workup

- **CXR:** To help diagnose pneumonia (ie, to see infiltrates and effusion), although a normal film does not necessarily rule it out.

- **CBC with differential:** In acute infection, can reveal leukopenia or leukocytosis.

- **Sputum Gram stain and culture:** Often low yield (due to contamination by oral flora and often discordant results between Gram stain and culture in pneumococcal pneumonia), but may help identify a microbiologic diagnosis in pneumonia.

- **Urine *Legionella* antigen, serum *Mycoplasma* PCR, cold agglutinin measurement:** To help diagnose specific causes of atypical pneumonia. Seldom useful in the initial evaluation of patients with community-acquired pneumonia.

- **Bronchoscopy with bronchoalveolar lavage:** An invasive test that is rarely necessary to diagnose community-acquired pneumonia, but a gold standard that is often used early when *P jiroveci* infection is suspected.

- **Pulse oximetry or ABG:** May help determine the need for hospitalization.

- **HIV antibody:** Although HIV is less likely in this scenario, an antibody test should be offered to all patients with risk factors for this infection.

Opening Scenario

Gail Abbott, a 52-year-old female, comes to the office complaining of yellow eyes and skin.

Vital Signs

BP: 130/80 mm Hg

Temp: 98.3°F (36.8°C)

RR: 15/minute

HR: 70/minute, regular

Examinee Tasks

1. Take a focused history.

2. Perform a focused physical exam (do not perform rectal, genitourinary, or female breast exam).

3. Explain your clinical impression and workup plan to the patient.

4. Write the patient note after leaving the room.

Checklist/SP Sheet

Patient Description

Patient is a 52 yo F.

Notes for the SP

- Sit up on the bed.
- Show signs of scratching.
- Exhibit RUQ tenderness on palpation.
- If ERCP, ultrasound, or MRI is mentioned, ask for an explanation.

Challenging Questions to Ask

"My father had pancreatic cancer. Could I have it too?"

Sample Examinee Response

"It's possible; that's why we always rule it out in patients with yellow eyes or skin. Your family history does put you at slightly increased risk. However, we won't know anything for certain until we run some tests."

Examinee Checklist

Building the Doctor-Patient Relationship

Entrance

☐ Examinee knocked on the door before entering.

☐ Examinee introduced self by name.

☐ Examinee identified his/her role or position.

☐ Examinee correctly used patient's name.

☐ Examinee made eye contact with the SP.

Reflective Listening

☐ Examinee asked an open-ended question and actively listened to the response.

☐ Examinee asked the SP to list his/her concerns and listened to the response without interrupting.

☐ Examinee summarized the SP's concerns, often using the SP's own words.

Information Gathering

☐ Examinee elicited data efficiently and accurately.

☑ Question	Patient Response
☐ Chief complaint	Yellow eyes and skin.
☐ Onset	Three weeks ago.
☐ Color of stool	Light.
☐ Color of urine	Dark.
☐ Pruritus	I started itching 2 months ago; Benadryl used to help, but not anymore.
☐ Severity of pruritus on a scale	Sometimes it's 7/10.
☐ Abdominal pain	Sometimes.
☐ Onset	It was around the same time that I noticed the change in the color of my eyes and skin.
☐ Constant/intermittent	Well, I don't have the pain all the time. It comes and goes.
☐ Frequency	At least once every day.
☐ Progression	It is the same.
☐ Severity of pain on a scale	When I have the pain, it is 3/10, and then it may go down to 0.
☐ Location	It is here (points to the RUQ).
☐ Radiation	No.
☐ Quality	Dull.
☐ Alleviating factors	Tylenol. I take 4 pills every day just to make sure I do not feel the pain.
☐ Exacerbating factors	None.
☐ Relationship of food to pain	None.
☐ Previous episodes of similar pain	No.
☐ Nausea/vomiting	Sometimes I feel nauseated when I am in pain, but no vomiting.
☐ Diarrhea/constipation	No.

☑ Question	Patient Response
☐ Colonoscopy	Never.
☐ Blood transfusion	Yes, when I had a C-section 20 years ago.
☐ Fever, night sweats	No.
☐ Fatigue	Yes, recently.
☐ Weight changes	No.
☐ Appetite changes	I have no appetite.
☐ Joint pain	No.
☐ Travel history	I went to Mexico for a brief vacation about 2 months ago.
☐ Immunization before travel	No.
☐ Current medications	Tylenol, Synthroid.
☐ Similar episodes	No.
☐ Past medical history	Hypothyroidism.
☐ Past surgical history	I had 2 C-sections at ages 25 and 30 and a tubal ligation at age 35.
☐ Family history	My father died at 55 of pancreatic cancer. My mother is alive and healthy.
☐ Occupation	I work in a travel agency.
☐ Illicit drug use	No.
☐ Tobacco	No.
☐ Sexual activity	Yes, with my husband.
☐ Drug allergies	Penicillin, causes rash.
☐ How much alcohol do you drink?	I have had 1 or 2 glasses of wine every day for the past 30 years.
☐ CAGE questions	No (to all 4).
☐ Affecting job/relationships/legal problems	No.

Connecting with the Patient

☐ Examinee recognized the SP's emotions and responded with PEARLS.

Physical Examination

☐ Examinee washed his/her hands.

☐ Examinee asked permission to start the exam.

☐ Examinee used respectful draping.

☐ Examinee did not repeat painful maneuvers.

☑ Exam Component	Maneuver
☐ HEENT	Inspected sclerae, under tongue
☐ CV exam	Auscultation
☐ Pulmonary exam	Auscultation
☐ Abdominal exam	Inspection, auscultation, palpation (including Murphy's sign), percussion, measurement of liver span, palpation or percussion for splenomegaly, fluid wave for shifting dullness
☐ Extremities	Checked for asterixis, edema
☐ Skin	Looked for spider nevi, cutaneous telangiectasias, palmar erythema

Closure

☐ Examinee discussed initial diagnostic impressions.

☐ Examinee discussed initial management plans:

    ☐ Follow-up tests.

☐ Examinee asked if the SP had any other questions or concerns.

Sample Closure

Mrs. Abbott, the symptoms you describe are usually due to a disorder either in the liver itself or in the bile ducts, which are physically close to your liver. We will have to run some blood tests and conduct imaging studies such as ultrasound to get a better idea of what is going on. Once we find the cause of your problem, we can come up with an appropriate treatment plan. Until then, I recommend that you stop drinking and limit your use of Tylenol, as both may harm your liver. Do you have any questions for me?

Patient Note

History

Physical Examination

Patient Note

Differential Diagnosis

Diagnosis #1

History Finding(s):	Physical Exam Finding(s):

Diagnosis #2

History Finding(s):	Physical Exam Finding(s):

Diagnosis #3

History Finding(s):	Physical Exam Finding(s):

Diagnostic Workup

History

HPI: *52 yo F c/o yellow skin and eyes × 3 weeks.*

- *Light-colored stool and dark urine.*
- *3/10 RUQ pain, dull, intermittent (daily), no radiation, unrelated to meals, relieved by Tylenol.*
- *Fatigue.*
- *Anorexia.*
- *Pruritus up to 7/10 in severity.*
- *Nausea.*
- *Recent travel to Mexico.*
- *History of blood transfusion 20 years ago.*
- *No diarrhea, constipation, or weight loss.*

ROS: *Negative except as above.*

Allergies: *Penicillin, causes rash.*

Medications: *Tylenol, Synthroid.*

PMH: *Hypothyroidism.*

PSH: *2 C-sections, tubal ligation.*

SH: *No smoking, 1–2 glasses of wine/day for 30 years, CAGE 0/4, no illicit drugs. Sexually active with husband only.*

FH: *Father died of pancreatic cancer at age 55. No other FH of GI cancer.*

Physical Examination

Patient is in no acute distress.

VS: *WNL.*

HEENT: *Sclerae icteric.*

Chest: *Clear breath sounds bilaterally.*

Heart: *RRR; normal S1/S2; no murmurs, rubs, or gallops.*

Abdomen: *Soft, nondistended, C-section scar. Mild RUQ tenderness without rebound or guarding, ⊖ Murphy's sign, ⊕ BS, no organomegaly or masses. No evidence of fluid wave suggestive of ascites.*

Skin: *Jaundice, excoriations due to scratching, no spiders/telangiectasias/palmar erythema.*

Extremities: *No asterixis, no edema.*

Differential Diagnosis

Diagnosis #1: Extrahepatic biliary obstruction (eg, pancreatic cancer, cholangiocarcinoma, ampullary carcinoma, sphincter of Oddi dysfunction)	
History Finding(s):	**Physical Exam Finding(s):**
Light stools, dark urine	Jaundice, scleral icterus
Pruritus	RUQ tenderness
Father with pancreatic cancer	

Diagnosis #2: Viral hepatitis	
History Finding(s):	**Physical Exam Finding(s):**
History of blood transfusion	Jaundice, scleral icterus
Recent travel to Mexico	RUQ tenderness

Diagnosis #3: Acetaminophen hepatotoxicity	
History Finding(s):	**Physical Exam Finding(s):**
Frequent acetaminophen use	Jaundice, scleral icterus
Concomitant alcohol use	RUQ tenderness

Diagnostic Workup

AST/ALT/bilirubin/alkaline phosphatase
U/S—RUQ abdomen
Viral hepatitis serologies

CASE DISCUSSION

Patient Note Differential Diagnoses

Jaundice results from hyperbilirubinemia, the cause of which may be hepatic or nonhepatic. The presence of a change in stool and urine color excludes unconjugated hyperbilirubinemia (eg, that associated with hemolysis or Gilbert's syndrome). Thus, the predominantly conjugated hyperbilirubinemia suspected in this patient may be due to hepatocellular disease, drugs, sepsis, hereditary disorders such as Dubin-Johnson syndrome, or extrahepatic biliary obstruction. Cholangitis is ruled out by the absence of fever and chills associated with episodes of abdominal pain.

- **Extrahepatic biliary obstruction:** The patient's family history puts her at increased risk for pancreatic cancer, which classically presents with painless jaundice. However, her intermittent pain (suggesting intermittent biliary obstruction) narrows the differential to choledocholithiasis (stone in the common bile duct), cholangiocarcinoma, carcinoma of the ampulla, or sphincter of Oddi dysfunction.

- **Viral hepatitis:** The patient is at risk for hepatitis A (in light of her trip to Mexico) and chronic hepatitis C (given her remote blood transfusion). However, the intermittent nature of her RUQ pain makes acute hepatitis less likely.

- **Acetaminophen hepatotoxicity:** This should be suspected in acute liver injury, as even moderate amounts of acetaminophen may overwhelm the metabolic capacity of a damaged liver (usually in alcoholics and in patients with chronic hepatitis or cirrhosis).

Additional Differential Diagnoses

- **Alcoholic hepatitis:** The patient's symptoms are consistent with this diagnosis. Hepatomegaly is often present. Although she reports drinking only one or two glasses of wine daily, patients often underreport alcohol consumption.

- **Primary biliary cirrhosis:** This usually occurs in women 40–60 years of age, often with pruritus as a presenting symptom. It is commonly found in patients with other autoimmune diseases, such as hypothyroidism (as in this case). However, jaundice is usually a late finding and is not associated with RUQ pain.

Diagnostic Workup

- **AST/ALT/bilirubin/alkaline phosphatase:** These levels can help differentiate a hepatocellular process (primarily associated with increased AST and ALT) from a cholestatic process (primarily associated with increased bilirubin and alkaline phosphatase).

- **U/S—RUQ abdomen:** Used to diagnose biliary obstruction, stones, and intrahepatic tumors.

- **Viral hepatitis serologies:** Hepatitis A IgM antibody should be checked to document recent infection. Other screening tests include hepatitis B surface antigen and hepatitis C antibody.

- **CBC:** Patients with chronic liver disease often exhibit a low platelet count as a result of portal hypertension and subsequent splenomegaly.

- **PT/PTT:** A coagulopathy is often seen in advanced liver disease and is attributable to synthetic dysfunction and subsequent clotting factor deficiencies.

- **Acetaminophen level:** Used to diagnose acetaminophen overdose.

- **CT—abdomen:** A CT scan provides information similar to that above but is more expensive.

- **MRCP/ERCP:** Can identify the cause, location, and extent of biliary obstruction. ERCP is invasive but has the advantage of being both a diagnostic and a therapeutic tool in many cases. MRCP is a noninvasive MRI-based diagnostic substitute.

Opening Scenario

Edward Albright, a 53-year-old male, comes to the ED complaining of dizziness.

Vital Signs

BP: 135/90 mm Hg

Temp: 98.0°F (36.7°C)

RR: 16/minute

HR: 76/minute, regular

Examinee Tasks

1. Take a focused history.

2. Perform a focused physical exam (do not perform rectal, genitourinary, or female breast exam).

3. Explain your clinical impression and workup plan to the patient.

4. Write the patient note after leaving the room.

Checklist/SP Sheet

Patient Description

Patient is a 53 yo M, married with 3 children.

Notes for the SP

- Ask the examinee to speak loudly. Pretend that you have difficulty hearing in your left ear and that you hear better when the examinee moves closer to your right ear.

- Refuse to walk if the examinee asks you to. Pretend that you are afraid of falling down. Walk only if the examinee explains why he/she would like to see your gait.

Challenging Questions to Ask

"I am really scared about my hearing, doctor. Do you think this will be permanent?"

Sample Examinee Response

"I understand your concern, Mr. Albright. A variety of permanent and nonpermanent conditions can cause your symptoms, but before I can confidently answer your question, I would like to do a few more tests to better understand why you have been dizzy and why your hearing is affected. After that, we can discuss possible reasons for your hearing problems."

Examinee Checklist

Building the Doctor-Patient Relationship

Entrance

☐ Examinee knocked on the door before entering.

☐ Examinee introduced self by name.

☐ Examinee identified his/her role or position.

☐ Examinee correctly used patient's name.

☐ Examinee made eye contact with the SP.

Reflective Listening

☐ Examinee asked an open-ended question and actively listened to the response.

☐ Examinee asked the SP to list his/her concerns and listened to the response without interrupting.

☐ Examinee summarized the SP's concerns, often using the SP's own words.

Information Gathering

☐ Examinee elicited data efficiently and accurately.

☑ Question	Patient Response
☐ Chief complaint	I feel dizzy.
☐ Describe the meaning of dizziness	Well, I feel as if the room were spinning around me.
☐ Onset	Two days ago.
☐ Progression	It is getting worse.
☐ Constant/intermittent	It comes and goes.
☐ Duration	It lasts for 20–30 minutes.
☐ Timing	It can happen anytime.
☐ Positions that can elicit the dizziness (lying down, sitting, standing up)	When I get up from bed or lie down to sleep, but as I said, it can happen anytime.
☐ Positions that can relieve the dizziness	None.
☐ Tinnitus	No.
☐ Hearing loss (which ear, when)	Yes, I have difficulty hearing you in my left ear. This started yesterday.
☐ Fullness or pressure in the ears	No.
☐ Discharge from the ears	No.
☐ Falls	No, sometimes I feel unsteady as if I were going to fall down, but I don't fall.
☐ Nausea/vomiting	Yes, I feel nauseated, and I vomited several times.
☐ Recent infections	I have had really bad diarrhea. I've had it for the past 3 days, but it is much better today.
☐ Fever	No.
☐ Description of stool	It was a watery diarrhea with no blood.
☐ Abdominal pain	No.
☐ URI (runny nose, sore throat, cough)	No.
☐ Headaches	No.
☐ Head trauma	No.

☑ Question	Patient Response
☐ Current medications	Furosemide, captopril.
☐ Past medical history	High blood pressure, diagnosed 7 years ago.
☐ Past surgical history	Appendectomy.
☐ Family history	No similar problem in the family.
☐ Occupation	Executive director of an insurance company.
☐ Alcohol use	Yes, I drink 2–3 beers a week.
☐ Illicit drug use	No.
☐ Tobacco	No.
☐ Sexual activity	Yes, with my wife.
☐ Drug allergies	No.

Connecting with the Patient

☐ Examinee recognized the SP's emotions and responded with PEARLS.

Physical Examination

☐ Examinee washed his/her hands.

☐ Examinee asked permission to start the exam.

☐ Examinee used respectful draping.

☐ Examinee did not repeat painful maneuvers.

☑ Exam Component	Maneuver
☐ HEENT	Inspected for nystagmus, funduscopic exam, otoscopy, assessed hearing, Rinne and Weber tests, inspected mouth and throat
☐ CV exam	Auscultation, orthostatic vital signs
☐ Neurologic exam	Cranial nerves, motor exam, DTRs, gait, Romberg's sign, tilt test (eg, Dix-Hallpike maneuver)

Closure

☐ Examinee discussed initial diagnostic impressions.

☐ Examinee discussed initial management plans:

    ☐ Follow-up tests.

☐ Examinee asked if the SP had any other questions or concerns.

Sample Closure

Mr. Albright, the dizziness you are experiencing may be due to a problem in your ears or brain, or it may result from low blood pressure. We will have to run some tests to pinpoint the source of your symptoms. These may include blood tests, a hearing evaluation, and an MRI that will provide detailed images of your brain. Until we find the cause of your problem, you should be careful when you stand up quickly or walk unaccompanied, and you should use hand railings whenever possible. Do you have any questions for me?

USMLE STEP 2 CS **Patient Note**

History

Physical Examination

PRACTICE CASES

Differential Diagnosis

Diagnosis #1

History Finding(s):   **Physical Exam Finding(s):**

Diagnosis #2

History Finding(s):   **Physical Exam Finding(s):**

Diagnosis #3

History Finding(s):   **Physical Exam Finding(s):**

Diagnostic Workup

History

HPI: *53 yo M c/o intermittent dizziness × 2 days.*

- *Sensation of room spinning around him.*
- *Occurs during day when getting up or lying down.*
- *Episodes last 20–30 minutes and are progressively getting worse.*
- *Left-sided hearing loss since yesterday.*
- *Nausea and vomiting.*
- *Watery, nonbloody diarrhea × 3 days that has since resolved.*
- *No tinnitus, fullness in ear, ear discharge, headache, or head trauma.*
- *No recent URI.*

ROS: *Negative except as above.*
Allergies: *NKDA.*
Medications: *Furosemide, captopril.*
PMH: *Hypertension, diagnosed 7 years ago.*
PSH: *Appendectomy.*
SH: *No smoking, 2–3 beers/week, no illicit drugs.*
FH: *Noncontributory.*

Physical Examination

Patient is in no acute distress.

VS: *WNL, no orthostatic changes.*
HEENT: *NC/AT, PERRLA, EOMI without nystagmus, no papilledema, no cerumen, TMs normal, mouth and oropharynx normal.*
Heart: *RRR; normal S1/S2; no murmurs, rubs, or gallops.*
Neuro: *Cranial nerves: 2–12 grossly intact except for decreased hearing acuity in the left ear. ⊕ Rinne (air conduction > bone conduction on the left), Weber no lateralization, ⊖ tilt test. Motor: Strength 5/5 throughout. DTRs: 2+ intact, symmetric, ⊖ Babinski bilaterally. Cerebellar: ⊖ Romberg, finger to nose normal. Gait: Normal.*

Differential Diagnosis

Diagnosis #1: Ménière's disease	
History Finding(s):	**Physical Exam Finding(s):**
Sensation of room spinning	Decreased hearing acuity on the left
Left-sided hearing loss	Positive Rinne test

Diagnosis #2: Benign paroxysmal positional vertigo	
History Finding(s):	**Physical Exam Finding(s):**
Sensation of room spinning	
Onset with positional changes	
Duration 20–30 minutes	

Diagnosis #3: Orthostatic hypotension causing dizziness	
History Finding(s):	**Physical Exam Finding(s):**
History of diarrhea	
Taking antihypertensive medication	

Diagnostic Workup

Dix-Hallpike maneuver
Audiometry
MRI—brain

CASE DISCUSSION

Patient Note Differential Diagnoses

Vertigo signals vestibular disease, whereas lightheadedness and dysequilibrium are usually nonvestibular in origin. A central vestibular system lesion (eg, vertebrobasilar insufficiency, brain stem and cerebellar tumors, MS) is unlikely in this patient given the presence of hearing loss and an otherwise normal neurologic exam. Vertigo syndromes due to peripheral lesions are discussed below. These cases are often accompanied by nausea and vomiting, and vertigo may be so severe that the patient is unable to walk or stand.

- **Ménière's disease:** This classically presents with episodic vertigo (usually lasting 1–8 hours) and low-frequency hearing loss as well as with features not seen in this case, such as tinnitus and a sensation of aural fullness. Symptoms result from distention of the endolymphatic compartment of the inner ear. Syphilis and head trauma are two known causes.

- **Benign paroxysmal positional vertigo (BPPV):** This describes transient vertigo following changes in head position, but it is not associated with hearing loss.

- **Orthostatic hypotension due to dehydration:** Risk factors for dehydration in this case include diarrhea and loop diuretic use. However, the patient does not complain of lightheadedness and is not objectively orthostatic.

Additional Differential Diagnoses

- **Labyrinthitis:** This frequently follows a viral infection (usually URI) and is accompanied by hearing loss and tinnitus, but vertigo is usually continuous and lasts several days to a week.

- **Perilymphatic fistula:** This is a rare cause of vertigo and sensorineural hearing loss that usually results from head trauma or extensive barotrauma. Episodes of vertigo are fleeting, generally lasting seconds.

- **Acoustic neuroma:** Acoustic neuroma more commonly causes continuous dysequilibrium rather than episodic vertigo. As noted above, central lesions are unlikely in patients with vertigo, hearing loss, and an otherwise normal neurologic exam. However, an intracranial mass lesion must be ruled out in any patient with unilateral hearing loss.

Diagnostic Workup

- **Dix-Hallpike maneuver:** Used to diagnose BPPV (look for nystagmus and reproduction of vertigo).

- **Audiometry:** Used to assess hearing function.

- **MRI—brain:** Required for the evaluation of central vestibular lesions.

- **VDRL/RPR:** To rule out syphilis, which can cause Ménière's disease.

- **Brain stem auditory evoked potentials:** Used to help diagnose central vestibular disease.

- **Electronystagmography:** Used to document characteristics of nystagmus that may differentiate central from peripheral vestibular system lesions.

Opening Scenario

Kathleen Moore, a 33-year-old female, comes to the clinic complaining of knee pain.

Vital Signs

BP: 130/80 mm Hg

Temp: 99.9°F (37.7°C)

RR: 16/minute

HR: 76/minute, regular

Examinee Tasks

1. Take a focused history.

2. Perform a focused physical exam (do not perform rectal, genitourinary, or female breast exam).

3. Explain your clinical impression and workup plan to the patient.

4. Write the patient note after leaving the room.

Checklist/SP Sheet

Patient Description

Patient is a 33 yo F, divorced with 2 daughters.

Notes for the SP

- Pretend to have pain when the examinee moves your left knee in all directions.
- Do not allow the examinee to fully flex or extend your left knee.
- Paint your left knee red to make it look inflamed.

Challenging Questions to Ask

"Do you think I will be able to walk on my knee like before?"

Sample Examinee Response

"Most likely, but that depends on the underlying problem and your response to treatment. I need to perform a physical examination before we can figure out an appropriate course of treatment."

Examinee Checklist

Building the Doctor-Patient Relationship

Entrance

☐ Examinee knocked on the door before entering.

☐ Examinee introduced self by name.

☐ Examinee identified his/her role or position.

☐ Examinee correctly used patient's name.

☐ Examinee made eye contact with the SP.

Reflective Listening

☐ Examinee asked an open-ended question and actively listened to the response.

☐ Examinee asked the SP to list his/her concerns and listened to the response without interrupting.

☐ Examinee summarized the SP's concerns, often using the SP's own words.

Information Gathering

☐ Examinee elicited data efficiently and accurately.

☑ Question	Patient Response
☐ Chief complaint	Left knee pain.
☐ Onset	Two days ago.
☐ Function	I can't move it. I use a cane to walk.
☐ Redness	Yes.
☐ Swelling of the joint	Yes.
☐ Alleviating factors	Rest and Tylenol help a little bit.
☐ Exacerbating factors	Moving my knee and walking.
☐ History of trauma to the knee	No.
☐ Other joint pain	Yes, my wrists and fingers are always painful and stiff. Five years ago I had a painful, swollen big toe on my left foot, but the swelling went away after the doctor at the urgent clinic gave me some medicine.
☐ Duration of the pain in the fingers	Six months.
☐ Stiffness in the morning/duration	Yes, for an hour.
☐ Photosensitivity	No.
☐ Rashes	No.
☐ Oral ulcers	I had many in my mouth last month, but they've resolved now. They seem to come and go.
☐ Fatigue	Yes, I've had no energy to work and have felt tired all the time for the past 6 months.
☐ Fever/chills	I feel hot now, but I have no chills.
☐ Hair loss	No.
☐ Cold temperature causing problems with the fingers	Sometimes my fingers become pale and then blue when they are exposed to cold weather or cold water.
☐ Heart symptoms (chest pain, palpitations)	No.
☐ Pulmonary complaints (shortness of breath, cough)	No.

✓ Question	Patient Response
☐ Neurologic complaints (seizures, weakness, numbness)	No.
☐ Urinary problems (hematuria)	No.
☐ Abdominal pain	No.
☐ History of recent tick bite	No.
☐ Pregnancies	I have 2 daughters. Both were delivered by C-section.
☐ Miscarriages/abortions	I had 2 spontaneous abortions a long time ago.
☐ Last menstrual period	Two weeks ago.
☐ Weight changes	I've lost about 10 pounds over the past 6 months.
☐ Appetite changes	I don't have a good appetite.
☐ Current medications	I used Tylenol to relieve my pain, but it is not working as well anymore.
☐ Past medical history	None.
☐ Past surgical history	Two C-sections at ages 23 and 25.
☐ Family history	My mother has rheumatoid arthritis and is living in a nursing home. I don't know my father.
☐ Occupation	Waitress.
☐ Alcohol use	I don't drink a lot, usually 2–4 beers a week except for weekends, when I don't count.
☐ CAGE questions	No (to all 4).
☐ Last alcohol ingestion	Four days ago.
☐ Illicit drug use	No.
☐ Tobacco	Yes, a pack a day for the past 20 years.
☐ Sexual activity	I am sexually active with a new boyfriend whom I met 2 months ago.
☐ Use of condoms	Occasionally.
☐ Number of sexual partners during the past year	Four.
☐ Active with men, women, or both	Men only.
☐ Vaginal discharge	No.
☐ History of STDs	Yes, I had gonorrhea a year ago. I took antibiotics and was fine.
☐ Drug allergies	No.

Connecting with the Patient

☐ Examinee recognized the SP's emotions and responded with PEARLS.

Physical Examination

☐ Examinee washed his/her hands.

☐ Examinee asked permission to start the exam.

☐ Examinee used respectful draping.

☐ Examinee did not repeat painful maneuvers.

☑ *Exam Component*	*Maneuver*
☐ Mouth exam	Inspection
☐ Musculoskeletal exam	Inspection and palpation (compared both knees, including range of motion); examined other joints (shoulders, elbows, wrists, hands, fingers, hips, ankles)
☐ Hair and skin exam	Inspection
☐ CV exam	Auscultation
☐ Pulmonary exam	Auscultation
☐ Abdominal exam	Auscultation, palpation, percussion

Closure

☐ Examinee discussed initial diagnostic impressions.

☐ Examinee discussed initial management plans:

    ☐ Follow-up tests: Examinee mentioned the need for a pelvic exam.

    ☐ Examinee discussed safe sex practices.

☐ Examinee asked if the SP had any other questions or concerns.

Sample Closure

Ms. Moore, there are a few things that could be causing your knee pain, such as gout, an infection, or rheumatoid arthritis. To find out, I would like to obtain fluid from your knee and then draw some blood. Sometimes infections from the pelvis can spread to other parts of your body, such as your knee, and for that reason I would also like to do a pelvic exam. These tests will likely reveal the source of your pain. You mentioned earlier that you don't always use condoms. I know condoms may be difficult to use regularly, but they are important in helping control the spread of STDs. Do you have any questions for me?

Patient Note

History

Physical Examination

Patient Note

Differential Diagnosis

Diagnosis #1

History Finding(s):

Physical Exam Finding(s):

Diagnosis #2

History Finding(s):

Physical Exam Finding(s):

Diagnosis #3

History Finding(s):

Physical Exam Finding(s):

Diagnostic Workup

History

HPI: *33 yo F c/o left knee pain that started 2 days ago and is causing difficulty walking. She has swelling and redness in her left knee and mild fever but no chills. She denies trauma. She has a history of fatigue and painful wrists and fingers and has experienced 1-hour morning stiffness over the past 6 months. She also recalls multiple oral ulcers that resolved last month. She describes Raynaud's phenomenon but denies rash, photosensitivity, hair loss, or recent tick bites. She recalls a 10-lb weight loss over the past 6 months and has no appetite.*

ROS: *Negative except as above.*

Allergies: *NKDA.*

Medications: *Tylenol.*

PMH: *Episode of acute left big toe arthritis 5 years ago; gonorrhea 1 year ago.*

PSH: *Two C-sections, 2 spontaneous abortions.*

SH: *1 PPD for 20 years. Usually drinks 2–4 beers/week; on weekends drinks more; last ingestion 4 days ago; CAGE 0/4. No illicit drugs. Sexually active with multiple partners; inconsistent condom use.*

FH: *Mother has rheumatoid arthritis and lives in a nursing home.*

Physical Examination

Patient is in no acute distress but favors the left knee.

VS: *WNL except for low-grade fever.*

HEENT: *No oral lesions.*

Chest: *Clear breath sounds bilaterally.*

Heart: *RRR; normal S1/S2; no murmurs, rubs, or gallops.*

Abdomen: *Soft, nondistended, ⊕ BS, no hepatosplenomegaly.*

Extremities: *Erythema, tenderness, pain, and restricted range of motion on flexion and extension of left knee compared to right knee. ⊕ swelling at left knee. Fingers and hands with stiffness bilaterally. Shoulder, elbow, wrist, hip, and ankle joints WNL bilaterally.*

Differential Diagnosis

Diagnosis #1: Gout	
History Finding(s):	**Physical Exam Finding(s):**
Monoarticular joint pain and tenderness	Joint tenderness and stiffness
History of swollen toe	Swelling at left knee
Occasional alcohol use	

Diagnosis #2: Rheumatoid arthritis

History Finding(s):	Physical Exam Finding(s):
Morning joint stiffness	Joint tenderness and stiffness
Family history of rheumatoid arthritis	Temperature 99.9°F
Systemic symptoms (anorexia, weight loss, fatigue, fever)	

Diagnosis #3: Systemic lupus erythematosus

History Finding(s):	Physical Exam Finding(s):
Systemic symptoms (anorexia, weight loss, fatigue)	Joint tenderness and stiffness
History of multiple oral ulcers	
History of 2 spontaneous abortions	
Raynaud's phenomenon	

Diagnostic Workup

CBC with differential
Immunologic testing (eg, ANA titer, anti-dsDNA, RF, anti-CCP)
Knee aspiration with Gram stain, culture, and inspection for crystals
XR—left knee and both hands

CASE DISCUSSION

Patient Note Differential Diagnoses

- **Gout:** This acute, usually monoarticular, crystal-induced arthritis rarely occurs in premenopausal women, but the patient's history of first MTP arthritis ("podagra") is classic for gout. Alcohol ingestion causes hyperuricemia and may precipitate an acute attack. Foot, ankle, and knee joints are also commonly affected. Gout does not explain her hand arthralgias, but osteoarthritis is common and may coexist.

- **Rheumatoid arthritis (RA):** This is suggested in a patient with a positive family history, symmetric small joint arthritis (eg, fingers, wrists), prolonged morning stiffness, and systemic symptoms (low-grade fever, anorexia, weight loss, fatigue, and weakness). However, this patient's hand joints were not red, warm, swollen, or tender on exam. Monoarthritis is also uncommon but is occasionally seen early in the course of the disease.

- **Systemic lupus erythematosus (SLE):** Joint symptoms (usually symmetric peripheral arthralgias), constitutional symptoms, and Raynaud's phenomenon may be early manifestations of this disease. Unilateral knee involvement is not typical. The diagnosis requires at least four of the following 11 criteria: malar ("butterfly") rash, discoid rash, symmetric arthritis, photosensitivity, oral ulcers, serositis, renal disease, CNS involvement, hematologic disorders (her fatigue may be due to anemia), immunologic abnormalities (her history of spontaneous abortions may signal the presence of antiphospholipid antibodies), or ANA positivity. More testing needs to be done before SLE can be diagnosed in this case.

Additional Differential Diagnoses

- **Pseudogout:** Another crystal-induced arthritis, pseudogout frequently involves the knees and wrists but is usually seen in patients older than 60 years of age.

- **Gonococcal septic arthritis:** This occurs in healthy hosts, most commonly young women (women are much more likely than men to have asymptomatic genitourinary gonococcal infection, which allows the bacteria to mutate and disseminate). The knee is the most frequently involved joint, but the monoarthritis (or tenosynovitis) is usually preceded by a few days of migratory polyarthralgias. Also, this patient does not have the characteristic rash, which consists of small necrotic pustules on the extremities (including the palms and soles).

- **Nongonococcal septic arthritis:** This occurs suddenly, usually affects the knee or wrist, and is most commonly caused by S aureus. However, it is a disease of an abnormal host; previous joint damage and IV drug use are key risk factors not present in this case.

- **Osteoarthritis:** Onset is insidious, joint stiffness brief, and joint inflammation minimal, all of which are incongruent with this patient's presentation. Also, osteoarthritis spares the wrist and MCP joints and is not associated with constitutional symptoms.

Diagnostic Workup

- **CBC:** To look for anemia, leukopenia, and/or thrombocytopenia in SLE or for leukocytosis in acute gout and septic arthritis.

- **Immunologic tests:** ANA is a highly sensitive but nonspecific screening test for SLE. A negative test essentially excludes the disease. If ANA is positive, antibody against double-stranded DNA (anti-dsDNA), antibody against the Smith antigen, anticardiolipin antibodies, and lupus anticoagulant should be investigated to help confirm the diagnosis of SLE. RF is present in > 75% of patients with RA. Anti–cyclic citrullinated peptide (anti-CCP) antibody has high specificity (up to 96%) for RA and is frequently sent when RA is suspected as the diagnosis.

- **Knee aspiration, Gram stain, culture, and inspection for crystals:** In most cases of acute monoarthritis, joint aspiration must be performed to rule out septic arthritis. Inflammatory joint synovial fluid contains > 3000 WBCs/μL, and septic joint fluid often contains > 50,000 cells/μL. The demonstration of needle-shaped, negatively birefringent crystals or rhomboid-shaped, weakly positively birefringent crystals confirms gout or pseudogout, respectively.

- **XR—left knee and both hands:** Specific changes in RA include symmetric joint space narrowing, marginal bony erosions, and periarticular demineralization. However, x-rays are usually normal during the first six months of illness. In gout, look for punched-out cortical erosions and a sclerotic joint margin. In pseudogout, look for calcified articular cartilage ("chondrocalcinosis"). In osteoarthritis, look for joint space narrowing, marginal osteophytes, subchondral osteosclerosis, and occasionally subchondral cysts.

- **Pelvic exam and cervical cultures:** Necessary to investigate gonococcal infection and often positive in the absence of symptoms (urine, anorectal, and throat cultures may also be necessary).

- **Blood culture:** An important test in septic arthritis if systemic symptoms are present.

Opening Scenario

Will Foreman, a 31-year-old male, comes to his primary care physician complaining of heel pain.

Vital Signs

BP: 125/80 mm Hg

Temp: 99.0°F (37.2°C)

RR: 14/minute

HR: 69/minute, regular

Examinee Tasks

1. Take a focused history.

2. Perform a focused physical exam (do not perform rectal, genitourinary, or female breast exam).

3. Explain your clinical impression and workup plan to the patient.

4. Write the patient note after leaving the room.

Checklist/SP Sheet

Patient Description

Patient is a 31 yo M.

Notes for the SP

- Pretend to have pain on the bottom of your right heel and into the arch of your right foot when the examinee extends your toes (moves them up).

- Exhibit pain when the examinee palpates the arch of your right foot and the bottom of your right heel.

- Give the appearance of pain with the first few steps you take after sitting.

Challenging Questions to Ask

"Doctor, can you just give me some powerful pain meds so that I can keep running? I am training for a marathon."

Sample Examinee Response

"First we need to do a complete evaluation to determine the cause of your pain. Then we can discuss the nature of your treatment."

Examinee Checklist

Building the Doctor-Patient Relationship

Entrance

☐ Examinee knocked on the door before entering.

☐ Examinee introduced self by name.

☐ Examinee identified his/her role or position.

☐ Examinee correctly used patient's name.

☐ Examinee made eye contact with the SP.

Reflective Listening

☐ Examinee asked an open-ended question and actively listened to the response.

☐ Examinee asked the SP to list his/her concerns and listened to the response without interrupting.

☐ Examinee summarized the SP's concerns, often using the SP's own words.

Information Gathering

☐ Examinee elicited data efficiently and accurately.

☑ Question	Patient Response
☐ Chief complaint	Right heel pain.
☐ Location	It hurts the most at my heel.
☐ Onset	It came on gradually over the past 2 weeks.
☐ Precipitating events	Not really, but I have been training for a marathon.
☐ Constant/intermittent	Intermittent.
☐ Frequency	It usually hurts every day. It seems to be worse in the morning.
☐ When does it hurt in the morning?	It hurts the most with the first few steps I take after I get out of bed.
☐ Progression	It has stayed about the same.
☐ Severity on a scale	When it hurts, it can get up to a 7/10.
☐ Radiation	It occasionally radiates into the arch of my foot.
☐ Radiation proximally (up the leg or down from the back)	No.
☐ Quality	Stretching/tearing pain.
☐ Burning, tingling, numbness	No.
☐ Alleviating factors	Massaging the arch of my foot and applying ice.
☐ Exacerbating factors	Walking barefoot or walking after sitting for a prolonged period of time.
☐ Other joint pain	No.
☐ Previous episodes of similar pain	No.
☐ Previous injury to your feet or ankles.	No.
☐ Constitutional symptoms (nausea/vomiting, weight/appetite changes, fever/chills, diarrhea/constipation, fatigue)	No.
☐ Current medications	Occasionally I take ibuprofen for the pain.
☐ Past medical history (be sure to address diabetes, rheumatologic disorders, and cancer)	No.

☑ Question	Patient Response
☐ Past surgical history	None.
☐ Family history (be sure to address diabetes, rheumatologic disorders, and cancer)	My father has arthritis.
☐ Occupation	I work as an accountant.
☐ Avocation	Runner.
☐ Alcohol use	I have approximately 1–2 beers a week.
☐ Illicit drug use	No.
☐ Tobacco	No.
☐ Sexual activity	I am sexually active with my wife of 10 years.
☐ Drug allergies	No.

Connecting with the Patient

☐ Examinee recognized the SP's emotions and responded with PEARLS.

Physical Examination

☐ Examinee washed his/her hands.

☐ Examinee asked permission to start the exam.

☐ Examinee used respectful draping.

☐ Examinee did not repeat painful maneuvers.

☑ Exam Component	Maneuver
☐ CV exam	Auscultation, distal pulses (posterior tibialis, dorsalis pedis), capillary refill of the toes
☐ Pulmonary exam	Auscultation
☐ Abdominal exam	Auscultation, palpation
☐ Extremities	■ Inspection of both feet and ankles—non–weight bearing, weight bearing, and with ambulation ■ Palpation of medial calcaneal tuberosity, Achilles tendon, plantar fascia, retrocalcaneal bursae ■ Passive range of motion and general strength of ipsilateral knee and hip ■ Ankle dorsiflexion and great toe extension and passive range of motion; strength testing of ankle dorsiflexion and plantar flexion
☐ Neurologic exam	Checked sensation to light touch for dermatomes of foot and ankle; assessed Achilles tendon reflex

Closure

☐ Examinee discussed initial diagnostic impressions.

☐ Examinee discussed initial management plans:

    ☐ Follow-up tests: X-ray of right ankle.

☐ Examinee asked if the SP had any other questions or concerns.

Sample Closure

Mr. Foreman, the most likely cause of your heel pain is plantar fasciitis, which is the most common cause of pain on the bottom of the heel. It typically resolves over a few months, with conservative treatment consisting of stretching, massage, NSAIDs, and avoidance of painful activities. I would highly suggest that you decrease the amount of running you do and avoid walking barefoot on hard surfaces until this improves. We will get an x-ray today to help confirm that there is no obvious fracture or foreign body and to look for possible bone spurs. If you would like, I can send you to physical therapy to help you get started on these exercises. If your symptoms are not responsive to this treatment over the next 2 months, we may consider a bone scan to rule out a stress fracture. Do you have any questions for me?

Patient Note

History

Physical Examination

Patient Note

Differential Diagnosis

Diagnosis #1

History Finding(s):

Physical Exam Finding(s):

Diagnosis #2

History Finding(s):

Physical Exam Finding(s):

Diagnosis #3

History Finding(s):

Physical Exam Finding(s):

Diagnostic Workup

History

HPI: *31 yo M c/o pain on the plantar surface of his right heel. The pain started gradually about 2 weeks ago and has not progressed. The patient denies trauma or a specific inciting event but admits to training for a marathon. He describes the pain as intermittent and states that it is worse after getting out of bed in the morning and after prolonged sitting. He reports that the pain has a tearing/stretching quality and that it can get as high as 7/10. He has used ice, massage, and occasional ibuprofen for the pain, with limited relief. The patient denies any tingling, burning, or numbness. He denies proximally radiating symptoms but does report occasional pain radiating into his arch.*

ROS: *Denies nausea/vomiting, weight/appetite changes, fever/chills, diarrhea/constipation, or fatigue.*

Allergies: *NKDA.*

Medications: *Occasional ibuprofen.*

PMH: *None. Denies cancer, rheumatologic disorders, or diabetes.*

PSH: *None.*

SH: *No smoking, 1–2 beers/week, no illicit drugs. Works as an accountant; sexually active with wife of 10 years. Marathon runner.*

FH: *Father with arthritis. Denies FH of cancer, rheumatologic disorders, or diabetes.*

Physical Examination

Patient is pleasant and in no acute distress.

VS: *WNL.*

Chest: *Clear to auscultation bilaterally.*

Heart: *RRR; normal S1/S2; no murmurs, rubs, or gallops.*

Abdomen: *Soft, nontender, nondistended, ⊕ BS.*

Extremities: *Posterior tibialis and dorsalis pedis pulses 2+ bilaterally; mild bilateral rear/midfoot pronation; range of motion of hip/knee/ankle and foot WNL. Tender to palpation over medial calcaneal tuberosity and plantar fascia; plantar heel and arch pain with dorsiflexion of toes.*

Neuro: *Motor: Strength 5/5 in hip/knee/ankle and foot. Sensation: Intact to light tough in saphenous, sural, and deep/superficial peroneal nerve distributions (dermatomes L4–S1). DTRs: 1+ in Achilles tendon. Gait: Non-antalgic gait pattern.*

Differential Diagnosis

Diagnosis #1: Plantar fasciitis	
History Finding(s):	**Physical Exam Finding(s):**
Training for a marathon	Tenderness over medial calcaneal tuberosity
Pain is gradual	Pain with toe dorsiflexion
Pain worsens with first few steps in morning and after prolonged sitting	

Patient Note

Diagnosis #2: Calcaneal stress fracture

History Finding(s):	Physical Exam Finding(s):
Training for a marathon	Tenderness over plantar heel and arch
Diffuse pain over heel	
Refractory to conservative management	

Diagnosis #3: Achilles tendinitis

History Finding(s):	Physical Exam Finding(s):
Training for a marathon	Pain with toe dorsiflexion

Diagnostic Workup

XR—right ankle/foot
Bone scan
MRI—right ankle/foot

CASE DISCUSSION

Patient Note Differential Diagnoses

Heel pain in adults can be caused by several distinct entities. For this reason, it is essential that the examiner ascertain the precise location of the symptoms, as this is the first step in determining the most likely diagnosis.

- **Plantar fasciitis:** The most common cause of plantar heel pain in adults, plantar fasciitis typically results from repetitive use or excessive loading (eg, training for a marathon). Pes planus, pes cavus, decreased subtalar joint mobility, and a tight Achilles tendon can all predispose to plantar fasciitis. The pain is typically gradual in onset and worse with the first few steps in the morning and after prolonged sitting. Examination reveals marked tenderness over the medial calcaneal tuberosity and increased pain with passive dorsiflexion of the toes. Conservative management includes analgesics, stretching, exercise, orthotics, and night splinting.

- **Calcaneal stress fracture:** The calcaneus is second only to the metatarsals in terms of stress fractures of the foot. Stress fractures are common in athletes who are involved in running or jumping sports as well as in patients who have risk factors for osteopenia. Patients typically have diffuse heel pain that is made worse by medial and lateral compression. A calcaneal stress fracture may be considered in this patient if his symptoms prove refractory to conservative management. Follow-up diagnostic testing (eg, x-ray, bone scan) may then be warranted.

- **Achilles tendinitis:** Patients with Achilles tendinitis typically complain of posterior heel pain either on the Achilles tendon insertion site or on the tendon itself during running, jumping, and harsh activities. Tenderness to palpation, swelling, and nodules along the Achilles tendon are common. Pain may also increase with passive dorsiflexion of the ankle. Again, this condition is commonly due to overuse or to poor biomechanics. Conservative management includes rest, analgesics, and stretching/strengthening exercises.

Additional Differential Diagnoses

- **Retrocalcaneal bursitis:** Patients with this condition usually complain of posterior heel pain secondary to chronic irritation of the underlying bursae. The bursae are located between the posterior calcaneus and the Achilles tendon and between the Achilles tendon and the skin. The condition is commonly caused by ill-fitting footwear that has a poorly fitting, rigid heel cup. It can also be associated with Haglund's deformity (a bony spur on the posterosuperior aspect of the calcaneus), which may exacerbate the condition. Conservative management includes analgesics, proper shoe wear, and heel padding.

- **Tarsal tunnel syndrome:** The tarsal tunnel is on the medial aspect of the heel and is formed by the flexor retinaculum traversing over the talus and calcaneus. Compression of the tibial nerve in the tunnel can lead to pain, burning, tingling, or numbness that can radiate to the plantar heel and even to the distal sole and toes. Symptoms may be exacerbated by percussion of the tarsal tunnel or with dorsiflexion and eversion of the foot. Conservative management includes analgesics and correction of foot mechanics with orthotics.

- **Foreign body:** If a foreign body is suspected, the foot should be inspected for signs of an entrance wound. The patient may or may not describe a mechanism of injury. Signs of local infection such as warmth, erythema, pain, induration, or a fluctuant mass should also be sought. Conservative management includes foreign body removal, topical antimicrobials, and appropriate dressing.

- **Ankle sprain:** Ankle ligament injuries are the most common musculoskeletal injury, with the lateral collateral ligament complex most commonly involved. Patients typically describe an injury pattern consistent with "rolling" the ankle, often in the plantarflexed and inverted position. Examination reveals tenderness to palpation over the involved ligaments and increased laxity on stress testing. Significant edema and ecchymosis are often present in the acute/subacute stages. Conservative treatment involves rest, ice, compression, elevation, NSAIDs, and bracing.

Diagnostic Workup

- **XR—right ankle/foot:** X-rays in this region may demonstrate calcaneal spur formation (calcification) at the proximal plantar fascia (as in this patient) or at the Achilles tendon insertion. Care must be taken to correlate these findings with symptoms and with the physical examination, as such calcification can also be seen in asymptomatic patients. Increased prominence of the posterosuperior calcaneus (Haglund's deformity) may also be demonstrated.

- **Bone scan:** If conservative treatment fails in this patient, follow-up with a bone scan is recommended in two months to rule out calcaneal stress fracture, as would be demonstrated by an increased area of uptake.

- **MRI—right ankle/foot:** Reserved for suspected soft tissue involvement, which could include the degree of Achilles tendon degeneration, rupture of the Achilles tendon, or articular cartilage defects.

Opening Scenario

The mother of Maria Sterling, an 18-month-old female child, comes to the office complaining that her child has a fever.

Examinee Tasks

1. Take a focused history.

2. Explain your clinical impression and workup plan to the mother.

3. Write the patient note after leaving the room.

Checklist/SP Sheet

Patient Description

The patient's mother offers the history; the child is at home.

Notes for the SP

Show concern regarding your child's situation.

Challenging Questions to Ask

- "Do you think that I did the right thing by coming here and telling you about my child's fever?"

- "Is my child going to be okay?"

Sample Examinee Response

"You certainly did the right thing by coming in today. Maria may have an infection that is causing her fever, so we need to examine her here in the office and then decide whether she needs any tests and/or treatment."

Examinee Checklist

Building the Doctor-Patient Relationship

Entrance

☐ Examinee knocked on the door before entering.

☐ Examinee introduced self by name.

☐ Examinee identified his/her role or position.

☐ Examinee correctly used patient's name.

☐ Examinee made eye contact with the SP.

Reflective Listening

☐ Examinee asked an open-ended question and actively listened to the response.

☐ Examinee asked the SP to list his/her concerns and listened to the response without interrupting.

☐ Examinee summarized the SP's concerns, often using the SP's own words.

Information Gathering

☐ Examinee elicited data efficiently and accurately.

☑ Question	Patient Response
☐ Chief complaint	My child has a fever.
☐ Onset	Two days ago.
☐ Temperature	I measured it, and it was 101°F on her forehead.
☐ Runny nose	Not currently, but she did have a runny nose for a few days about a week ago.
☐ Ear pulling/ear discharge	Yes, she has been pulling at her right ear for 2 days.
☐ Cough	Not currently, but she was coughing for a few days about a week ago.
☐ Shortness of breath	No.
☐ Difficulty swallowing	She seems to have trouble swallowing, but I'm not sure.
☐ Rash	Yes, she has a rash on her face and chest.
☐ Description of the rash	Tiny red dots, some slightly elevated, over the chest, back, belly, and face. There is no rash on her arms or legs.
☐ Onset of rash and progression	It started 2 days ago on her face and then spread to her chest, back, and belly.
☐ Nausea/vomiting	Yes, she had an episode of vomiting last night
☐ Change in bowel habits or in stool color or consistency	No.
☐ Change in urinary habits or in urine smell or color	No.
☐ Shaking (seizures)	No.
☐ How has the child looked (lethargic, irritated, playful, etc.)?	She looks tired. She is not playing with her toys today and is not watching TV the way she usually does.
☐ Appetite changes	She is not eating much but is able to drink milk.
☐ Ill contacts	No.
☐ Day care center	Yes.
☐ Ill contacts in day care center	I don't know.
☐ Vaccinations	Up to date.
☐ Last checkup	One month ago, and everything was normal.
☐ Birth history	It was a 40-week vaginal delivery with no complications.
☐ Child weight, height, and language development	Normal.
☐ Eating habits	Whole milk and solid food; I did not breast-feed my child.
☐ Sleeping habits	She has not slept well for 2 days.
☐ Hearing problems	No.

☑ Question	Patient Response
☐ Vision problems	No.
☐ Current medications	Tylenol.
☐ Past medical history	Three months ago she had an ear infection that was treated successfully with amoxicillin.
☐ Past surgical history	None.
☐ Drug allergies	No.

Connecting with the Patient

☐ Examinee recognized the SP's emotions and responded with PEARLS.

Physical Examination

None.

Closure

☐ Examinee discussed initial diagnostic impressions.

☐ Examinee discussed initial management plans:

  ☐ Follow-up tests.

☐ Examinee asked if the SP had any other questions or concerns.

Sample Closure

Mrs. Sterling, it appears that your child is suffering from an infection that may be viral or bacterial. She may be suffering from an ear infection or something more serious. A physical exam and some blood tests will be needed to identify the source of infection and the type of virus or bacteria involved. Although viral infections generally clear on their own, most bacterial infections require antibiotics; however, such infections generally respond well to treatment. Do you have any questions for me?

Patient Note

History

_____
_____
_____
_____
_____
_____
_____
_____
_____
_____
_____
_____
_____
_____
_____

Physical Examination

_____
_____
_____
_____
_____
_____
_____
_____
_____
_____
_____
_____
_____
_____

Patient Note

Differential Diagnosis

Diagnosis #1

History Finding(s): | **Physical Exam Finding(s):**

Diagnosis #2

History Finding(s): | **Physical Exam Finding(s):**

Diagnosis #3

History Finding(s): | **Physical Exam Finding(s):**

Diagnostic Workup

Patient Note

History

HPI: *History obtained from mother. Patient is 18-month-old F with fever × 2 days.*

- *Temperature recorded at home, 101°F.*
- *Tired and not playing with toys or watching TV as usual.*
- *Pulling at right ear.*
- *Difficulty swallowing and sleeping × 2 days.*
- *Loss of appetite.*
- *One episode of vomiting.*
- *Maculopapular facial rash that spread over the chest, back, and abdomen, sparing the arms and legs.*
- *Attends day care center, no known history of sick contacts.*
- *No ear discharge.*
- *History of cough and runny nose for a few days last week.*

ROS: *Negative except as above.*
Allergies: *NKDA.*
Medications: *Tylenol.*
PMH: *Otitis media 3 months ago, treated with amoxicillin.*
Birth history: *40-week vaginal delivery with no complications.*
Dietary history: *Formula milk and solid food. She was not breast-fed.*
Immunization history: *UTD.*
Developmental history: *Last checkup was 1 month ago and showed normal weight, height, hearing, vision, and developmental milestones.*

Physical Examination

None.

Differential Diagnosis

Diagnosis #1: Acute otitis media	
History Finding(s):	**Physical Exam Finding(s):**
Fever (101°F)	
Pulling at right ear; fatigued and not watching TV as usual	
History of otitis media	
Runny nose and cough that have subsided	

Patient Note

Diagnosis #2: Meningococcal meningitis

History Finding(s):	Physical Exam Finding(s):
Maculopapular facial rash that spread to the chest, back, and abdomen	
Fever (101°F)	
Difficulty sleeping for 2 days	
Recent episode of vomiting	

Diagnosis #3: Scarlet fever

History Finding(s):	Physical Exam Finding(s):
Maculopapular facial rash that spread to the chest, back, and abdomen	
Fever (101°F)	
Difficulty swallowing for 2 days	

Diagnostic Workup

Pneumatic otoscopy
LP—CSF analysis
CBC with differential, blood culture, UA and urine culture
Throat culture
Platelets, PT/PTT, D-dimer, fibrin split products, fibrinogen

CASE DISCUSSION

Patient Note Differential Diagnoses

- **Acute otitis media:** Infections of the middle ear are more common in younger children because of their shorter and more horizontal Eustachian tubes. Fever, otalgia, loss of appetite, temporary hearing loss, and general irritability suggest this diagnosis but are not always present. Upper respiratory viral infection is a common risk factor for developing acute otitis media. This patient has a recent history of cough and runny nose, both of which are suggestive of a viral URI. In addition, patients with a prior history of otitis media are more prone to having another episode.

- **Meningococcal meningitis:** Fever, lethargy, and a possible petechial rash suggest meningococcemia. Patients may also have headache, vomiting, photophobia, neck stiffness, and seizures. This patient had a single episode of vomiting. Although her immunizations are up to date, meningococcal vaccinations are typically not given until 11–12 years of age; therefore, at 18 months, the patient would not yet have been immunized. Treatment is critical, as meningococcal meningitis is a severe, rapidly progressive, and sometimes fatal infection.

- **Scarlet fever:** This patient has fever, difficulty swallowing (possible pharyngitis), and a rash that started on her face and spread to her trunk. However, the history does not indicate whether the rash consists of a diffuse erythema with punctate, sandpaper-like elevations that spare the area around the mouth. In addition, scarlet fever is more common among school-age children. However, the patient does attend day care, where she may potentially have been exposed to sick contacts. Left untreated, *Streptococcus pyogenes* infection can lead to rheumatic heart disease. A throat culture would aid in identifying this illness.

Additional Differential Diagnoses

- **Fifth disease or other viral exanthem:** In children, viruses commonly present with low-grade fever and rash. In general, viral exanthems are nonspecific in their appearance and are usually maculopapular and diffuse. Parvovirus B19 infection, or fifth disease, usually presents as intense red facial flushing (a "slapped cheek" appearance) that spreads over the trunk and becomes more diffuse. However, almost any virus can be accompanied by rash in a pediatric patient, and it is not always necessary to ascertain which virus is causing the illness. If the illness is prolonged or particularly troublesome, viral cultures, molecular tests (PCR), and/or antibody titers can be ordered to determine the exact etiology.

- **Varicella:** Fever and rash, along with day care attendance, are consistent with this infection. In varicella, lesions are present in various stages of development at any given time (eg, red macules, vesicles, pustules, crusting), and the rash is intensely pruritic. Because the patient's immunizations are up to date, it is unlikely that she has varicella.

Diagnostic Workup

- **Pneumatic otoscopy:** Key to look for the tympanic membrane (TM) erythema and decreased mobility seen in otitis media.

- **LP—CSF analysis:** Should be performed if there is any concern for meningitis. CSF analysis includes cell count and differential, glucose, protein, Gram stain, culture, latex agglutination for common bacterial antigens, and occasionally PCR for specific viruses.

- **CBC with differential, blood culture, UA and urine culture:** To isolate *Neisseria meningitidis* and to screen for occult bacteremia or UTI.

- **Throat culture:** To isolate *S pyogenes*, which causes scarlet fever. The rash is pathognomonic for this diagnosis.

- **Platelets, PT/PTT, D-dimer, fibrin split products, fibrinogen:** Evidence of DIC is often seen in meningococcemia.

- **Tympanometry:** Useful in infants older than six months of age; confirms abnormal TM mobility in otitis media.

- **Parvovirus B19 IgM antibody:** The best marker of acute or recent infection in suspected fifth disease.

- **Skin lesion scrapings:** Varicella antigens are identified by PCR or direct immunofluorescence (DFA) of skin lesions. A Tzanck smear (more of a historic test and no longer recommended) may show multinucleated giant cells in varicella infection.

- **Varicella antibody titer:** May be useful in uncertain cases (look for a fourfold rise in antibody titer following acute infection).

Opening Scenario

Marilyn McLean, a 54-year-old female, comes to the office complaining of persistent cough.

Vital Signs

BP: 120/80 mm Hg

Temp: 99.5°F (37.5°C)

RR: 15/minute

HR: 75/minute, regular

Examinee Tasks

1. Take a focused history.

2. Perform a focused physical exam (do not perform rectal, genitourinary, or female breast exam).

3. Explain your clinical impression and workup plan to the patient.

4. Write the patient note after leaving the room.

Checklist/SP Sheet

Patient Description

Patient is a 54 yo F.

Notes for the SP

- Cough as the examinee enters the room.

- Continue coughing every 3–4 minutes during the encounter.

- Hold a red-stained tissue in your hand to simulate blood. Don't show it to the examinee unless he/she asks you.

- During the encounter, pretend to have a severe attack of coughing. Note whether the examinee offers you a glass of water or a tissue.

Challenging Questions to Ask

"Will I get better if I stop smoking?"

Sample Examinee Response

"Well, we still have to sort out exactly what is causing your cough. If you stop smoking, your chronic cough should improve. But regardless of what is causing your cough, smoking cessation will significantly decrease your cancer risk in the long term."

Examinee Checklist

Building the Doctor-Patient Relationship

Entrance

☐ Examinee knocked on the door before entering.

☐ Examinee introduced self by name.

☐ Examinee identified his/her role or position.

☐ Examinee correctly used patient's name.

☐ Examinee made eye contact with the SP.

Reflective Listening

☐ Examinee asked an open-ended question and actively listened to the response.

☐ Examinee asked the SP to list his/her concerns and listened to the response without interrupting.

☐ Examinee summarized the SP's concerns, often using the SP's own words.

Information Gathering

☐ Examinee elicited data efficiently and accurately.

☐ Examinee offered the SP a glass of water or a tissue during the severe bout of coughing.

☑ Question	Patient Response
☐ Chief complaint	Persistent cough.
☐ Onset	I've had a cough for years, especially in the morning. This past month, the cough has gotten worse, and it is really annoying me.
☐ Changes in the cough during the day	No.
☐ Progression of the cough during the past month	It is getting worse.
☐ Do you cough at night?	Yes, sometimes I can't sleep because of it.
☐ Alleviating/exacerbating factors	Nothing.
☐ Sputum production	Yes.
☐ Amount	Two teaspoonfuls, stable.
☐ Color	Yellowish mucus.
☐ Odor	None.
☐ Consistency	Thick and viscous.
☐ Blood	Yes, recently.
☐ Amount of blood	Streaks.
☐ Preceding symptoms/events	None.
☐ Fever/chills	Mild fever, especially at night. I didn't take my temperature. I have had no chills.
☐ Night sweats	Yes.
☐ Chest pain	No.

☑ Question	Patient Response
☐ Shortness of breath	Yes, when I walk up the stairs.
☐ Exposure to TB	Yes, I work in a nursing home, and several of our residents are under treatment for TB.
☐ Recent travel	None.
☐ Last PPD	Last year, before I started working in the nursing home. It was negative.
☐ Associated symptoms (wheezing, abdominal pain, nausea/vomiting, diarrhea/constipation)	None.
☐ Appetite changes	Yes, I no longer have an appetite.
☐ Weight changes	I've lost 6 pounds in the past 2 months without intending to.
☐ Fatigue	Yes, I don't have the energy that I had before.
☐ Since when	Two months ago.
☐ Current medications	Cough syrup "over the counter," multivitamins, albuterol inhaler.
☐ Past medical history	Chronic bronchitis.
☐ Past surgical history	Tonsillectomy and adenoidectomy, age 11.
☐ Family history	My father died of old age. My mother is alive and has Alzheimer's.
☐ Occupation	Nurse's aide.
☐ Alcohol use	None.
☐ Illicit drug use	Never.
☐ Tobacco	No, I stopped smoking 2 weeks ago.
☐ Duration	I've smoked for the past 35 years.
☐ Amount	One to two packs a day.
☐ Sexual activity	With my husband.
☐ Drug allergies	No.

Connecting with the Patient

☐ Examinee recognized the SP's emotions and responded with PEARLS.

Physical Examination

☐ Examinee washed his/her hands.

☐ Examinee asked permission to start the exam.

☐ Examinee used respectful draping.

☐ Examinee did not repeat painful maneuvers.

☑ Exam Component	Maneuver
☐ Head and neck exam	Inspected mouth, throat, lymph nodes
☐ CV exam	Auscultation
☐ Pulmonary exam	Auscultation, palpation, percussion
☐ Abdominal exam	Auscultation, palpation
☐ Extremities	Inspection

Closure

☐ Examinee discussed initial diagnostic impressions.

☐ Examinee discussed initial management plans:

    ☐ Follow-up tests.

☐ Examinee asked if the SP had any other questions or concerns.

Sample Closure

Mrs. McLean, your cough may be due to a lung infection that can be treated with antibiotics, or it may result from something more serious, such as cancer. We will need to obtain some blood and sputum tests as well as a chest x-ray to identify the source of your cough. In addition, we may find it necessary to conduct more sophisticated tests in the future. The fact that you work in a nursing home puts you at risk for acquiring tuberculosis, so we are going to test you for that as well. I would also recommend that you adhere to standard respiratory precautions while working with patients who are infected with TB. Do you have any questions for me?

USMLE STEP 2 CS **Patient Note**

History

Physical Examination

PRACTICE CASES

Patient Note

Differential Diagnosis

Diagnosis #1

History Finding(s):   *Physical Exam Finding(s):*

Diagnosis #2

History Finding(s):   *Physical Exam Finding(s):*

Diagnosis #3

History Finding(s):   *Physical Exam Finding(s):*

Diagnostic Workup

Patient Note

History

HPI: *54 yo F with PMH of chronic bronchitis c/o worsening cough × 1 month.*

- *Chronic cough for years.*
- *2 teaspoons of yellowish phlegm with streaks of blood.*
- *Dyspnea on exertion.*
- *Fever and sweats at night.*
- *Fatigue.*
- *Decreased appetite, 6-lb unintentional weight loss over 2 months.*
- *Exposure to TB as nurse's aide working in nursing home.*
- *Last PPD: 1 year ago and negative.*
- *No chest pain, chills, or wheezing.*
- *No recent travel.*

ROS: *Negative except as above.*
Allergies: *NKDA.*
Medications: *OTC cough syrup, multivitamins, albuterol inhaler.*
PMH: *Per HPI.*
PSH: *Tonsillectomy and adenoidectomy, age 11.*
SH: *1–2 PPD for 35 years; stopped smoking 2 weeks ago. No EtOH. Sexually active with husband only.*
FH: *Noncontributory.*

Physical Examination

Patient is in no acute distress.

VS: *WNL.*
HEENT: *Mouth and pharynx WNL.*
Neck: *No JVD, no lymphadenopathy.*
Chest: *Clear breath sounds bilaterally; no rhonchi, rales, or wheezing; tactile fremitus normal.*
Heart: *Apical impulse not displaced; RRR; normal S1/S2; no murmurs, rubs, or gallops.*
Abdomen: *Soft, nontender, ⊕ BS, no hepatosplenomegaly.*
Extremities: *No clubbing, cyanosis, or edema.*

Differential Diagnosis

Diagnosis #1: Pulmonary tuberculosis	
History Finding(s):	**Physical Exam Finding(s):**
Fever and night sweats with fatigue; worsening cough of 1 month's duration	Blood-tinged mucus
Close contact with patients with active TB	
Decreased appetite with unintentional weight loss of 6 lbs over 2 months	

Patient Note

Diagnosis #2: Lung cancer

History Finding(s):	**Physical Exam Finding(s):**
Fever and night sweats with fatigue	Blood-tinged mucus
Decreased appetite with unintentional weight loss of 6 lbs over 2 months	
History of heavy smoking and chronic bronchitis	

Diagnosis #3: Typical pneumonia

History Finding(s):	**Physical Exam Finding(s):**
Fever	Sputum production
Mucus production	
History of heavy smoking and chronic bronchitis	

Diagnostic Workup

PPD or QuantiFERON Gold
CBC
Blood cultures
Sputum Gram stain, AFB smear, routine and mycobacterial sputum cultures, and cytology
CXR—PA and lateral
CT—chest
Bronchoscopy
Lung biopsy

CASE DISCUSSION

Patient Note Differential Diagnoses

- **Pulmonary tuberculosis:** Clinical suspicion is high for this diagnosis given the patient's constitutional symptoms (fever and night sweats, unintentional weight loss) coupled with hemoptysis and recent exposure to active TB. The patient should be placed in respiratory isolation immediately. In those who have had recent contact with TB patients, a PPD is considered positive if it shows ≥ 5 mm of induration.

- **Lung cancer:** As noted above, constitutional symptoms and hemoptysis in a long-time smoker are worrisome for cancer. Although not found on this patient's physical exam, clubbing can be found in COPD patients with underlying lung malignancy.

- **Typical pneumonia:** Classic bacterial pneumonia begins with abrupt onset of fever, chills, pleuritic chest pain, and productive cough. Signs of pulmonary consolidation on physical exam are absent in up to two-thirds of documented cases. The more subacute time course seen here makes this diagnosis less likely.

Additional Differential Diagnoses

- **Lung abscess:** A lung abscess due to anaerobic bacteria is usually associated with gradual onset of fatigue, fever, night sweats, and cough producing a foul-smelling expectoration. Symptoms evolve over a period of weeks or months (the time course in this case favors abscess over uncomplicated pneumonia). Other bacterial causes of lung abscess typically present more acutely.

- **Atypical pneumonia:** Refers to infection by *Mycoplasma pneumoniae*, *Chlamydia pneumoniae*, and *Legionella* species. These can all present similarly with an insidious onset of fever, malaise, headache, myalgia, sore throat, hoarseness, chest pain, and nonproductive cough. Sputum may be blood-streaked. GI symptoms may be prominent in *Legionella* infection, and severe ear pain due to bullous myringitis may complicate up to 5% of *Mycoplasma* infections. The presence of weight loss, night sweats, and productive cough makes atypical pneumonia less likely in this case.

- **COPD exacerbation:** This patient's baseline productive cough is due to COPD/chronic bronchitis secondary to tobacco exposure. Exacerbations of chronic bronchitis are more acute and involve increased sputum production and/or increased wheezing and dyspnea. Night sweats and weight loss are not typical features of this diagnosis.

- **Other etiologies:** Other common, benign causes of chronic cough include postnasal drip, GERD, asthma, and ACE inhibitors.

Diagnostic Workup

- **PPD (tuberculin skin test) or QuantiFERON Gold:** The PPD test is a screening tool for *Mycobacterium tuberculosis* infection. The QuantiFERON Gold test is a newer and more specific test for prior *M tuberculosis* infection, but its availability varies depending on the testing center.

- **CBC:** To identify leukocytosis in infection (nonspecific).

- **Blood cultures:** May be useful in severe pneumonia to identify causative pathogenic bacteria.

- **Sputum Gram stain, AFB smear, routine and mycobacterial sputum cultures, and cytology:** To identify a causative agent of infection or to help detect malignancy.

- **CXR—PA and lateral:** To look for apical cavitary disease in TB reactivation, noncalcified nodules in lung cancer, a cavity with an air-fluid level in lung abscess, a patchy infiltrative pattern in atypical pneumonia, and lobar consolidation in typical pneumonia.

- **CT—chest:** May demonstrate lesions unseen on CXR, and aids in characterizing the size, shape, and composition of lung and mediastinal pathology. Any nodules found on CT require comparison to a previous scan if available. A chest CT can also guide diagnostic procedures (eg, percutaneous transthoracic biopsies) and assist in staging.

- **Bronchoscopy:** Useful in diagnosing and staging lung cancer as well as in diagnosing infections.

- **Lung biopsy:** Can lead to definitive diagnosis. A range of techniques can be used depending on the location of the tumor.

Opening Scenario

William Jordan, a 61-year-old male, comes to the office complaining of fatigue.

Vital Signs

BP: 135/85 mm Hg

Temp: 98.6°F (37°C)

RR: 13/minute

HR: 70/minute, regular

Examinee Tasks

1. Take a focused history.

2. Perform a focused physical exam (do not perform rectal, genitourinary, or female breast exam).

3. Explain your clinical impression and workup plan to the patient.

4. Write the patient note after leaving the room.

Checklist/SP Sheet

Patient Description

Patient is a 61 yo M, married with 3 children.

Notes for the SP

- Look weak and sad, and lean forward while seated.
- Exhibit abdominal discomfort that increases when you lie on your back.
- Show pain on palpation of the epigastric area.

Challenging Questions to Ask

"I want to go on a trip with my wife. Can we do the tests after I come back?"

Sample Examinee Response

"It doesn't sound as though you're feeling well enough to be able to enjoy a trip. Let's do some initial blood tests, and then we can see how you're feeling and decide whether we're comfortable letting you go away."

Examinee Checklist

Building the Doctor-Patient Relationship

Entrance

☐ Examinee knocked on the door before entering.

☐ Examinee introduced self by name.

☐ Examinee identified his/her role or position.

☐ Examinee correctly used patient's name.

☐ Examinee made eye contact with the SP.

Reflective Listening

☐ Examinee asked an open-ended question and actively listened to the response.

☐ Examinee asked the SP to list his/her concerns and listened to the response without interrupting.

☐ Examinee summarized the SP's concerns, often using the SP's own words.

Information Gathering

☐ Examinee elicited data efficiently and accurately.

☑ Question	Patient Response
☐ Chief complaint	Feeling tired, weak, low energy.
☐ Onset	Six months ago.
☐ Associated events	None.
☐ Progression of the fatigue during the day	The same throughout the day.
☐ Affecting job/performance	Yes, I don't have energy for my daily 30-minute walk with my dog, and even at work I am not as energetic as I was before.
☐ Appetite changes	I have a poor appetite.
☐ Weight changes	I have lost 8 pounds during the past 6 months. I did not intend to do so.
☐ Change in bowel habits	I have a bowel movement 2–3 times a week. It has been like this for the past 10 years. Recently I've noticed more foul-smelling and greasy-looking stools.
☐ Blood in stool	No.
☐ Abdominal pain or discomfort	Yes, I do feel some discomfort here (points to the epigastric area).
☐ Onset of discomfort	Four months ago; it increased gradually.
☐ Quality	Vague, deep.
☐ Severity on a scale	4/10.
☐ Alleviating/exacerbating factors	Nothing makes it worse, but I feel better when I lean forward.
☐ Relationship to food	No.
☐ Radiation	I feel the discomfort reaching my back.
☐ Nausea/vomiting	Sometimes I feel nauseated.
☐ Feeling of depression	Yes, I feel sad.
☐ Reason for feeling sad	I don't know, really.
☐ Suicidal thoughts/plans/attempts	No.

☑ Question	Patient Response
☐ Feelings of blame, guilt, worthlessness	No.
☐ Sleeping problems (falling asleep, staying asleep, early waking, snoring)	I wake up unusually early in the morning. It has been like this for the past 2 months.
☐ Loss of concentration	Yes, I can't concentrate anymore while watching the news or playing cards with my friends.
☐ Loss of interest	I don't enjoy playing cards with my friends anymore. I feel that life is boring.
☐ Associated symptoms (fever/chills, chest pain, cough, shortness of breath, cold intolerance, skin/hair changes)	None.
☐ Current medications	Tylenol, but it is not helping.
☐ Past psychiatric history	No.
☐ Past medical history	No.
☐ Past surgical history	Appendectomy at age 16.
☐ Family history	My father died in a car accident and had diabetes, and my mother died of breast cancer.
☐ Occupation	Police officer, retired 1 year ago.
☐ Alcohol use	Two beers daily and 3–4 on weekends. It's been like this for many years now. It helps me relax.
☐ Illicit drug use	Never.
☐ Tobacco	I stopped it 6 months ago after 30 years of smoking a pack a day (because I felt disgusted, and smoking made me feel sick).
☐ Exercise	I walk 30 minutes every day.
☐ Diet	Regular; I like junk food.
☐ Sexual activity	Sexually active with my wife.
☐ Drug allergies	No.

Connecting with the Patient

☐ Examinee recognized the SP's emotions and responded with PEARLS.

Physical Examination

☐ Examinee washed his/her hands.

☐ Examinee asked permission to start the exam.

☐ Examinee used respectful draping.

☐ Examinee did not repeat painful maneuvers.

☑ Exam Component	Maneuver
☐ Head and neck exam	Inspected conjunctivae, mouth and throat, lymph nodes; examined thyroid gland
☐ CV exam	Auscultation
☐ Pulmonary exam	Auscultation
☐ Abdominal exam	Auscultation, percussion, palpation (including rebound tenderness and Murphy's sign)
☐ Extremities	Inspection, palpation

Closure

☐ Examinee discussed initial diagnostic impressions.

☐ Examinee discussed initial management plans:

    ☐ Follow-up tests.

    ☐ Depression counseling:

        ☐ Support system at home (friends, family).

        ☐ Support systems in the hospital and community.

    ☐ Coping skills: Exercise, relaxation techniques, spending more time with family and friends.

☐ Examinee asked if the SP had any other questions or concerns.

Sample Closure

Mr. Jordan, your symptoms are consistent with a few different diagnoses. They may be caused by an ulcer that would resolve with a course of antibiotics and acid suppressors, or they may have a more serious cause, such as pancreatic cancer. I am going to schedule you for an abdominal CT scan that may reveal the source of your pain, and I will also run some blood tests. I know you are concerned about your upcoming vacation, but the results of your tests should be back within a few days, and they should give us a good idea what is wrong with you. In the meantime, our social worker can meet with you to help you find ways to cope with the stress you have been experiencing in your life. Do you have any questions for me?

Patient Note

History
_____
_____
_____
_____
_____
_____
_____
_____
_____
_____
_____
_____
_____
_____
_____
_____

Physical Examination
_____
_____
_____
_____
_____
_____
_____
_____
_____
_____
_____
_____
_____
_____
_____

Patient Note

Differential Diagnosis

Diagnosis #1

History Finding(s):

Physical Exam Finding(s):

Diagnosis #2

History Finding(s):

Physical Exam Finding(s):

Diagnosis #3

History Finding(s):

Physical Exam Finding(s):

Diagnostic Workup

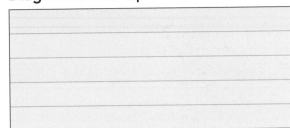

History

HPI: *61 yo M c/o fatigue and weakness. The patient notes that the fatigue and weakness started 6 months ago. He feels tired all day. He has poor appetite and unintentionally lost 8 lbs in the past 6 months. He also complains of occasional nausea and of a vague, deep epigastric discomfort that radiates to the back. This discomfort started 4 months ago and has gradually increased to a severity of 4/10. The discomfort decreases when he leans forward and increases when he lies on his back. There is no relationship of the pain to food. No changes in bowel movement regularity, but he has recently noticed more foul-smelling, greasy-looking stools. He denies blood in the stool. He feels sad sometimes, has lost interest in things that he used to enjoy, wakes up unusually early in the morning, and complains of low energy and concentration that have affected his daily activities and work. The patient denies suicidal ideation or plans. No feelings of guilt or worthlessness.*

ROS: *Negative except as above.*
Allergies: *NKDA.*
Medications: *Tylenol.*
PMH: *None.*
PSH: *Appendectomy at age 16.*
SH: *1 PPD for 30 years; stopped 6 months ago. Drinks 2 beers daily and 3–4 beers on weekends. Sexually active with his wife.*
FH: *Father with diabetes, died accidentally. Mother died from breast cancer.*

Physical Examination

Patient is in no acute distress, looks sad.

VS: *WNL.*
HEENT: *No conjunctival pallor, mouth and pharynx normal.*
Neck: *Supple, no JVD, no lymphadenopathy, thyroid normal.*
Chest: *Clear breath sounds bilaterally.*
Heart: *RRR; normal S1/S2; no murmurs, rubs, or gallops.*
Abdomen: *Soft, nondistended, mild epigastric tenderness, no rebound tenderness, ⊖ Murphy's sign, ⊕ BS, no hepatosplenomegaly.*
Extremities: *No edema.*

Differential Diagnosis

Diagnosis #1: Pancreatic cancer	
History Finding(s):	**Physical Exam Finding(s):**
History of smoking and eating foods that are high in fat content	Mild epigastric tenderness
Unintentional weight loss of 8 lbs over past 6 months	
Foul-smelling, greasy-looking stools	

Diagnosis #2: Depression

History Finding(s):	Physical Exam Finding(s):
Feelings of sadness	
Loss of interest in activities; early awakening; impaired concentration; low energy	
Decreased appetite and unintentional weight loss	

Diagnosis #3: Chronic pancreatitis

History Finding(s):	Physical Exam Finding(s):
History of alcohol use	Mild epigastric tenderness
Worsening epigastric discomfort that radiates to the back	
Foul-smelling, greasy-looking stools	

Diagnostic Workup

CBC, stool for occult blood
Glucose
Fecal fat studies
Amylase, lipase
AST/ALT/bilirubin (direct, indirect, and total)/ alkaline phosphatase
CT—abdomen

CASE DISCUSSION

Patient Note Differential Diagnoses

- **Pancreatic cancer:** The pattern and location of the patient's pain are worrisome for pancreatic disease, and his weight loss raises concern for malignancy. Smoking is among the most significant risk factors for pancreatic cancer; others include chronic pancreatitis, diabetes mellitus, and a high-fat diet. Depression may be the initial manifestation of pancreatic cancer, and diarrhea—presumably due to malabsorption—is an occasional early finding. Malabsorption is suggested by the patient's foul-smelling, greasy-looking stools.

- **Depression:** The patient has many classic symptoms of depression (**SIG E CAPS**; see Case 33). Although it may be a somatic symptom of depression, his abdominal pain is of significant concern and warrants a thorough medical evaluation.

- **Chronic pancreatitis:** The pattern and location of pain are consistent with this diagnosis, but usually there is a history of recurrent episodes of similar pain. The patient's alcohol use should be explored further, as alcoholism accounts for 70–80% of cases of chronic pancreatitis (the patient consumes more than 14 drinks a week, which is considered the limit for males). Moreover, his history of foul-smelling, greasy-looking stools may suggest pancreatic insufficiency, which is a manifestation of chronic pancreatitis.

Additional Differential Diagnoses

- **Peptic ulcer disease:** Suspect this diagnosis in any patient with epigastric pain, although the complaint is neither sensitive nor specific enough to make a reliable diagnosis. It is important to note that many patients deny any relationship of the pain to meals. Weight loss, however, is unusual in uncomplicated ulcer disease and may suggest gastric malignancy.

- **Hypothyroidism:** Nonspecific symptoms such as fatigue and weakness may suggest this common diagnosis. Abdominal pain is unusual.

Diagnostic Workup

- **CBC, stool for occult blood:** A fecal occult blood test is a useful means of screening for potential blood loss. A CBC can determine hemoglobin levels, which, when compared to a known baseline level, can confirm the presence of significant blood loss.

- **Glucose:** To screen for pancreatic endocrine dysfunction (eg, diabetes mellitus, which is a risk factor for pancreatic cancer).

- **Fecal fat studies:** Ordered in suspected cases of pancreatic insufficiency. Fecal elastase and chymotrypsin would likely be decreased in the setting of pancreatic insufficiency.

- **Amylase, lipase:** Nonspecific, but can be elevated in chronic pancreatitis or malignancy.

- **AST/ALT/bilirubin (direct, indirect, and total)/alkaline phosphatase:** To look for evidence of obstructive jaundice (often seen in pancreatic cancer). Alkaline phosphatase and bilirubin levels would be elevated in obstruction, whereas AST and ALT are generally normal unless the liver is involved.

- **CT—abdomen:** To diagnose pancreatic cancer or other pathology and to look for pancreatic calcifications suggestive of chronic pancreatitis.

- **TSH:** Thyroid disease must be ruled out in a patient with symptoms of depression.

- **U/S—abdomen:** To diagnose gallstones as the underlying cause of pancreatitis. This test is particularly useful if acute pancreatitis is suspected. Ultrasound is routinely performed on patients with acute pancreatitis to help determine if gallstones are the cause.

- **Upper endoscopy:** To diagnose ulcer disease.

Opening Scenario

James Miller, a 54-year-old male, comes to the clinic for hypertension follow-up.

Vital Signs

BP: 135/88 mm Hg

Temp: 98.0°F (36.7°C)

RR: 16/minute

HR: 70/minute, regular

Examinee Tasks

1. Take a focused history.

2. Perform a focused physical exam (do not perform rectal, genitourinary, or female breast exam).

3. Explain your clinical impression and workup plan to the patient.

4. Write the patient note after leaving the room.

Checklist/SP Sheet

Patient Description

Patient is a 54 yo M who appears anxious.

Notes for the SP

Don't mention impotence unless the examinee asks whether you are having any side effects from your medications or whether you have any other concerns.

Challenging Questions to Ask

"I think it is my age. Isn't that right, doctor?"

Sample Examinee Response

"No, I don't think it's because of your age. I worry more about your medications. However, testosterone levels can decrease with age, and we will check for that."

Examinee Checklist

Building the Doctor-Patient Relationship

Entrance

☐ Examinee knocked on the door before entering.

☐ Examinee introduced self by name.

☐ Examinee identified his/her role or position.

☐ Examinee correctly used patient's name.

☐ Examinee made eye contact with the SP.

Reflective Listening

☐ Examinee asked an open-ended question and actively listened to the response.

☐ Examinee asked the SP to list his/her concerns and listened to the response without interrupting.

☐ Examinee summarized the SP's concerns, often using the SP's own words.

Information Gathering

☐ Examinee elicited data efficiently and accurately.

☑ Question	Patient Response
☐ Chief complaint	I am here to check on my blood pressure.
☐ Onset	Last year I found out that I have hypertension.
☐ Treatment	The doctor started me on hydrochlorothiazide, but my blood pressure has remained high. He added propranolol 6 months ago.
☐ Compliance with medications	Well, sometimes I forget to take the pills, but in general I take them regularly.
☐ Last blood pressure checkup	Six months ago.
☐ How he is feeling today	Good.
☐ Home monitoring of blood pressure	No.
☐ Any other symptoms (fatigue, headaches, dizziness, blurred vision, nausea, palpitations, chest pain, shortness of breath, urinary changes, weakness, bowel movement changes, sleep problems, hair loss)	I've been losing more hair than usual from my head. I think I'm starting to go bald.
☐ Medication side effects	Over the past 4 months I have started to experience problems with my sexual performance. A friend told me it is the propranolol, but I think it is my age. Isn't that right, doctor?
☐ Description of the problem	I have a weak erection. Sometimes I can't get an erection at all.
☐ Severity on 1–10 scale, where 1 is flaccid and 6 is adequate for penetration	About a 4.
☐ Early-morning or nocturnal erections	No.
☐ Libido	That's weak, too, doc. I'm just not as interested in sex as I used to be.
☐ Marital or work problems	No, my wife is great, and I am very happy in my job.
☐ Feelings of depression	No.
☐ Feelings of anxiety or stress	No.
☐ Any leg or buttock pain while walking or resting	No.
☐ Weight changes	No.
☐ Appetite changes	No.
☐ Diabetes	No.

✓ Question	Patient Response
☐ History of hypercholesterolemia	Yes, it was diagnosed last year.
☐ Previous heart problems	No.
☐ History of TIA or stroke	No.
☐ Current medications	Propranolol, hydrochlorothiazide, lovastatin.
☐ Past medical history	None.
☐ Past surgical history	None.
☐ Family history	My father died at age 50 of a heart attack. My mother is healthy, but she has Alzheimer's disease. She is in a nursing home now.
☐ Occupation	Schoolteacher.
☐ Diet	I eat a lot of junk food.
☐ Exercise	No.
☐ Alcohol use	Yes, 3–4 beers a week for the past 10 years.
☐ Illicit drug use	No.
☐ Tobacco	No.
☐ Social history	I am married and live with my wife.
☐ Sexual activity	I had a wonderful sex life with my wife until 4 months ago, when I started having this problem that I told you about. I think I am getting old.
☐ Drug allergies	No.

Connecting with the Patient

☐ Examinee recognized the SP's emotions and responded with PEARLS.

Physical Examination

☐ Examinee washed his/her hands.

☐ Examinee asked permission to start the exam.

☐ Examinee used respectful draping.

☐ Examinee did not repeat painful maneuvers.

✓ Exam Component	Maneuver
☐ Head and neck exam	Funduscopic exam, carotid auscultation
☐ CV exam	Palpation, auscultation
☐ Pulmonary exam	Auscultation
☐ Abdominal exam	Auscultation, palpation
☐ Extremities	Inspection, palpation of peripheral pulses
☐ Neurologic exam	DTRs, Babinski's sign, sensation and strength in bilateral lower extremities

Closure

☐ Examinee discussed initial diagnostic impressions.

☐ Examinee discussed initial management plans:

    ☐ Follow-up tests: Examinee mentioned the need for genital and rectal exams.

    ☐ Lifestyle modification (diet, exercise, alcohol cessation).

    ☐ Changing propranolol to another antihypertensive medication that does not cause erectile dysfunction.

☐ Examinee asked if the SP had any other questions or concerns.

Sample Closure

Mr. Miller, your blood pressure level was 135/88 when we measured it earlier today, which is close to our target of 130/80. However, it would be even better if we could get it down to around 120/80. Fortunately, that should be feasible with lifestyle changes such as decreasing your salt and fat intake and increasing the amount of exercise you are doing. As for your problems with your erection, this is a very common side effect of one of the blood pressure medications you are taking. For this reason, I would like to give you a medication other than propranolol to control your blood pressure. I am also going to order some blood tests to make sure that your problem is not due to any other medical condition. In addition, I would like to perform a genital exam as well as a rectal exam to assess your prostate. Do you have any questions for me?

Patient Note

History

Physical Examination

Patient Note

Differential Diagnosis

Diagnosis #1

History Finding(s):   Physical Exam Finding(s):

Diagnosis #2

History Finding(s):   Physical Exam Finding(s):

Diagnosis #3

History Finding(s):   Physical Exam Finding(s):

Diagnostic Workup

Patient Note

History

HPI: *54 yo M presents for follow-up of his hypertension that was diagnosed last year. He was initially started on HCTZ; propranolol was added 6 months ago. He is fairly compliant with his medications. He does not monitor his blood pressure at home. His last blood pressure checkup was 6 months ago. He is feeling well except for erectile dysfunction and decreased libido noted 4 months ago. No leg claudication or any previous history of heart problems, stroke, TIA, or diabetes. No marital or work problems. No depression, anxiety, appetite or weight changes, or history of trauma.*

ROS: *Negative except as above.*

Allergies: *NKDA.*

Medications: *HCTZ, propranolol, lovastatin.*

PMH: *Hypertension, hypercholesterolemia diagnosed 1 year ago.*

PSH: *None.*

SH: *No smoking, 3–4 beers/week, no illicit drugs. Works as a schoolteacher; married and lives with his wife.*

FH: *Father died of a heart attack at age 50. Mother is in a nursing home due to Alzheimer's disease.*

Physical Examination

Patient is in no acute distress.

VS: *WNL.*

HEENT: *No funduscopic abnormalities.*

Neck: *No carotid bruits, no JVD.*

Chest: *Clear breath sounds bilaterally.*

Heart: *Apical impulse not displaced; RRR; normal S1/S2; no murmurs, rubs, or gallops.*

Abdomen: *Soft, nondistended, nontender, ⊕ BS, no bruits, no organomegaly.*

Extremities: *No edema, no hair loss or skin changes. Radial, brachial, femoral, dorsalis pedis, and posterior tibialis 2+ and symmetric.*

Neuro: *Motor: Strength 5/5 in bilateral lower extremities. Sensation: Intact to pinprick and soft touch in lower extremities. DTRs: Symmetric 2+ in lower extremities, ⊖ Babinski bilaterally.*

Differential Diagnosis

Diagnosis #1: Medication-induced erectile dysfunction	
History Finding(s):	**Physical Exam Finding(s):**
Taking propranolol	
Onset of ED coincides with propranolol use	
No early-morning or nocturnal tumescence	

Diagnosis #2: Erectile dysfunction secondary to vascular disease

History Finding(s):	Physical Exam Finding(s):
History of hypertension	
History of hyperlipidemia	
No early-morning or nocturnal tumescence	

Diagnosis #3: Hypogonadism

History Finding(s):	Physical Exam Finding(s):
Loss of libido and ED	
Hair loss	
No early-morning or nocturnal tumescence	

Diagnostic Workup

Genital and rectal exams
Serum glucose
Testosterone level
Prolactin, TSH, LH/FSH
Ferritin
MRI—brain
Doppler U/S—penis
Dynamic cavernosography

CASE DISCUSSION

Patient Note Differential Diagnoses

- **Medication-induced erectile dysfunction (ED):** Antihypertensives (but rarely diuretics) and alcohol are commonly associated with ED. β-blockers can often cause loss of libido and ED. This patient's ED began two months after he was started on propranolol. In addition, his lack of early-morning and nocturnal tumescence suggests an organic rather than a psychological etiology.

- **ED secondary to vascular disease:** Hypertension and hyperlipidemia are risk factors for atherosclerotic vascular disease, but there are no historical or physical findings to suggest its presence in this case (eg, angina, leg claudication, diminished pulses, hair loss in the legs, or thin, shiny skin).

- **Hypogonadism:** Testosterone deficiency has many underlying etiologies but, as with other endocrine problems, is attributable to either central (due to insufficient gonadotropin secretion by the pituitary) or end-organ disease (pathology in the testes themselves). In addition to diminished libido and possible ED, there are often associated symptoms such as hot flashes, fatigue, hair loss, and depression. This patient has hair loss, which is suggestive of testosterone deficiency.

Additional Differential Diagnoses

- **Depression:** Psychogenic causes can lead to loss of libido and loss of erections and are suggested when nocturnal or early-morning erections are preserved (not seen in this case). This patient denies other depressive symptoms, but further exploration of his feelings about his nursing-home-bound mother may be more revealing.

- **Peyronie's disease:** Fibrous plaque of the tunica albuginea can lead to penile scarring and ED.

Diagnostic Workup

- **Genital exam:** To rule out Peyronie's disease (eg, to look for penile scarring or plaque formation).

- **Rectal exam:** To detect masses or prostatic abnormalities.

- **Serum glucose:** To screen for diabetes, a possible contributor to ED.

- **Testosterone level:** To screen for hypogonadism.

- **Prolactin, TSH:** To screen for other abnormalities of pituitary function in patients with hypogonadotropic hypogonadism.

- **LH/FSH:** Gonadotropin levels should be checked in patients with low or borderline testosterone levels. Levels are elevated ("hypergonadotropic") in the setting of testicular pathology and are low ("hypogonadotropic") in the setting of pituitary or hypothalamic disease.

- **Ferritin:** To screen for hemochromatosis, a common condition; ED can be an early manifestation due to iron deposition in the pituitary gland causing hypogonadotropic hypogonadism.

- **MRI—brain:** To rule out a pituitary or hypothalamic lesion in patients presenting with hypogonadotropic hypogonadism.

- **Doppler U/S—penis:** To assess blood flow in the cavernous arteries.

- **Dynamic cavernosography:** To determine the site and extent of venous leak (suspected in patients with normal arterial inflow).

- **BUN/Cr, electrolytes, cholesterol, UA, ECG:** Useful in the longitudinal care of hypertension and hyperlipidemia. Can be used to screen for kidney disease, for LVH or prior silent MIs, for response to cholesterol-lowering medication, and for complications of medical therapy (eg, diuretic-induced hypokalemia).

Opening Scenario

Gwen Potter, a 20-year-old female, comes to the clinic complaining of sleeping problems.

Vital Signs

BP: 120/80 mm Hg

Temp: 98.6°F (37°C)

RR: 18/minute

HR: 102/minute

Examinee Tasks

1. Take a focused history.

2. Perform a focused physical exam (do not perform rectal, genitourinary, or female breast exam).

3. Explain your clinical impression and workup plan to the patient.

4. Write the patient note after leaving the room.

Checklist/SP Sheet

Patient Description

Patient is a 20 yo F of average height and weight.

Notes for the SP

- Look anxious and irritable.
- Pretend that you are worried about performing well in college.
- Exhibit a fine tremor on outstretched fingertips and brisk reflexes.

Challenging Questions to Ask

"Will I ever be able to sleep well again, doctor?"

Sample Examinee Response

"First we need to run some tests to rule out underlying medical problems. In the meantime, I recommend some lifestyle changes. If you drink coffee, I strongly recommend that you cut down on your caffeine intake. You could also benefit from exercising, preferably during the day and not right before bedtime. Finally, you should get into the habit of going to bed early—for example, at 10 P.M. each night. It would help if you went to sleep around the same time each night and woke up around the same time each morning. I would also encourage you to abstain from drinking alcohol several hours before bedtime."

Examinee Checklist

Building the Doctor-Patient Relationship

Entrance

☐ Examinee knocked on the door before entering.

☐ Examinee introduced self by name.

☐ Examinee identified his/her role or position.

☐ Examinee correctly used patient's name.

☐ Examinee made eye contact with the SP.

Reflective Listening

☐ Examinee asked an open-ended question and actively listened to the response.

☐ Examinee asked the SP to list his/her concerns and listened to the response without interrupting.

☐ Examinee summarized the SP's concerns, often using the SP's own words.

Information Gathering

☐ Examinee elicited data efficiently and accurately.

☑ Question	Patient Response
☐ Chief complaint	Difficulty falling asleep.
☐ Duration	It has been going on for more than 6 months now but has worsened over the past month.
☐ Total hours of sleep per night	I sleep around 4 hours a night. After I wake up, I have trouble falling back asleep. Usually I need 8 hours of sleep to feel refreshed.
☐ Time you fall asleep	I usually get in bed around midnight, but I don't fall asleep until around 2 A.M.
☐ Activities before sleep	I watch TV.
☐ Sleep interruptions	Yes, I wake up a couple of times during the night.
☐ Early spontaneous awakening	No, the alarm goes off and wakes me up at 6 A.M.
☐ Snoring	I do snore. My boyfriend told me about my snoring a few months ago, but he said that he is fine with it.
☐ Daytime sleepiness	I feel very sleepy during class and while driving to school at 7 A.M.
☐ Daytime naps	I feel the need to take naps but have no time for them. My final exams are coming up soon, and I need to study. I'm worried about how I'll do on them.
☐ Recent stressful events/illnesses	Well, I am stressed out about getting good grades in college. I have been working hard to get an A in all of my classes. I'm taking a heavier course load this semester to finish school on time.
☐ Relationship	My boyfriend is very understanding but has a hard time waking me up in the mornings for class. We have a good relationship.
☐ Sadness, depression, loss of interest in hobbies	No.
☐ Exercise	Before I started college, I worked out an hour a day every evening, but lately it has become harder and harder for me to find the time to hit the gym.
☐ Caffeine intake	I drink at least 5–6 cups of coffee or energy drinks every day to stay awake.
☐ Tremors	None.

☑ Question	Patient Response
☐ Shortness of breath	No.
☐ Palpitations	Yes, I feel my heart racing most of the time, especially after I drink coffee.
☐ Sweating	Not really, but lately I have noticed that my palms are wet most of the time.
☐ Irritability	Yes.
☐ Intolerance to heat/cold	No.
☐ Weight changes	I have lost 6 pounds over the past month despite having a good appetite and eating more than usual.
☐ Frequency of menstrual period	Regular. I have been on oral contraceptive pills for the past 2 years.
☐ Contraceptives	Condoms and oral contraceptive pills.
☐ Fever	No.
☐ Change in bowel habits or in stool color or consistency	I used to go once a day, but lately I've been going 2 or 3 times each day. I have no loose stools or blood in my stool.
☐ Urinary habits	Normal.
☐ Neck pain	No.
☐ Skin changes	No.
☐ Any pain in joints/muscle	No.
☐ Hair loss/thinning	No.
☐ Current medications (antidepressants, antihistamines, pain medication)	All I take are multivitamins and oral contraceptive pills.
☐ Past medical history	None.
☐ Past surgical history	I had a tonsillectomy when I was 12.
☐ Family history	None.
☐ Occupation	College student.
☐ Alcohol use	Occasionally 1 or 2 beers a week, and only on the weekends, never immediately before bed.
☐ Illicit drug use	None.
☐ Tobacco	None.
☐ Drug allergies	None.

Connecting with the Patient

☐ Examinee recognized the SP's emotions and responded with PEARLS.

Physical Examination

☐ Examinee washed his/her hands.

☐ Examinee asked permission to start the exam.

☐ Examinee used respectful draping.

☐ Examinee did not repeat painful maneuvers.

☑ Exam Component	Maneuver
☐ HEENT exam	Inspection, palpation, auscultation of thyroid for lymphadenopathy
☐ CV exam	Auscultation
☐ Pulmonary exam	Auscultation
☐ Abdominal exam	Inspection, auscultation, palpation
☐ Extremities	Checked for tremor on outstretched fingertips; looked for edema
☐ Skin exam	Inspection
☐ Neurologic exam	Looked for brisk reflexes

Closure

☐ Examinee discussed initial diagnostic impressions.

☐ Examinee discussed initial management plans.

    ☐ Follow-up tests.

☐ Examinee asked if the SP had any other questions or concerns.

Sample Closure

Ms. Potter, on the basis of your history and my examination, I think there are a few factors that might be contributing to your sleeping problems. The first is the anxiety and stress you've been experiencing over performing well in college. Although this is perfectly understandable, you may not be able to perform at your best if you don't get a good night's sleep. On the other hand, your problems could stem from your caffeine use, which I urge you to reduce or stop completely. Another possibility has to do with your thyroid function. Sometimes hyperactivity of the thyroid gland can cause some of the symptoms you describe, and the only way to rule this out is through a blood test. In light of your history of snoring, we may need to do a sleep study in the future to rule out sleep apnea. At this point, I encourage you to proceed with the lifestyle changes I have recommended, and I will see you for follow-up to find out how you are doing. Do you have any questions or concerns?

Patient Note

History

Physical Examination

Patient Note

Differential Diagnosis

Diagnosis #1

History Finding(s):   **Physical Exam Finding(s):**

Diagnosis #2

History Finding(s):   **Physical Exam Finding(s):**

Diagnosis #3

History Finding(s):   **Physical Exam Finding(s):**

Diagnostic Workup

History

HPI: *20 yo F college student c/o inability to sleep. She has difficulty falling asleep until 2 A.M. and also has difficulty staying asleep. She used to get 8 hours of sleep, but for the past month she has been getting a total of only 4 hours per night. She has difficulty getting up after hearing the alarm and feels tired while at school. She notes inability to concentrate during classes and while driving. The patient appears to be stressed about her coursework and about her performance at school. She has also been snoring for the past few months and has had palpitations, especially after drinking caffeine. She has a history of drinking 4–5 cups of coffee per day. She has lost weight (6 lbs in 1 month) and has sweaty palms. There is an increase in the frequency of her bowel movements. She lives with her boyfriend, and they use condoms and OCPs for contraception. There is no history of sexual abuse, recent infection, or recent tragic events in her life.*

ROS: *Negative except as above.*

Allergies: *NKDA.*

Medications: *Multivitamins, OCPs.*

PMH: *None.*

PSH: *Tonsillectomy at age 12.*

SH: *No smoking, 1–2 beers/week, no illicit drugs.*

FH: *Not significant.*

Physical Examination

Patient appears anxious and restless.

VS: *HR 102/minute.*

Chest: *Clear breath sounds bilaterally.*

Heart: *Tachycardic; normal S1/S2; no murmurs, rubs, or gallops.*

Abdomen: *Soft, nontender, nondistended, ⊕ BS, no guarding, no hepatosplenomegaly.*

Skin: *Normal, no rashes, palms moist.*

Neuro: *Brisk reflexes.*

Differential Diagnosis

Diagnosis #1: Anxiety	
History Finding(s):	**Physical Exam Finding(s):**
Impaired concentration, irritability, difficulty sleeping, muscle tension, sweating, and palpitations	Tachycardia (HR 102/minute)
Anxiety over academic achievement	
No history of substance use	

Diagnosis #2: Caffeine-induced insomnia

History Finding(s):	Physical Exam Finding(s):
Drinks 4–5 cups of caffeine per day	Tachycardia (HR 102/minute)
Spends 2 hours awake before falling asleep	
History of palpitations that are more pronounced after drinking caffeine	

Diagnosis #3: Hyperthyroidism

History Finding(s):	Physical Exam Finding(s):
Anxiety	Tachycardia (HR 102/minute)
History of unintentional weight loss, fatigue, sweating, palpitations, and increased bowel movements	Brisk reflexes

Diagnostic Workup

TSH, FT_3, FT_4

CASE DISCUSSION

Patient Note Differential Diagnoses

- **Anxiety:** Fatigue and sleep disturbances are common in anxiety states. The clinical manifestations of anxiety can be both psychological (eg, tension, fears, difficulty concentrating) and somatic (eg, tachycardia, sweating, hyperventilation, palpitations, tremor). This patient describes irritability, trouble concentrating, and difficulty sleeping for more than six months, which supports a diagnosis of generalized anxiety disorder. The source of her anxiety is likely her desire to excel in college. Although not required for an official diagnosis of generalized anxiety disorder, somatic manifestations of anxiety are many and include tachycardia, sweating, hyperventilation, palpitations, and tremor.

- **Caffeine-induced insomnia:** The most common pharmacologic cause of insomnia, caffeine use produces increased latency to sleep onset, more frequent arousals during sleep, and a reduction in total sleep time several hours after ingestion. Even small amounts of caffeine can significantly disturb sleep in some patients. This patient's high intake of coffee makes caffeine-induced insomnia a possible diagnosis.

- **Hyperthyroidism:** Clinical hyperthyroidism is associated with anxiety, tremor, palpitations, sweating, frequent bowel movements, fatigue, menstrual irregularities, unintentional weight loss, and heat intolerance. The patient presented in this case has anxiety, palpitations, sweating, increased bowel movements, fatigue, and weight loss, suggesting the need to rule out hyperthyroidism.

Additional Differential Diagnoses

- **Insomnia due to depression:** Several mood disorders are associated with insomnia. Depression can be associated with sleep onset insomnia, sleep maintenance insomnia, or early-morning wakefulness. Hypersomnia occurs in some depressed patients, especially adolescents and those with either bipolar or seasonal (fall/winter) depression.

- **Insomnia secondary to adjustment disorder:** Any significant life event, such as a change of occupation, loss of a loved one, illness, or examinations, can be a significant stressful event in people's lives. Behavioral or mood changes associated with adjustment disorder typically start within three months of the stressful event, end six months after the stressor, and cause significant impairment in one's life. Increased sleep latency, frequent awakenings from sleep, and early-morning awakening can all result. Recovery is rapid, usually occurring within a few weeks.

- **Illicit drug use:** Drugs such as cocaine and amphetamine increase sympathetic activity and can thus cause insomnia.

- **Obstructive sleep apnea (OSA):** More than 50% of patients evaluated for OSA complain of symptoms of insomnia, including difficulty in initiating and maintaining sleep and early-morning awakening. OSA has a higher association with obesity and large tonsils. However, given that this patient has had a tonsillectomy, it is unlikely that enlarged tonsils secondary to OSA are the cause of her disorder.

Diagnostic Workup

- **TSH, FT_3, FT_4:** The patient gives a history of weight loss, increased frequency of bowel movements, palpitations, and sweaty palms, all of which suggest hyperthyroidism. An elevated FT_4 with suppressed TSH is diagnostic.

- **Urine toxicology:** Although this patient denies illicit drug use, a toxicology screen will help rule out the use of CNS stimulants that can cause insomnia (eg, cocaine, amphetamine).

- **CBC:** Can help detect anemia, hidden infection, or malignancy, all of which can cause the fatigue and weight loss seen in this patient.

- **Polysomnography:** A diagnostic test for OSA syndrome that can also help assess the severity of the disease as well as any comorbidities with which it might be associated.

- **ECG:** Nonspecific changes can be seen with hyperthyroidism and anxiety disorders.

CASE 30
DOORWAY INFORMATION

Opening Scenario

The mother of Angelina Harvey, a 2-year-old female child, calls the office complaining that her child has noisy and strange breathing.

Examinee Tasks

1. Take a focused history.

2. Explain your clinical impression and workup plan to the mother.

3. Write the patient note after leaving the room.

Checklist/SP Sheet

Patient Description

The patient's mother offers the history over the phone.

Notes for the SP

Show concern about your child's health, but add that you don't want to come to the office unless you have to because you do not have transportation.

Challenging Questions to Ask

- "Can you explain to me exactly what is going on with my child and what can be done for it?"
- "How will I be able to get a ride to the office?"

Sample Examinee Response

"It is hard for me to give you an accurate answer over the phone. I would like you to bring your child here so that I can examine her and perhaps run some tests. After that, I will be able to give you a more accurate assessment of her condition. We will arrange for the social worker to speak with you about arranging transportation to the office."

Examinee Checklist

Building the Doctor-Patient Relationship

Entrance

☐ Examinee introduced self by name.

☐ Examinee identified his/her role or position.

☐ Examinee correctly used patient's name and identified caller and relationship of caller to patient.

Reflective Listening

☐ Examinee asked an open-ended question and actively listened to the response.

☐ Examinee asked the SP to list his/her concerns and listened to the response without interrupting.

☐ Examinee summarized the SP's concerns, often using the SP's own words.

Information Gathering

☐ Examinee elicited data efficiently and accurately.

☑ Question	Patient Response
☐ Chief complaint	My baby has noisy and strange breathing.
☐ Onset	It started suddenly about an hour ago.
☐ Progression	It is getting worse.
☐ Description of the activity that preceded the event	She was playing with toys.
☐ Description of the sound	It is a noisy sound, as if she swallowed a washing machine.
☐ Consistency	The sound is always the same.
☐ Best heard on inhalation or exhalation	On inhalation.
☐ Can you identify anything that may have caused it?	None.
☐ Alleviating/exacerbating factors (feeding, crying, supine position, sleep)	None.
☐ Associated problems (cough, fever)	Yes, there is some coughing, but it was present earlier. She had a low-grade fever for the past week, but her temperature today was normal. It was 101.2°F at its worst.
☐ Is the cough barking in nature?	No.
☐ Is it productive?	No.
☐ Any blood in cough?	No.
☐ Is she crying?	Yes.
☐ Is her crying muffled or weak?	Weak with occasional muffling.
☐ Breathing fast	I can't tell, but it seems as though she's trying hard to breathe.
☐ Nausea/vomiting	No.
☐ Drooling	No.
☐ Blueness of skin or fingers	No.
☐ Difficulty in swallowing food	No.
☐ Similar episodes in the past	No.
☐ Hoarseness of voice	There is occasional hoarseness.
☐ Snoring at night	No.
☐ History of allergies in the family	No.
☐ Psychological or social stress in the recent past	No.
☐ Day care center	Yes.
☐ Ill contacts in day care center	Not to my knowledge.
☐ Vaccinations	Up to date.

✓ Question	Patient Response
☐ Last checkup	Two weeks ago, and everything was normal.
☐ Growth, development, and milestones	All were fine. She met all milestones in a timely manner.
☐ Birth history	It was an uncomplicated spontaneous vaginal delivery.
☐ Eating habits	Normal.
☐ Current medications	None.
☐ Past medical history	Nothing of note.
☐ Past surgical history	None.
☐ Family history	None.

Connecting with the Patient

☐ Examinee recognized the SP's emotions and responded with PEARLS.

Physical Examination

None.

Closure

☐ Examinee discussed initial diagnostic impressions.

☐ Examinee discussed initial management plans:

    ☐ Follow-up tests.

☐ Examinee asked if the SP had any other questions or concerns.

Sample Closure

Mrs. Harvey, on the basis of the information I have gathered from you, I'm considering the possibility that your daughter might have swallowed a foreign body. However, the possibility that an infection might be causing her problem needs to be ruled out. Right now, I feel that your daughter needs emergency medical attention. Since you do not have access to transportation, I strongly suggest that you call 911 immediately and bring her to the medical center. In the meantime, I suggest that you avoid putting a finger in her mouth or performing any blind finger sweep, as doing so may cause the foreign body to become more deeply lodged if it is actually present. If you observe significant respiratory compromise or choking, perform the Heimlich maneuver by thrusting your daughter's tummy with sudden pressure. I hope you understood what we have discussed. Do you have any questions or concerns? Okay, I will see you once you get to the hospital.

Patient Note

History

Physical Examination

Differential Diagnosis

Diagnosis #1

History Finding(s):

Physical Exam Finding(s):

Diagnosis #2

History Finding(s):

Physical Exam Finding(s):

Diagnosis #3

History Finding(s):

Physical Exam Finding(s):

Diagnostic Workup

History

HPI: *The source of information is the patient's mother. The mother of a 2 yo F c/o her child suddenly developing noisy breathing that is getting progressively worse. The child was playing with her toys when she developed the noisy breathing. The sound is consistent, best heard on inhalation, and similar to that of a washing machine. There is no relation to posture. It is associated with a nonproductive cough without any associated hemoptysis, tachypnea, drooling, or bluish discoloration of the skin. Her vaccinations are up to date.*

ROS: *Negative.*
Allergies: *NKDA.*
Medications: *None.*
PMH: *Uncomplicated spontaneous vaginal delivery.*
PSH: *None.*
FH: *Noncontributory.*

Physical Examination

None.

Differential Diagnosis

Diagnosis #1: Foreign body aspiration	
History Finding(s):	**Physical Exam Finding(s):**
Sudden onset while playing with toys	
Noisy breathing	

Diagnosis #2: Croup	
History Finding(s):	**Physical Exam Finding(s):**
Noisy breathing	
Difficulty breathing	
Fever for the past week	

Diagnosis #3: Epiglottitis	
History Finding(s):	**Physical Exam Finding(s):**
Occasional voice hoarseness	
Occasional muffling	

Diagnostic Workup

ABG
CXR—PA and lateral
XR—neck, AP and lateral
CBC with differential
Bronchoscopy
Direct laryngoscopy

CASE DISCUSSION

Patient Note Differential Diagnoses

There are three types of stridor: **inspiratory stridor,** which indicates obstruction at the level of the larynx or superior to it; **expiratory stridor,** which points to obstruction inferior to the larynx; and **biphasic stridor,** which suggests obstruction in the trachea. Stridor that presents with hoarseness suggests involvement of the vocal cords.

- **Foreign body aspiration:** The sudden and dramatic onset of symptoms, especially when a foreign body (usually a toy or peanuts) is in the vicinity before the patient develops symptoms, helps support this diagnosis. The patient is breathing noisily and is experiencing some shortness of breath, both of which are consistent with aspiration of a foreign body.

- **Croup:** Croup is common in children six months to three years of age, usually developing insidiously as a URI. The most likely culprit for croup is parainfluenza. This patient has had a low-grade fever for the past week, which is suggestive of a viral infection. Although not found in this patient, a characteristic barking cough is often present in croup.

- **Epiglottitis:** Occurs more frequently in children 2–6 years of age, and begins with a short prodrome. Its hallmark feature, significant drooling with symptomatic relief while bending forward, is not present in this patient. However, the patient has experienced voice hoarseness. The most common etiology of epiglottitis is *Haemophilus influenzae* type b, but given that this patient's immunizations are up to date, it is unlikely that this is the cause of her disorder.

Additional Differential Diagnoses

- **Laryngitis:** Occurs in children older than five years of age. The absence of stridor and the presence of a hoarse voice are characteristic.

- **Retropharyngeal abscess:** Patients are usually younger than six years of age. They lack stridor, their voice is muffled, and drooling is often present.

- **Angioedema:** Can occur at any age, and may be an allergic response or hereditary (congenital). Congenital angioedema does not appear to apply to this patient, as she would likely have exhibited some manifestation of immune compromise. Onset is sudden, and the clinical features of stridor and facial edema are found. Respiration is laborious.

- **Peritonsillar abscess:** Typically occurs in children older than 10 years of age. Onset is gradual, with a history of a sore throat and tonsillitis. There is no stridor.

- **Laryngeal papilloma:** A chronic condition characterized by a hoarse voice; most commonly diagnosed in children three months to three years of age.

Diagnostic Workup

- **ABG:** It is essential to determine blood gas concentrations in order to indirectly assess ventilation and gaseous exchange in the lung.

- **CXR—PA and lateral:** It is noteworthy that the majority of foreign bodies are not visible on CXR PA plain films. Therefore, a normal radiograph cannot rule out an aspirated foreign body. However, when a foreign body obstructs the lower airway and causes air trapping, the expiratory film may sometimes reveal air trapping as a result of the ball-and-valve effect.

- **XR—neck, AP and lateral:** May show narrowing of the trachea (steeple sign) in croup, extrinsic pressure, or a classic swollen glottis (thumbprint sign) in epiglottitis.

- **CBC with differential:** To rule out or rule in an underlying infective pathology.

- **Bronchoscopy:** Used as a diagnostic and therapeutic modality in cases of foreign body aspiration.

- **Direct laryngoscopy:** Useful when differentials of laryngomalacia or laryngeal lesions such as papilloma are suspected.

Opening Scenario

Jessica Anderson, a 21-year-old female, comes to the ED complaining of abdominal pain.

Vital Signs

BP: 120/80 mm Hg

Temp: 100.5°F (38.1°C)

RR: 20/minute

HR: 88/minute, regular

Examinee Tasks

1. Take a focused history.

2. Perform a focused physical exam (do not perform rectal, genitourinary, or female breast exam).

3. Explain your clinical impression and workup plan to the patient.

4. Write the patient note after leaving the room.

Checklist/SP Sheet

Patient Description

Patient is a 21 yo F, single with 1 child.

Notes for the SP

- Exhibit right lower abdominal tenderness on palpation.
- Show rebound tenderness (pain when the examinee removes his palpating hand).
- Demonstrate guarding (contraction of the abdominal muscles when palpating the RLQ).
- Experience pain in the RLQ when the examinee presses on the LLQ (Rovsing's sign).
- Manifest pain when the examinee extends your right hip (psoas sign).

Challenging Questions to Ask

- "My child is in the house alone. I must leave now."
- "I can't afford to stay in the hospital. Please give me a prescription for antibiotics so that I can leave."

Sample Examinee Response

"Ms. Anderson, I understand your concern for your child's safety. However, it is most important that we make sure your illness isn't life threatening. Our social worker would be happy to work with you to ensure that your child is taken care of, as well as to address any financial concerns you may have."

Examinee Checklist

Building the Doctor-Patient Relationship

Entrance

☐ Examinee knocked on the door before entering.

☐ Examinee introduced self by name.

☐ Examinee identified his/her role or position.

☐ Examinee correctly used patient's name.

☐ Examinee made eye contact with the SP.

Reflective Listening

☐ Examinee asked an open-ended question and actively listened to the response.

☐ Examinee asked the SP to list his/her concerns and listened to the response without interrupting.

☐ Examinee summarized the SP's concerns, often using the SP's own words.

Information Gathering

☐ Examinee elicited data efficiently and accurately.

☑ Question	Patient Response
☐ Chief complaint	Abdominal pain.
☐ Onset	This morning.
☐ Frequency	Strong, steady pain.
☐ Progression	It is getting worse.
☐ Severity on a scale	7/10.
☐ Location	It is here (points to the right lower abdomen).
☐ Radiation	No.
☐ Quality	Cramping.
☐ Alleviating factors	None.
☐ Exacerbating factors	Movement.
☐ Pain with ride to hospital	Yes.
☐ Precipitating events	None.
☐ Fever/chills	I've been a little hot since this morning, but no chills.
☐ Nausea/vomiting	I feel nauseated and vomited once 2 hours ago.
☐ Description of vomitus	It was a sour, yellowish fluid.
☐ Blood in vomitus	No.
☐ Diarrhea/constipation	Loose bowel movements this morning.
☐ Description of stool	Brown.
☐ Blood in stool	No.

☑ Question	Patient Response
☐ Urinary frequency/burning	No.
☐ Last menstrual period	Five weeks ago.
☐ Vaginal spotting	Yes, today is the first day of my menstrual period.
☐ Color of the spotting	Brownish.
☐ Vaginal discharge	No.
☐ Frequency of menstrual periods	Every 4 weeks; lasts for 7 days.
☐ Started menses	Age 13.
☐ Pads/tampons changed this day	One, but usually 2–3 a day.
☐ Pregnancies	Three years ago.
☐ Problems during pregnancy/delivery	No, it was a normal delivery, and my child is healthy.
☐ Miscarriages/abortions	None.
☐ Current medications	Ibuprofen.
☐ Sexual activity	Yes.
☐ Contraceptives	Oral contraceptive pills. My boyfriend refuses to use condoms.
☐ Sexual partners	One partner; I met him 6 months ago.
☐ Over the past year	I had 3 sexual partners.
☐ History of STDs	Yes, I had some kind of infection 6 months ago, but I can't remember the name of it. The doctor gave me a shot and some pills for 1 week, and then it was over.
☐ Treatment of the partner	He refused the treatment.
☐ HIV test	No.
☐ Past medical history	None except for what I've mentioned.
☐ Past surgical history	None.
☐ Occupation	Waitress.
☐ Alcohol use	Two or three beers a week.
☐ Illicit drug use	No.
☐ Tobacco	One pack a day for the past 6 years.
☐ Drug allergies	No.

Connecting with the Patient

☐ Examinee recognized the SP's emotions and responded with PEARLS.

Physical Examination

☐ Examinee washed his/her hands.

☐ Examinee asked permission to start the exam.

☐ Examinee used respectful draping.

☐ Examinee did not repeat painful maneuvers.

☑ Exam Component	Maneuver
☐ CV exam	Auscultation
☐ Pulmonary exam	Auscultation
☐ Abdominal exam	Inspection, auscultation, palpation, percussion, psoas sign, obturator sign, Rovsing's sign, CVA tenderness

Closure

☐ Examinee discussed initial diagnostic impressions.

☐ Examinee discussed initial management plans:

    ☐ Follow-up tests: Examinee mentioned the need for rectal and pelvic exams.

    ☐ Safe sex practices.

    ☐ Help with smoking cessation.

    ☐ Assistance of social workers to help the patient identify available financial resources.

☐ Examinee asked if the SP had any other questions or concerns.

Sample Closure

Ms. Anderson, your symptoms may be due to a problem with your reproductive organs, such as an infection in your fallopian tube or a cyst on your ovary. They might also result from a complicated pregnancy, which could be indicated if your pregnancy test comes back positive. Another possibility is an infection in your appendix, which could require surgery. To ensure an accurate diagnosis, we will need to run some tests, including a blood test, a urinalysis, a pregnancy test, and possibly a CT scan of your abdomen and pelvis. I will also need to perform rectal and pelvic exams. Since cigarette smoking is associated with a variety of diseases, I advise you to quit smoking; we have many ways to help you if you are interested. I also recommend that you use a condom every time you have intercourse to prevent STDs, including HIV, and to avoid pregnancy. Our social worker can meet with you to discuss your social situation, and she can offer you a variety of resources. Do you have any questions for me?

USMLE STEP 2 CS **Patient Note**

History

Physical Examination

Patient Note

Differential Diagnosis

Diagnosis #1

History Finding(s):   **Physical Exam Finding(s):**

Diagnosis #2

History Finding(s):   **Physical Exam Finding(s):**

Diagnosis #3

History Finding(s):   **Physical Exam Finding(s):**

Diagnostic Workup

Patient Note

History

HPI: *21 yo G1P1 F c/o right lower abdominal pain that started this morning. The pain is 7/10, crampy, nonradiating, and constant. It is exacerbated by movement and accompanied by fever, nausea, vomiting, and loose stools. The patient noticed some brownish spotting this morning. No urinary symptoms; no abnormal vaginal discharge.*

OB/GYN: *LMP 5 weeks ago. Regular periods every 4 weeks lasting 7 days. Menarche at age 13. Uncomplicated NSVD at full term 3 years ago.*

ROS: *Negative except as above.*

Allergies: *NKDA.*

Medications: *Ibuprofen.*

PMH: *STD 1 month ago, possibly treated with ceftriaxone and doxycycline.*

PSH: *None.*

SH: *1 PPD for 6 years, 2–3 beers/week, no illicit drugs. Unprotected sex with multiple partners over the past year.*

Physical Examination

Patient is in pain.

VS: *WNL except for temperature of 100.5°F.*

Chest: *No tenderness, clear breath sounds bilaterally.*

Heart: *RRR; normal S1/S2; no murmurs, rubs, or gallops.*

Abdomen: *Soft, nondistended, hypoactive BS, no hepatosplenomegaly. Direct and rebound RLQ tenderness, RLQ guarding, ⊕ psoas sign, ⊕ Rovsing's sign, ⊖ obturator sign, no CVA tenderness.*

Differential Diagnosis

Diagnosis #1: Appendicitis	
History Finding(s):	**Physical Exam Finding(s):**
Right lower abdominal pain	RLQ direct and rebound tenderness
Pain is exacerbated by movement	RLQ guarding
Nausea and vomiting	Temperature 100.5°F
Low-grade fever	Positive Rovsing's sign
	Positive psoas sign

Diagnosis #2: Pelvic inflammatory disease	
History Finding(s):	**Physical Exam Finding(s):**
STD 6 months ago with untreated partner	RLQ tenderness
Nausea and vomiting	Temperature 100.5°F
Spotting	
Unprotected sex with multiple partners	
Low-grade fever	

Diagnosis #3: Ruptured ectopic pregnancy	
History Finding(s):	**Physical Exam Finding(s):**
Last menstrual period 5 weeks ago and spotting	RLQ rebound tenderness
Crampy lower abdominal pain	RLQ guarding
Pain is exacerbated by movement	
Nausea and vomiting	
Pain is of recent onset	

Diagnostic Workup

Urine hCG
Pelvic exam
Cervical cultures
U/S—abdomen/pelvis
CT—abdomen/pelvis
CBC

CASE DISCUSSION

Patient Note Differential Diagnoses

This case is written primarily to elicit the differential diagnosis of RLQ pain in a woman of childbearing age. The presentation of gynecologic diseases commonly mimics appendicitis.

- **Appendicitis:** In a patient presenting with RLQ pain, low-grade fever, nausea and vomiting, and peritoneal signs (pain exacerbated by movement), appendicitis should certainly be in the differential. The abdominal exam revealed direct and rebound RLQ tenderness, RLQ guarding, a positive psoas sign, and a positive Rovsing's sign—all of which are associated with appendicitis. However, the onset of pain in appendicitis is usually gradual.

- **Pelvic inflammatory disease (PID):** Suspicion is high for this diagnosis in a patient who presents with recent-onset lower abdominal pain and low-grade fever in the setting of a recent STD and unprotected sex with an untreated partner. The standard treatment for gonorrhea and chlamydia consists of ceftriaxone and doxycycline. Left untreated, these infections can progress to PID. Other findings suggestive of PID include abnormal menstrual bleeding, nausea and vomiting, and a history of multiple sex partners.

- **Ruptured ectopic pregnancy:** Although this patient does not have previously documented PID (or a previous tubal pregnancy), the crampy lower abdominal pain, nausea and vomiting, and vaginal spotting that she is experiencing after a five-week period of amenorrhea suggest this diagnosis. However, positive psoas and Rovsing's signs are not typical of an ectopic pregnancy.

Additional Differential Diagnoses

- **Ruptured ovarian cyst:** The patient's sudden-onset, unilateral lower abdominal pain, rebound tenderness, and guarding are consistent with this diagnosis. Rupture may occur at any time during the menstrual cycle, and symptoms may resemble a ruptured ectopic pregnancy as described above. However, this diagnosis is less common than appendicitis and PID. In addition, given the patient's history of having her last menstrual period five weeks ago, ruptured ectopic pregnancy must be placed higher on the differential, as a ruptured ovarian cyst would not be associated with a late menstrual period.

- **Adnexal torsion:** This presentation may be due to adnexal torsion, an uncommon complication that is most often associated with ovarian enlargement due to a benign mass.

- **Gastroenteritis:** Viral gastroenteritis presents with crampy abdominal pain, nausea and vomiting, low-grade fever, and diarrhea. It can be difficult to distinguish from appendicitis and gynecologic etiologies but is less likely in this case given the presence of rebound tenderness.

- **Abortion:** The fact that the patient's last menstrual period was only five weeks ago makes this diagnosis less likely, but the crampy abdominal pain and vaginal spotting may signal an abortion. Furthermore, the presence of fever suggests possible septic abortion.

- **Endometriosis:** This is an unlikely diagnosis, in part because the patient has no history of chronic pelvic pain, dysmenorrhea, dyspareunia, or infertility, which are often associated. In the setting of established endometriosis, this presentation in a patient with acute, severe pain, including rebound tenderness, could be due to rupture of an endometrioma ("chocolate cyst").

Diagnostic Workup

- **Urine hCG:** Positive in both ectopic and intrauterine pregnancies. Urine and serum tests are equally sensitive, but quantitative hCG levels (available only via serum test) may help diagnose and treat ectopic pregnancy.

- **Pelvic exam:** Look for cervical motion tenderness and discharge, uterine size, and adnexal masses or tenderness.

- **Cervical cultures:** *Neisseria gonorrhoeae* and *Chlamydia trachomatis*, the main causes of PID, are detected by means of DNA probes.

- **U/S—abdomen/pelvis:** Can help diagnose appendiceal or ovarian pathology. Transvaginal ultrasound can identify an intrauterine gestational sac when the time elapsed since the last menstrual period is 35 days (this corresponds to a β-hCG of approximately 1500 mIU/mL); fluid in the cul-de-sac is nonspecific and may suggest ectopic pregnancy or a ruptured ovarian cyst.

- **CT—abdomen/pelvis:** Can detect the presence of appendiceal inflammation, abscess in appendicitis, or signs of other GI or gynecologic pathology.

- **CBC:** Findings are nonspecific, but leukocytosis may be seen in infection or appendicitis.

- **UA:** To rule out UTI.

- **Laparoscopy:** Can diagnose ectopic pregnancy (gold standard), ruptured ovarian cyst, ovarian torsion, PID ± tubo-ovarian abscess, appendicitis, and the like.

Opening Scenario

Virginia Black, a 65-year-old female, comes to the clinic complaining of forgetfulness and confusion.

Vital Signs

BP: 135/85 mm Hg

Temp: 98.0°F (36.7°C)

RR: 16/minute

HR: 76/minute, regular

Examinee Tasks

1. Take a focused history.

2. Perform a focused physical exam (do not perform rectal, genitourinary, or female breast exam).

3. Explain your clinical impression and workup plan to the patient.

4. Write the patient note after leaving the room.

Checklist/SP Sheet

Patient Description

Patient is a 65 yo F, widowed with 1 daughter.

Notes for the SP

- The examinee will name 3 objects for you and ask you to recall them after a few minutes. Pretend that you are unable to do so.

- If asked, give the examinee a list of your current medications (a piece of paper with "nitroglycerin patch, hydrochlorothiazide, and aspirin" written on it).

- Pretend that you have some weakness in your left arm.

- Show an increase in DTRs of the left arm and leg.

Challenging Questions to Ask

"Do you think I have Alzheimer's disease?"

Sample Examinee Response

"At this time I don't know; we still need to run some tests. What makes you concerned about having Alzheimer's?"

Examinee Checklist

Building the Doctor-Patient Relationship

Entrance

☐ Examinee knocked on the door before entering.

☐ Examinee introduced self by name.

☐ Examinee identified his/her role or position.

☐ Examinee correctly used patient's name.

☐ Examinee made eye contact with the SP.

Reflective Listening

☐ Examinee asked an open-ended question and actively listened to the response.

☐ Examinee asked the SP to list his/her concerns and listened to the response without interrupting.

☐ Examinee summarized the SP's concerns, often using the SP's own words.

Information Gathering

☐ Examinee elicited data efficiently and accurately.

☑ Question	Patient Response
☐ Chief complaint	Difficulty remembering things.
☐ Onset	I can't remember exactly, but my daughter told me that I started forgetting last year.
☐ Progression	My daughter has told me that it is getting worse.
☐ Things that are difficult to remember	Turning off the stove, my phone number, my keys, the way home, the names of my friends.
☐ Daily activities (bathing, feeding, toileting, dressing, transferring into and out of chairs and bed)	I have some trouble with these, and I need help sometimes.
☐ Shopping	Well, I stopped shopping, since I've lost my way home so many times. My daughter shops for me.
☐ Cooking	I stopped cooking because I often leave the stove on and accidentally started a fire once.
☐ Housework	I live with my daughter, and she does most of it.
☐ Paying the bills	I used to do my own bills, but I couldn't keep up. My daughter does this for me now.
☐ Gait problems	No.
☐ Urinary incontinence	No.
☐ Feelings of sadness or depression	Since my husband died a year ago, I sometimes get sad. My forgetfulness makes me more upset.
☐ Difficulty sleeping	No.
☐ Headaches	No.
☐ Lightheadedness or feeling faint	Only if I stand up too quickly.
☐ Passing out	No.
☐ Falls	Yes, sometimes.
☐ Head trauma	I think so; I had a large bruise on the side of my head a while back. I don't remember what happened anymore.
☐ Did you see a doctor for that fall?	No, it was just a bruise.

☑ Question	Patient Response
☐ Any shaking or seizures	No.
☐ Visual changes	No.
☐ Weakness/numbness/paresthesias	Yes, I have weakness in my left arm from a stroke I had a long time ago.
☐ Speech difficulties	No.
☐ Heart problems	I had a heart attack a long time ago.
☐ Chest pain, shortness of breath, abdominal pain, nausea/vomiting, diarrhea/constipation	No.
☐ Weight changes	I've lost weight. I don't know how much.
☐ Appetite changes	I don't have an appetite.
☐ High blood pressure	Yes, for a long time.
☐ Current medications	I don't know their names. (Shows the list to the examinee.)
☐ Past medical history	I think that's enough, isn't it?
☐ Past surgical history	I had a bowel obstruction a long time ago, and they removed part of my intestine. I don't remember how long ago it was.
☐ Family history	My father and mother died healthy a long time ago.
☐ Occupation	I retired after the death of my husband.
☐ Alcohol use	No.
☐ Illicit drug use	No.
☐ Tobacco	No.
☐ Social history	I live with my daughter.
☐ Sexual activity	Not since the death of my husband a year ago.
☐ Support systems (family, friends)	I have many friends who care about me, besides my daughter.
☐ Drug allergies	No.

Connecting with the Patient

☐ Examinee recognized the SP's emotions and responded with PEARLS.

Physical Examination

☐ Examinee washed his/her hands.

☐ Examinee asked permission to start the exam.

☐ Examinee used respectful draping.

☐ Examinee did not repeat painful maneuvers.

☑ Exam Component	Maneuver
☐ Eye exam	Inspected pupils, fundus
☐ Neck exam	Carotid auscultation
☐ CV exam	Auscultation, orthostatic vital signs
☐ Pulmonary exam	Auscultation
☐ Abdominal exam	Palpation
☐ Neurologic exam	Mini-mental status exam, cranial nerves, motor exam, DTRs, gait, Romberg's sign, sensory exam

Closure

☐ Examinee discussed initial diagnostic impressions.

☐ Examinee discussed initial management plans:

  ☐ Follow-up tests.

  ☐ Need to obtain history directly from other family members.

  ☐ Need to evaluate home safety and supervision.

  ☐ Need to obtain community resources to help the patient at home.

☐ Examinee offered support throughout the illness.

☐ Examinee asked if the SP had any other questions or concerns.

Sample Closure

Mrs. Black, your symptoms may be due to a number of disorders that can affect the brain, many of which are treatable. We need to run some tests to identify the cause of your problem. I would also like to ask your permission to speak with your daughter. She can help me with your diagnosis, and I can answer any questions she might have about what is happening to you and how she can help. I would also like you and your family to meet with the social worker to assess at-home supervision and safety measures. The social worker will inform you of resources that are available in the community to help you. If you would like, I can remain in close contact with you and your family to provide additional help and support. Do you have any questions for me?

Patient Note

History

Physical Examination

Patient Note

Differential Diagnosis

Diagnosis #1

History Finding(s):   Physical Exam Finding(s):

Diagnosis #2

History Finding(s):   Physical Exam Finding(s):

Diagnosis #3

History Finding(s):   Physical Exam Finding(s):

Diagnostic Workup

History

HPI: *65 yo F c/o difficulty remembering × 1 year, after death of husband.*

- *Progressively worsening memory.*
- *Affects daily activities (bathing, feeding, toileting, dressing, transferring into and out of chairs and bed, shopping, cooking, managing money, using the telephone, cleaning the house).*
- *Transient orthostatic lightheadedness with frequent falls, 1 head injury without medical attention.*
- *Upset due to memory difficulty.*
- *Weight loss, no appetite.*
- *No headache, visual changes, gait problems, difficulty sleeping, or urinary incontinence.*

ROS: *Residual weakness in left arm after a stroke.*

Allergies: *NKDA.*

Medications: *HCTZ, aspirin, transdermal nitroglycerin.*

PMH: *Hypertension, stroke, MI. The patient cannot remember exactly when she had them.*

PSH: *Partial bowel resection due to obstruction many years ago. Patient does not remember how long ago this occurred.*

SH: *No smoking, no EtOH, no illicit drugs. She is a widow (husband died 1 year ago), is retired, lives with her daughter, and has a good support system (family, friends).*

FH: *Noncontributory.*

Physical Examination

Patient is in no acute distress.

VS: *WNL, no orthostatic changes.*

HEENT: *Normocephalic, atraumatic, PERRLA, no funduscopic abnormalities.*

Neck: *Supple, no carotid bruits.*

Chest: *Clear breath sounds bilaterally.*

Heart: *RRR; normal S1/S2; no murmurs, rubs, or gallops.*

Abdomen: *Soft, nondistended, nontender, no hepatosplenomegaly.*

Neuro: *Mental status: Alert and oriented × 3, spells backward but can't recall 3 items. Cranial nerves: 2–12 intact. Motor: Strength 5/5 in all muscle groups except 3/5 in left arm. DTRs: Asymmetric 3+ in left upper and lower extremities, 1+ in the right, ⊕ Babinski bilaterally. Cerebellar: ⊖ Romberg. Gait: Normal. Sensation: Intact to pinprick and soft touch.*

Differential Diagnosis

Diagnosis #1: Alzheimer's disease	
History Finding(s):	**Physical Exam Finding(s):**
Steady cognitive decline	Failed 3-item recall
Memory impairment	
Impaired executive functioning	
Decline in activities of daily living	

Diagnosis #2: Vascular ("multi-infarct") dementia

History Finding(s):	Physical Exam Finding(s):
Previous stroke	Decreased strength in left upper extremity
History of coronary artery disease (MI)	DTRs 3+ in left upper and lower extremities
Hypertension	Positive Babinski bilaterally
Impaired executive functioning	Failed 3-item recall

Diagnosis #3: Dementia syndrome of depression

History Finding(s):	Physical Exam Finding(s):
Dysphoria after husband's death	Failed 3-item recall
Impaired executive functioning	
Memory impairment	

Diagnostic Workup

CT—head or MRI—brain
EEG or SPECT
CBC
Serum B_{12}, TSH, RPR
Electrolytes, calcium, glucose, BUN/Cr

CASE DISCUSSION

Dementia is an acquired, progressive impairment in cognitive function that includes amnesia accompanied by some degree of aphasia, apraxia, agnosia, and/or impaired executive function. Additional historical information must be sought from other family members to establish an accurate time course of cognitive decline. The dementia syndromes are primarily clinical diagnoses, and therefore the initial diagnostic workup should be directed toward the exclusion of partially reversible causes of dementia. Moreover, the top three diagnoses for this patient encounter may coexist, further complicating treatment.

Patient Note Differential Diagnoses

- **Alzheimer's disease:** This patient presents with a steady decline in cognitive function that is most consistent with Alzheimer's disease, the most common cause of dementia. Alzheimer's disease usually has an insidious onset characterized by a steady, progressive decline in cognitive function over a period of years. The earliest findings are impairment in memory and visuospatial abilities. Alzheimer's disease is a clinical diagnosis.

- **Vascular ("multi-infarct") dementia:** Vascular dementia often coexists with Alzheimer's disease, and given the patient's history of atherosclerotic vascular disease (eg, stroke, MI), it could certainly be contributing in this case. In vascular dementia, there is classically more of a fluctuating, stepwise cognitive deterioration that is temporally related to a recent stroke. This patient's stroke is not recent, and the pattern of her cognitive decline is more consistent with that of Alzheimer's disease. In addition, vascular dementia may be characterized by an earlier loss of executive function and personality changes.

- **Dementia syndrome of depression (DSD):** The time course of cognitive decline following the death of the patient's husband may indicate depression. In the elderly, depression can present atypically with symptoms of neurocognitive decline (vs. young patients, in whom dysphoria predominates). These symptoms may mimic or, more commonly, coexist with dementia. In contrast to Alzheimer's disease, DSD presents primarily as a dysexecutive syndrome and is a reversible cause of dementia. A thorough screening for depression should be conducted. However, it is more likely that this patient's cognitive decline has been progressive for several years but became more noticeable to her children after her husband died.

Additional Differential Diagnoses

- **Subdural hematoma:** This should be ruled out given the patient's history of falls and head trauma. Although her cognitive decline spans at least a year, it is possible that a comorbid chronic subdural hematoma could have exacerbated her mental status changes in recent weeks or months.

- **Vitamin B$_{12}$ deficiency:** A prior bowel resection (eg, resection of the terminal ileum) may put the patient at risk for this deficiency. It can cause depression, irritability, paranoia, confusion, and dementia but is usually associated with other neurologic symptoms, such as paresthesias and leg weakness. On occasion, dementia may precede the characteristic megaloblastic anemia.

- **Hypothyroidism:** This can cause neuropsychiatric symptoms (often a late finding) and must be ruled out in patients with dementia. However, there are no classic signs or symptoms to suggest hypothyroidism in this case.

Diagnostic Workup

The goal of the diagnostic workup for cognitive decline is to rule out potentially reversible causes of dementia and search for causes such as electrolyte disturbances, neoplasms, or infarcts.

- **CT—head:** Used to look for a crescent-shaped, hyperdense extra-axial mass in subdural hematoma, intracerebral masses, strokes, or dilated ventricles (as in normal pressure hydrocephalus).

- **MRI—brain:** The most sensitive exam with which to look for focal CNS lesions or atrophy.

- **EEG or SPECT:** Used in rare cases to help differentiate delirium from depression or dementia.

- **CBC:** Used to look for macrocytic anemia in vitamin B_{12} deficiency.

- **Serum B_{12}, TSH, RPR:** To screen for partially reversible causes of dementia (RPR can be restricted to patients who manifest signs of neurosyphilis).

- **Electrolytes, calcium, glucose, BUN/Cr:** To screen for medical conditions that can present with cognitive dysfunction (eg, hypernatremia, hypercalcemia, hyperglycemia, uremia).

Opening Scenario

Gary Mitchell, a 46-year-old male, comes to the office complaining of fatigue.

Vital Signs

BP: 120/85 mm Hg

Temp: 98.2°F (36.8°C)

RR: 12/minute

HR: 65/minute, regular

Examinee Tasks

1. Take a focused history.

2. Perform a focused physical exam (do not perform rectal, genitourinary, or female breast exam).

3. Explain your clinical impression and workup plan to the patient.

4. Write the patient note after leaving the room.

Checklist/SP Sheet

Patient Description

Patient is a 46 yo M.

Notes for the SP

- Look sad, and don't smile.

- Speak and move slowly.

- Start yawning as the examinee enters the room.

Challenging Questions to Ask

- "I think that life is full of misery. Why do we have to live?"

- "I am afraid that I might have AIDS."

Sample Examinee Response

This patient clearly has more to say. Silence is appropriate here, or the patient should be subtly encouraged to continue. Alternatively, you can say, "It sounds as though you're losing hope. Have you thought about hurting yourself or tried to do so?" Or "Tell me more about your concern about AIDS. Everything that you tell me is confidential and will not leave this room."

Examinee Checklist

Building the Doctor-Patient Relationship

Entrance

☐ Examinee knocked on the door before entering.

☐ Examinee introduced self by name.

☐ Examinee identified his/her role or position.

☐ Examinee correctly used patient's name.

☐ Examinee made eye contact with the SP.

Reflective Listening

☐ Examinee asked an open-ended question and actively listened to the response.

☐ Examinee asked the SP to list his/her concerns and listened to the response without interrupting.

☐ Examinee summarized the SP's concerns, often using the SP's own words.

Information Gathering

☐ Examinee elicited data efficiently and accurately.

☐ Examinee explored the SP's concern about AIDS (eg, "Tell me more about that.").

☑ Question	Patient Response
☐ Chief complaint	Feeling tired, no energy.
☐ Onset	Three months ago.
☐ Associated events	I was in a car accident 3 months ago, and I failed to save my friend from the car before it blew up.
☐ Injuries related to the accident	No.
☐ Progression of the fatigue during the day	Same throughout the day.
☐ Affecting job/performance	Yes, I can't concentrate on my work anymore. I don't have the energy to work.
☐ Appetite changes	Loss of appetite.
☐ Weight changes	I have gained 6 pounds over the past 3 months.
☐ Feeling of depression	Yes, I feel sad all the time.
☐ Suicidal thoughts/plans/attempts	I think of suicide sometimes but have had no plans or attempts.
☐ Feelings of blame or guilt	I don't know. It was an accident. I tried to help my friend but couldn't.
☐ Sleeping problems (falling asleep, staying asleep, early waking)	Well, I don't have problems falling asleep, but I wake up sometimes because of nightmares. I always see the accident, my friend calling for help, and the car blowing up. I feel so scared and helpless. I wake up multiple times at night and feel sleepy all day.
☐ Avoidance of stimuli	No.

☑ Question	Patient Response
☐ Support system (friends, family)	My girlfriend and parents are very supportive. They know I've been having a hard time and suggested I come see you to sort it out.
☐ Loss of concentration	Yes, I can't concentrate on my work.
☐ Associated symptoms (fever, chills, chest pain, shortness of breath, abdominal pain, diarrhea/constipation)	No.
☐ Cold intolerance	Yes.
☐ Skin/hair changes	My hair is falling out more than usual.
☐ Current medications	None.
☐ Past medical history	Well, I had some burning during urination. I don't really remember the diagnosis that the doctor reached, but it started with the letter C. I took antibiotics for a week. This was 5 months ago.
☐ Past surgical history	None.
☐ Family history	My parents are alive and in good health.
☐ Occupation	Accountant.
☐ Alcohol use	I have 2 or 3 beers a month.
☐ Illicit drug use	Never.
☐ Tobacco	One pack a day for 25 years.
☐ Exercise	No.
☐ Diet	The usual. I haven't changed anything in my diet in more than 10 years.
☐ Sexual activity	Not interested anymore. I have a girlfriend, and we have been together for the past 6 months. I don't use condoms because they make me feel uncomfortable. I have had several sexual partners in the past.
☐ Drug allergies	No.

Connecting with the Patient

☐ Examinee recognized the SP's emotions and responded with PEARLS.

Physical Examination

☐ Examinee washed his/her hands.

☐ Examinee asked permission to start the exam.

☐ Examinee used respectful draping.

☐ Examinee did not repeat painful maneuvers.

☑ Exam Component	Maneuver
☐ Head and neck exam	Inspected conjunctivae, mouth and throat, lymph nodes; examined thyroid gland
☐ CV exam	Auscultation
☐ Pulmonary exam	Auscultation
☐ Abdominal exam	Auscultation, palpation, percussion
☐ Extremities	Inspection, checked DTRs

Closure

☐ Examinee discussed initial diagnostic impressions.

☐ Examinee discussed initial management plans:

☐ Follow-up tests.

☐ Lifestyle modification (diet, exercise, relaxation techniques, smoking cessation).

☐ Safe sex practices.

☐ HIV testing and consent.

☐ Depression counseling:

☐ Sources of support (eg, trusted friends and loved ones) and information about community groups.

☐ Possible need for referral to a psychiatrist.

☐ Suicide contract (ie, contact your physician or go to the ED for any suicidal thoughts or plans).

☐ Examinee asked if the SP had any other questions or concerns.

Sample Closure

Mr. Mitchell, it appears that your life has been very stressful lately, and my suspicion is that you may be clinically depressed. Before I make a definitive diagnosis, however, I would like to order some blood tests, including one for HIV, as you have risk factors for sexually transmitted diseases. Once we have completed these tests, we should have a better idea of what is causing your fatigue. In the meantime, I strongly recommend that you quit smoking, exercise regularly, and participate in activities that you find relaxing. I would also like you to promise me that if you feel like hurting yourself, you will call someone who can help you or go immediately to an emergency department. Do you have any questions for me?

Patient Note

History

Physical Examination

Patient Note

Differential Diagnosis

Diagnosis #1

History Finding(s):   **Physical Exam Finding(s):**

Diagnosis #2

History Finding(s):   **Physical Exam Finding(s):**

Diagnosis #3

History Finding(s):   **Physical Exam Finding(s):**

Diagnostic Workup

Patient Note

History

HPI: *46 yo M c/o fatigue × 3 months.*

- *Fatigue began after unsuccessful attempt to save his friend after a car accident.*
- *Constant fatigue throughout the day.*
- *Low energy.*
- *Decreased concentration that is negatively affecting job as accountant.*
- *Decreased appetite, but gained 6 lbs over 3 months.*
- *Multiple awakenings and difficulty staying asleep due to recurrent nightmares about accident.*
- *Feels sleepy throughout the day.*
- *Feelings of being depressed and helpless.*
- *Passive suicidal ideation but no suicide plans/attempts.*
- *Cold intolerance.*
- *Hair loss.*
- *Loss of interest in sex.*
- *No constipation.*

ROS: *Negative except as above.*
Allergies: *NKDA.*
Medications: *None.*
PMH: *Urethritis (possibly chlamydia), treated 5 months ago.*
PSH: *None.*
SH: *1 PPD for 25 years, 2 beers/month. History of unprotected sex with multiple female partners.*
FH: *Noncontributory.*

Physical Examination

Patient is in no acute distress, looks tired with a flat affect, speaks and moves slowly.

VS: *WNL.*
HEENT: *No conjunctival pallor, mouth and pharynx WNL.*
Neck: *No lymphadenopathy, thyroid normal.*
Chest: *Clear breath sounds bilaterally.*
Heart: *RRR; normal S1/S2; no murmurs, rubs, or gallops.*
Abdomen: *Soft, nondistended, nontender, ⊕ BS, no hepatosplenomegaly.*
Extremities: *No edema, normal DTRs in lower extremities.*

Patient Note

Differential Diagnosis

Diagnosis #1: Major depressive disorder	
History Finding(s):	**Physical Exam Finding(s):**
Dysphoria, anhedonia	
Loss of appetite	
Passive suicidal ideation	
Decreased energy/fatigue	
Impaired concentration	
Early awakening	

Diagnosis #2: Hypothyroidism	
History Finding(s):	**Physical Exam Finding(s):**
Fatigue for 3 months	
Cold intolerance	
Hair loss	
Weight gain	

Diagnosis #3: Posttraumatic stress disorder	
History Finding(s):	**Physical Exam Finding(s):**
Nightmares about the trauma	
Negative mood/anhedonia	
Decreased concentration	
Difficulty staying asleep	

Diagnostic Workup

TSH
CBC
HIV antibody

CASE DISCUSSION

Patient Note Differential Diagnoses

Fatigue is a common, nonspecific complaint with many etiologies ranging from simple overexertion to serious diseases such as cancer.

- **Major depressive disorder (MDD):** This patient meets the criteria for the diagnosis of MDD, exhibiting many classic symptoms. The mnemonic **SIG E CAPS** helps recall these symptoms: **S**leep disturbance, decreased **I**nterest, feelings of **G**uilt (worthlessness), decreased **E**nergy (fatigue), decreased **C**oncentration/**C**ognition, change in **A**ppetite/weight changes, **P**sychomotor agitation or slowing, and **S**uicidal ideation. In order to meet the criteria outlined in the *Diagnostic and Statistical Manual of Mental Disorders* (DSM-5), a patient must report at least five of the above symptoms, including depressed mood or anhedonia as one of the five, for two weeks, and symptoms must significantly impair daily functioning.

- **Hypothyroidism:** This should be ruled out in a patient with fatigue for months. The patient's cold intolerance, hair loss, and weight gain are additional nonspecific symptoms that suggest this diagnosis.

- **Posttraumatic stress disorder (PTSD):** PTSD usually occurs within three months of the traumatic experience, and the duration of symptoms is longer than a month. DSM-5 criteria include a history of exposure to a traumatic event that meets specific requirements and symptoms from each of four symptom clusters: intrusion, avoidance, negative alterations in cognition and mood, and alterations in arousal and reactivity. Although this patient has many of the symptoms of PTSD (nightmares about the trauma, decreased concentration, anhedonia, negative mood, and difficulty staying asleep), he does not avoid stimuli related to the accident and therefore does not meet the full criteria at this time.

Additional Differential Diagnoses

- **HIV infection:** Given his history of STDs and unprotected sex with multiple partners, this patient should also be tested for HIV. However, it is highly unlikely that HIV infection accounts for his current depression (unless there are frontal lobe lesions due to infection or malignancy).

Diagnostic Workup

- **TSH:** A screening test for hypothyroidism.
- **CBC:** To rule out anemia.
- **HIV antibody:** To rule out HIV infection.

CASE 34
DOORWAY INFORMATION

Opening Scenario

Jessica Lee, a 32-year-old female, comes to the office complaining of fatigue.

Vital Signs

BP: 120/85 mm Hg

Temp: 98.2°F (36.8°C)

RR: 13/minute

HR: 80/minute, regular

Examinee Tasks

1. Take a focused history.

2. Perform a focused physical exam (do not perform rectal, genitourinary, or female breast exam).

3. Explain your clinical impression and workup plan to the patient.

4. Write the patient note after leaving the room.

Checklist/SP Sheet

Patient Description

Patient is a 32 yo F, married with 2 children.

Notes for the SP

- Look anxious and pale.
- Exhibit bruises on the face and arms that elicit pain when touched.

Challenging Questions to Ask

"I am drinking a lot of water, doctor. What do you think the reason is?"

Sample Examinee Response

"At this point I don't know for sure, but I want to run some tests. Drinking a lot of water could be the first sign of diabetes, and we will need to check for that."

Examinee Checklist

Building the Doctor-Patient Relationship

Entrance

☐ Examinee knocked on the door before entering.

☐ Examinee introduced self by name.

☐ Examinee identified his/her role or position.

☐ Examinee correctly used patient's name.

☐ Examinee made eye contact with the SP.

Reflective Listening

☐ Examinee asked an open-ended question and actively listened to the response.

☐ Examinee asked the SP to list his/her concerns and listened to the response without interrupting.

☐ Examinee summarized the SP's concerns, often using the SP's own words.

Information Gathering

☐ Examinee elicited data efficiently and accurately.

☑ Question	Patient Response
☐ Chief complaint	Feeling tired, weak, no energy.
☐ Onset	Five months ago.
☐ Associated events	None.
☐ Progression of the fatigue during the day	I feel okay in the morning; then gradually I start feeling more and more tired and weak.
☐ Change in vision (double vision) during the day	No.
☐ Affecting job/performance	Yes, I don't have energy to work.
☐ Appetite changes	I have a very good appetite.
☐ Weight changes	No.
☐ Feeling of depression	Sometimes I feel sad.
☐ Cause of bruises	I fell down the stairs and hurt myself (looks anxious). It is my fault. I don't always pay attention.
☐ Being physically or emotionally hurt or abused by anybody	Well, sometimes when my husband gets angry with me, but he loves me very much, and he promises not to do it again.
☐ Feeling safe/afraid at home	Sometimes I feel afraid, especially when my husband gets drunk.
☐ Have you ever experienced any head trauma or accidents as a result of your husband?	No.
☐ Are the children being abused or threatened?	Well, he slapped my younger son the other day for breaking a glass. He should be more attentive.
☐ Suicidal thoughts/plans/attempts	No.
☐ Feelings of blame or guilt	Yes, I think I am being awkward. It is my fault.
☐ Presence of guns at home	No.
☐ Any family members who know about the abuse	No.
☐ Emergency plan	No.
☐ Sleeping problems (falling asleep, staying asleep, early waking, snoring)	No.
☐ Loss of concentration	Yes, I can't concentrate on my work.

☑ Question	Patient Response
☐ Menstrual period	Regular and heavy; lasts 7 days.
☐ Last menstrual period	Two weeks ago.
☐ Urinary symptoms	I recently started to wake up at night to urinate.
☐ Polyuria	Yes, I have to go to the bathroom more often during the day.
☐ Pain during urination or change in the color of urine	No.
☐ Polydipsia	Yes, I feel thirsty all the time, and I drink a lot of water.
☐ Associated symptoms (fever, chills, chest pain, shortness of breath, abdominal pain, diarrhea/constipation, cold intolerance, skin/hair changes)	None.
☐ Current medications	None.
☐ Past medical history	None.
☐ Past surgical history	I fell and broke my arm a year ago.
☐ Family history	My father had diabetes and died of a heart attack. My mother is in a nursing home with Alzheimer's.
☐ Occupation	Nurse.
☐ Alcohol use	No.
☐ Illicit drug use	Never.
☐ Tobacco	No.
☐ Exercise	No.
☐ Diet	I don't really have one, but I know that I am overweight and should eat healthier foods. I am trying to change because my dad had diabetes.
☐ Sexual activity	I don't feel any desire for sex, but we do it when my husband wants.
☐ Drug allergies	No.

Connecting with the Patient

☐ Examinee recognized the SP's emotions and responded with PEARLS.

Physical Examination

☐ Examinee washed his/her hands.

☐ Examinee asked permission to start the exam.

☐ Examinee used respectful draping.

☐ Examinee did not repeat painful maneuvers.

☑ Exam Component	Maneuver
☐ Head and neck exam	Inspected conjunctivae, mouth and throat, lymph nodes; examined thyroid gland
☐ CV exam	Auscultation
☐ Pulmonary exam	Auscultation
☐ Abdominal exam	Auscultation, palpation, percussion
☐ Extremities	Inspection, motor exam, DTRs

Closure

☐ Examinee discussed initial diagnostic impressions.

☐ Examinee discussed initial management plans:

    ☐ Follow-up tests.

    ☐ Domestic violence counseling:

        ☐ "I care about your safety, and I am always available for help and support."

        ☐ "Everything we discuss is confidential, but I must involve child protective services if your children are being harmed."

        ☐ Support group information, including contact numbers or Web sites.

        ☐ Safety planning.

☐ Examinee asked if the SP had any other questions or concerns.

Sample Closure

Ms. Lee, I am concerned about your safety and your relationship with your husband. I would like you to know that I am available for help and support whenever you need it. Although everything we discuss is confidential, I must involve child protective services if I have reason to believe that your children are being abused. I will bring back some telephone numbers and contact information for you regarding where to go for help if you or your children are in a crisis or if you just want someone to talk to. I am also concerned about your frequent urination and thirst. I will run a simple blood test to see if you have any problems with your blood sugar or your hormones. Do you have any questions?

Patient Note

History

Physical Examination

Differential Diagnosis

Diagnosis #1
History Finding(s): Physical Exam Finding(s):

Diagnosis #2
History Finding(s): Physical Exam Finding(s):

Diagnosis #3
History Finding(s): Physical Exam Finding(s):

Diagnostic Workup

History

HPI: *32 yo F c/o fatigue and weakness × 5 months.*

- *Fatigue increases throughout the day.*
- *Loss of energy and concentration, which is affecting job as nurse.*
- *Patient admits that husband, who is an alcoholic, has beaten her.*
- *At least 1 episode of physical abuse directed at youngest son.*
- *Patient attempts to defend husband's actions.*
- *Feels guilty.*
- *Self-blame.*
- *Has not reported abuse. No head trauma or accidents due to husband.*
- *No emergency plan.*
- *Feels sad but denies suicidal ideation.*
- *Polyuria, polydipsia, nocturia × 5 months.*
- *LMP 2 weeks ago, menstrual period is regular, q28 days, lasting 7 days of heavy flow.*
- *No dysuria or change in color of urine.*
- *No constipation, cold intolerance, or change in appetite or weight.*
- *No sleep problems.*

ROS: *Negative except as above.*
Allergies: *NKDA.*
Medications: *None.*
PMH/PSH: *None.*
SH: *No smoking, no EtOH. Sexually active with her husband; decreased sexual desire.*
FH: *Diabetic father died from a heart attack; mother is in a nursing home with Alzheimer's disease.*

Physical Examination

Patient is obese, in no acute distress, looks anxious.

VS: *WNL.*
HEENT: *Pale conjunctivae.*
Neck: *No lymphadenopathy, thyroid normal.*
Chest: *Clear breath sounds bilaterally.*
Heart: *RRR; normal S1/S2; no murmurs, rubs, or gallops.*
Abdomen: *Soft, nondistended, nontender, ⊕ BS, no hepatosplenomegaly.*
Extremities: *Muscle strength 5/5 throughout; DTRs 2+; symmetric, painful bruises on both arms.*

Differential Diagnosis

Diagnosis #1: Domestic violence

History Finding(s):	Physical Exam Finding(s):
Admits to physical abuse	Symmetrical bruises on extremities
Exhibits self-blame	
Attempts to defend husband	
Episode of abuse directed at child	

Diagnosis #2: Diabetes mellitus

History Finding(s):	Physical Exam Finding(s):
Polyuria, polydipsia	
Obesity	
Family history of diabetes	

Diagnosis #3: Anemia

History Finding(s):	Physical Exam Finding(s):
Fatigue/weakness	Conjunctival pallor
Heavy menstrual flow	

Diagnostic Workup

Serum glucose, HbA_{1c}
CBC
Serum iron, ferritin, TIBC, serum B_{12}
UA
Electrolytes

CASE DISCUSSION

Patient Note Differential Diagnoses

- **Domestic violence:** The patient is clearly a victim of domestic violence and of her husband's alcoholism. This can explain many of her symptoms but not the polyuria or polydipsia.

- **Diabetes mellitus (DM):** Aside from domestic violence issues, many of the patient's symptoms can be explained by new-onset diabetes. Her obesity and positive family history put her at risk. She should also be asked about any recent vaginal yeast infections, which are a frequent complication of hyperglycemia (and may be its initial presenting symptom).

- **Anemia:** This may also help explain her fatigue and weakness. Menstruating females often have an iron deficiency anemia. Conjunctival pallor on exam has a high likelihood ratio for predicting a hematocrit < 30% (Hb < 10 g/dL).

Additional Differential Diagnoses

- **Major depressive disorder (MDD):** This patient does not currently meet the criteria for MDD. However, her history of intimate partner violence increases her risk of developing a mental disorder, with the degree of risk directly related to the frequency of violent episodes.

- **Hypothyroidism:** Nonspecific symptoms such as fatigue and weakness may suggest this common diagnosis. However, the patient denies constipation, weight/appetite changes, or cold intolerance. Hypothyroidism does not explain polyuria, polydipsia, or the admitted physical abuse.

- **Diabetes insipidus (DI):** This is an uncommon disease characterized by polyuria (of low specific gravity) and polydipsia. It has many etiologies and is caused by a deficiency of or resistance to vasopressin. Central diabetes can be idiopathic or acquired (eg, post–head trauma, benign tumors, or surgery). The patient's obesity, family history of DM, and lack of acquired causes of DI support DM as a more probable explanation for her symptoms.

- **Myasthenia gravis:** Increasing fatigue as the day progresses is highly nonspecific. By contrast, this disease involves fluctuating muscle weakness and presents with ptosis, diplopia, difficulty chewing or swallowing, respiratory difficulties, and/or limb weakness—all of which the patient has denied.

Diagnostic Workup

- **Serum glucose, HbA$_{1c}$:** To screen for DM.

- **CBC:** To investigate anemia. If the CBC is suggestive of iron deficiency anemia, the next step would be to order a serum iron level, ferritin, and TIBC. Serum B$_{12}$ levels should also be ordered to check for B$_{12}$ deficiency anemia.

- **UA:** Glucose or protein may be present in DM.

- **Electrolytes:** Hypernatremia may be seen in DI.

- **MRI—brain (pituitary protocol):** To look for mass lesions in central DI.

- **DDAVP nasal spray test ("vasopressin challenge test"):** To confirm a clinical suspicion of central DI.

Opening Scenario

Jack Edwards, a 27-year-old male, comes to the ED complaining of seeing strange writing on the wall.

Vital Signs

BP: 140/80 mm Hg

Temp: 98.3°F (36.8°C)

RR: 15/minute

HR: 110/minute, regular

Examinee Tasks

1. Take a focused history.

2. Perform a focused physical exam (do not perform rectal, genitourinary, or female breast exam).

3. Explain your clinical impression and workup plan to the patient.

4. Write the patient note after leaving the room.

Checklist/SP Sheet

Patient Description

Patient is a 27 yo M.

Notes for the SP

- Sit up on the bed.
- Give the impression that you are staring at the wall.

Challenging Questions to Ask

"Do you think someone is trying to give me instructions through the writing I see on the wall?"

Sample Examinee Response

"I don't think anyone is trying to give you instructions. If you have been taking illicit drugs, it may be that the drugs are causing you to see this writing. In any case, we are going to do some tests to try to figure out what is going on."

Examinee Checklist

Building the Doctor-Patient Relationship

Entrance

☐ Examinee knocked on the door before entering.

☐ Examinee introduced self by name.

☐ Examinee identified his/her role or position.

☐ Examinee correctly used patient's name.

☐ Examinee made eye contact with the SP.

Reflective Listening

☐ Examinee asked an open-ended question and actively listened to the response.

☐ Examinee asked the SP to list his/her concerns and listened to the response without interrupting.

☐ Examinee summarized the SP's concerns, often using the SP's own words.

Information Gathering

☐ Examinee elicited data efficiently and accurately.

☑ Question	Patient Response
☐ Chief complaint	I have been seeing strange writing on the wall.
☐ Onset	It started yesterday.
☐ Content	It is not clear, and I can't read it most of the time.
☐ Duration	It lasts less than a minute.
☐ Constant/intermittent	It comes and goes.
☐ Frequency	It has happened 3–4 times since yesterday.
☐ Do you see the writing while your eyes are closed?	Sometimes.
☐ Alleviating factors	None.
☐ Exacerbating factors	None.
☐ Major life changes or stressors	Not really.
☐ Headache	None.
☐ Visual changes or vision loss	None.
☐ Hearing changes	I feel as though I hear strange voices when I see the writing.
☐ Hearing loss	No.
☐ Content of the voices	I can't understand them; the voices seem distant.
☐ Feeling of being controlled	No.
☐ Do the voices/writing order you to harm yourself or others?	No.
☐ Do you think about harming yourself or others?	No.
☐ Enjoyment of daily activities	Yes.
☐ Mental illness in family	No.
☐ Do you ever have these symptoms without drug use?	No.
☐ Sleeping problems	No, but sometimes I find it difficult to wake up in the morning.
☐ Do you fall asleep suddenly during the day?	No, but sometimes I feel very sleepy during the day.
☐ Fever	No.

☑ Question	Patient Response
☐ Weight changes	None.
☐ Current medications	None.
☐ Past medical history	None.
☐ Head trauma	No.
☐ Past surgical history	None.
☐ Family history	My father had high blood pressure.
☐ Occupation	I work as a bartender.
☐ Alcohol use	No.
☐ Illicit drug use	Occasionally.
☐ Which illicit drugs do you use?	Angel dust; sometimes Ecstasy.
☐ Last use of illicit drugs	Yesterday at a party at my friend's house.
☐ Tobacco	Yes, I have smoked a pack a day for 6 years.
☐ Exercise	No.
☐ Sexual activity	Yes, with my girlfriend.
☐ Use of condoms	Yes, I use them.
☐ Drug allergies	No.

Connecting with the Patient

☐ Examinee recognized the SP's emotions and responded with PEARLS.

Physical Examination

☐ Examinee washed his/her hands.

☐ Examinee asked permission to start the exam.

☐ Examinee used respectful draping.

☐ Examinee did not repeat painful maneuvers.

☑ Exam Component	Maneuver
☐ Eye exam	Inspected pupils; checked for reactivity
☐ CV exam	Auscultation, vital signs
☐ Pulmonary exam	Auscultation
☐ Abdominal exam	Palpation
☐ Neurologic exam	Mini-mental status exam, cranial nerves, motor exam, DTRs, gait, sensory exam

Closure

☐ Examinee discussed initial diagnostic impressions.

☐ Examinee discussed initial management plans.

    ☐ Follow-up tests.

☐ Examinee asked if the SP had any other questions or concerns.

Sample Closure

Mr. Edwards, your symptoms could be caused by your illicit drug use, or they may be the result of a mental problem or even a medical condition. We will run some tests to try to clarify your condition. In addition, I recommend that you stop using illicit drugs and quit smoking. Do you have any questions for me?

Patient Note

History

Physical Examination

Differential Diagnosis

Diagnosis #1

History Finding(s):   **Physical Exam Finding(s):**

Diagnosis #2

History Finding(s):   **Physical Exam Finding(s):**

Diagnosis #3

History Finding(s):   **Physical Exam Finding(s):**

Diagnostic Workup

Patient Note

History

HPI: *27 yo M c/o episodes of seeing strange writing on the wall since yesterday. These episodes last less than a minute and have happened 3–4 times. The patient states that the writing is not clear and he cannot read the messages, but he thinks he might be getting instructions from them. He denies any other visual changes or visual loss. The patient also mentions hearing strange voices associated with the writing, adding that he cannot understand them either. He admits to having used illicit drugs 1 day before these events. He denies any headache, seizures, head trauma, or previous similar episodes. No appetite or weight changes, fever, or sleep problems.*

ROS: *Negative except as above.*

Allergies: *NKDA.*

Medications: *None.*

PMH: *None.*

PSH: *None.*

SH: *1 PPD for 6 years; uses PCP ("angel dust") and MDMA (Ecstasy) occasionally; no EtOH. Works as a bartender.*

FH: *Noncontributory.*

Physical Examination

Patient seems anxious and in mild distress.

VS: *HR 110, BP 140/80*

HEENT: *Pupils dilated, vertical gaze nystagmus.*

Chest: *Clear breath sounds bilaterally.*

Heart: *Tachycardic; normal S1/S2; no murmurs, rubs, or gallops.*

Abdomen: *Soft, nontender, nondistended, no hepatosplenomegaly.*

Neuro: *Mental status: Alert and oriented × 3, spells backward and recalls 3 objects. Cranial nerves: 2–12 intact. Motor: Strength 5/5 in all muscle groups. DTRs: Symmetric. Gait: Normal.*

Differential Diagnosis

Diagnosis #1: PCP intoxication	
History Finding(s):	**Physical Exam Finding(s):**
Drug use 1 day before presentation	Tachycardia (HR 110/minute)
Visual hallucinations	Hypertension (BP 140/80)
Noncommand auditory hallucinations	Vertical gaze nystagmus
Delusions	

Diagnosis #2: Substance-induced psychosis	
History Finding(s):	**Physical Exam Finding(s):**
Drug use 1 day before presentation	Pupils dilated
Visual hallucinations	
Noncommand auditory hallucinations	
Delusions	
No history of non-drug-related psychosis	
Does not associate drug use with presentation	

Diagnostic Workup

Urine toxicology
Electrolytes
CPK
Urine myoglobin
Mental status exam

CASE DISCUSSION

Patient Note Differential Diagnoses

- **PCP intoxication:** This patient clearly shows signs of PCP intoxication. Hallucinations, delusions, nystagmus, tachycardia, and hypertension are common in PCP intoxication. The mnemonic **RED DANES** helps recall common symptoms of PCP intoxication: **R**age, **E**rythema, **D**ilated pupils, **D**elusions, **A**mnesia, **N**ystagmus, **E**xcitation, and **S**kin dryness. This patient does not complain of myalgias, although rhabdomyolysis can occur in cases of large ingestions. Serum CPK and urine myoglobin should be measured to rule out this complication.

- **Substance-induced psychosis:** It is important to note that patients with substance-induced psychosis lack the insight to identify their recent drug use as a cause of their symptoms. The presentation is consistent with this diagnosis. Substance-induced psychosis requires that the substance ingested (medications, alcohol, or illicit drugs) be capable of causing psychosis and that the symptoms be more severe than expected for intoxication or withdrawal. In contrast to intoxication with perceptual disturbances, hallucinations and delusions are more prominent than other symptoms.

Additional Differential Diagnoses

- **Brief psychotic disorder:** Symptoms of psychosis may be induced by stressful events and may resolve with removal of the stressor. Auditory hallucinations are more common and typically accompany visual hallucinations. This patient describes both visual and auditory hallucinations. However, according to the *Diagnostic and Statistical Manual of Mental Disorders* (DSM-5), a diagnosis of brief psychotic disorder cannot be contemplated here because the patient has recently ingested a substance known to induce psychosis.

- **Psychosis secondary to a medical condition:** A variety of medical conditions can lead to hallucinations. These include neurologic problems such as CNS infections and neoplasms; endocrine conditions such as thyroid, parathyroid, or adrenal abnormalities; and hepatic and renal disorders. However, there is nothing in this patient's history to support a secondary medical condition.

- **Narcolepsy:** The visual hallucinations of narcolepsy are complex, generally occurring immediately before falling asleep (hypnagogic) or just after waking up (hypnopompic). Auditory or tactile sensations can be associated with visual hallucinations as well. Although this patient complains of daytime sleepiness, his symptoms are not severe enough to merit this diagnosis. Narcolepsy without cataplexy (muscular weakness with or without an emotional trigger) is classified as major somnolence disorder in DSM-5.

- **Seizure:** Visual hallucinations of epileptic origin can be simple or complex. They are variable in frequency and usually last for a few seconds. This diagnosis is unlikely because the patient has no known history of seizures.

Diagnostic Workup

- **Urine toxicology:** To detect commonly used illicit drugs, such as amphetamines, barbiturates, benzodiazepines, cannabinoids, cocaine, opioids, and phencyclidine (PCP).

- **Electrolytes:** To detect any medical condition that may cause neurologic or mental changes.

- **CPK and urine myoglobin:** To evaluate for rhabdomyolysis.

- **Mental status exam:** To evaluate for a possible psychiatric disorder, although in the setting of a recent substance exposure, the diagnosis of psychopathology is not possible.

CASE 36
DOORWAY INFORMATION

Opening Scenario

Frank Emanuel, a 32-year-old male, comes to the office for a preemployment medical checkup as requested by his prospective employer.

Vital Signs

BP: 130/85 mm Hg

Temp: 98.3°F (36.8°C)

RR: 15/minute

HR: 70/minute, regular

Examinee Tasks

1. Take a focused history.

2. Perform a focused physical exam (do not perform rectal, genitourinary, or female breast exam).

3. Explain your clinical impression and workup plan to the patient.

4. Write the patient note after leaving the room.

Checklist/SP Sheet

Patient Description

Patient is a 32 yo M.

Notes for the SP

- Sit up on the bed.
- Hold the physical exam request form in your hand.

Challenging Questions to Ask

"Do you think they are going to give me the job?"

Sample Examinee Response

"Employers routinely request medical examinations to ensure that potential employees are fit for the job, as well as to determine if they have any medical conditions that may prove hazardous to others in the work environment. I will ask you a few questions and perform a physical examination, and on the basis of what I find, I may or may not order further tests. Hopefully everything will be fine."

Examinee Checklist

Building the Doctor-Patient Relationship

Entrance

☐ Examinee knocked on the door before entering.

☐ Examinee introduced self by name.

☐ Examinee identified his/her role or position.

☐ Examinee correctly used patient's name.

☐ Examinee made eye contact with the SP.

Reflective Listening

☐ Examinee asked an open-ended question and actively listened to the response.

☐ Examinee asked the SP to list his/her concerns and listened to the response without interrupting.

☐ Examinee summarized the SP's concerns, often using the SP's own words.

Information Gathering

☐ Examinee elicited data efficiently and accurately.

☑ Question	Patient Response
☐ Medical complaints or problems	No.
☐ Chest pain (current and past)	No.
☐ Shortness of breath (current and past)	No.
☐ Palpitations or slow heart rate	No.
☐ Swelling in legs	No.
☐ Loss of consciousness/seizures	No.
☐ Headache	No.
☐ Weakness/numbness	No.
☐ Cough	Yes.
☐ Onset of cough	I've had this cough for years.
☐ Changes in the cough during the day	None.
☐ Progression of the cough	It is the same.
☐ Wheezing	No.
☐ Do you cough at night?	No.
☐ Sputum production	Yes.
☐ Amount of sputum	I am not sure. Around half a teaspoonful; stable.
☐ Color	White mucus.
☐ Odor	None.
☐ Blood in sputum	No.

☑ Question	Patient Response
☐ Fever/chills	None.
☐ Night sweats	No.
☐ Exposure to TB	No.
☐ Recent travel	I emigrated from Africa a month ago.
☐ Last PPD	I have never had this test.
☐ Joint pain or swelling	No.
☐ Nausea/vomiting	No.
☐ Abdominal pain	No.
☐ Diarrhea/constipation	No.
☐ Weight changes	No.
☐ Appetite changes	No.
☐ Change in stool color	No.
☐ Current medications	None.
☐ Past medical history	None.
☐ Past surgical history	None.
☐ Medical problems or diseases in your family	None.
☐ Vaccinations	My immunizations are up to date. I have my papers at home; I can fax them to you.
☐ Occupation	I used to work in a coal mine back home. I am applying for a new job.
☐ Alcohol use	No.
☐ Illicit drug use	No.
☐ Tobacco	Yes, a pack a day for 10 years.
☐ Sexual activity	Yes, with my wife.
☐ Drug allergies	None.

Connecting with the Patient

☐ Examinee recognized the SP's emotions and responded with PEARLS.

Physical Examination

☐ Examinee washed his/her hands.

☐ Examinee asked permission to start the exam.

☐ Examinee used respectful draping.

☐ Examinee did not repeat painful maneuvers.

☑ Exam Component	Maneuver
☐ Head and neck exam	Inspected mouth, throat; palpated lymph nodes
☐ CV exam	Auscultation
☐ Pulmonary exam	Auscultation, palpation, percussion
☐ Abdominal exam	Auscultation, palpation
☐ Extremities	Inspection
☐ Neurologic exam	Cranial nerves, motor exam, DTRs, gait

Closure

☐ Examinee discussed initial diagnostic impressions.

☐ Examinee discussed initial management plans:

   ☐ Follow-up tests.

☐ Examinee asked if the SP had any other questions or concerns.

Sample Closure

Mr. Emanuel, your physical examination is normal, but your cough may raise concern for some possible medical problems. We need to order some tests to make sure you are free of any serious medical conditions, and if we find anything, we will treat it right away. Since you just came here from Africa and you have never been tested for TB, we need to rule out pulmonary tuberculosis, not only because it is harmful to you but also because you may transmit it to your future coworkers. The other issue I want to talk to you about is your smoking. It puts you at increased risk of heart and lung disease, and I strongly urge you to quit. Do you have any questions?

History

_____
_____
_____
_____
_____
_____
_____
_____
_____
_____
_____
_____
_____
_____
_____

Physical Examination

_____
_____
_____
_____
_____
_____
_____
_____
_____
_____
_____
_____
_____
_____
_____
_____

Patient Note

Differential Diagnosis

Diagnosis #1
History Finding(s):   **Physical Exam Finding(s):**

Diagnosis #2
History Finding(s):   **Physical Exam Finding(s):**

Diagnosis #3
History Finding(s):   **Physical Exam Finding(s):**

Diagnostic Workup

History

HPI: *32 yo M with no PMH presents for a preemployment medical examination. He has no medical complaints or problems. Nevertheless, he mentioned having a chronic cough for many years with no recent change in frequency or severity. The cough is productive of half a teaspoonful of white mucus with no blood. The patient denies any dyspnea, fever or chills, chest pain, or wheezing and has had no appetite or weight changes. The patient is an African immigrant who came to the United States 1 month ago and reports no TB exposure. He has never had a PPD test. However, he states that his immunizations are up to date, and he will be faxing us the report to review.*

ROS: *Negative except as above.*
Allergies: *NKDA.*
Medications: *None.*
PMH: *Per HPI.*
PSH: *None.*
SH: *1 PPD for 10 years, no EtOH, no illicit drugs. Sexually active with wife only.*
FH: *Noncontributory.*

Physical Examination

VS: *WNL.*
HEENT: *Mouth and pharynx WNL.*
Neck: *No JVD, no lymphadenopathy.*
Chest: *Clear breath sounds bilaterally; no rhonchi, rales, or wheezing; tactile fremitus normal.*
Heart: *RRR; normal S1/S2; no murmurs, rubs, or gallops.*
Abdomen: *Soft, nontender, nondistended, ⊕ BS, no hepatosplenomegaly.*
Extremities: *No clubbing, cyanosis, or edema.*
Neuro: *Cranial nerves: 2–12 intact. Motor: Strength 5/5 in all muscle groups. DTRs: Symmetric. Gait: Normal.*

Differential Diagnosis

Diagnosis #1: COPD/chronic bronchitis	
History Finding(s):	**Physical Exam Finding(s):**
Chronic cough	
Sputum production	
History of smoking 1 PPD × 10 years	
Worked as coal miner	

Diagnosis #2: Pneumoconiosis

History Finding(s):	Physical Exam Finding(s):
Worked as coal miner	
Chronic cough	

Diagnosis #3: Pulmonary tuberculosis

History Finding(s):	Physical Exam Finding(s):
Recent emigration from Africa	
Chronic cough	

Diagnostic Workup

CXR—PA and lateral
PPD or QuantiFERON Gold
CBC

CASE DISCUSSION

Patient Note Differential Diagnoses

- **COPD/chronic bronchitis:** This patient's chronic cough and sputum production might be due to COPD/chronic bronchitis secondary to his smoking history and occupational exposure. Patients who are smokers and work in coal mines are more likely to develop COPD in addition to inhalant-induced restrictive lung diseases. CXR and pulmonary function tests can help distinguish these causes of lung pathology and assess their severity.

- **Pneumoconiosis:** Considering his occupational history as a coal miner, this patient has been exposed to coal dust and crystalline silica and is at increased risk of coal worker's pneumoconiosis and pulmonary silicosis.

- **Pulmonary tuberculosis:** Active TB infection is unlikely, as the patient denies systemic symptoms, blood-tinged sputum, dyspnea, chest pain, or exposure to TB. However, TB infection should be ruled out in this patient before he starts a new job, as he is an immigrant and has never been tested for TB. Latent infection should be treated to decrease the risk of progression to active TB.

Additional Differential Diagnoses

There are other possible causes of the patient's chronic cough that may be benign, such as GERD and asthma.

Diagnostic Workup

- **CXR—PA and lateral:** A good initial test in evaluating chronic cough. It may demonstrate cavitary lesions in TB or may show nodular calcification in silicosis. It is usually normal in benign causes of cough, such as asthma or GERD.

- **PPD (tuberculin skin test) or QuantiFERON Gold:** The PPD test is a screening tool for determining if a patient has been infected with *Mycobacterium tuberculosis*. A QuantiFERON Gold test can also be considered in this case, as it is more specific for prior infection with *M tuberculosis*. However, its availability is variable and based on the testing center.

- **CBC:** To identify leukocytosis in infection (nonspecific).

- **Sputum Gram stain, AFB smear, routine and mycobacterial sputum cultures:** To identify a causative agent of possible infection. However, a PPD or QuantiFERON Gold test would typically be ordered as a screening test before the collection of a sputum sample or culture in an outpatient setting.

- **Pulmonary function tests:** May distinguish obstructive from restrictive disease but is not diagnostic for pneumoconiosis. More often used as a test to determine the severity of disease.

Opening Scenario

Kenneth Klein, a 55-year-old male, comes to the clinic complaining of blood in his stool.

Vital Signs

BP: 130/80 mm Hg

Temp: 98.5°F (36.9°C)

RR: 16/minute

HR: 76/minute, regular

Examinee Tasks

1. Take a focused history.

2. Perform a focused physical exam (do not perform rectal, genitourinary, or female breast exam).

3. Explain your clinical impression and workup plan to the patient.

4. Write the patient note after leaving the room.

Checklist/SP Sheet

Patient Description

Patient is a 55 yo M, married with 2 children.

Notes for the SP

If colonoscopy is mentioned by the examinee, ask, "What does that word mean?"

Challenging Questions to Ask

"My father had colon cancer. Could I have it too?"

Sample Examinee Response

"It is a possibility. Tell me more about the symptoms you're having that concern you with regard to cancer."

Examinee Checklist

Building the Doctor-Patient Relationship

Entrance

☐ Examinee knocked on the door before entering.

☐ Examinee introduced self by name.

☐ Examinee identified his/her role or position.

☐ Examinee correctly used patient's name.

☐ Examinee made eye contact with the SP.

Reflective Listening

☐ Examinee asked an open-ended question and actively listened to the response.

☐ Examinee asked the SP to list his/her concerns and listened to the response without interrupting.

☐ Examinee summarized the SP's concerns, often using the SP's own words.

Information Gathering

☐ Examinee elicited data efficiently and accurately.

☑ Question	Patient Response
☐ Chief complaint	Blood in my stool.
☐ Onset	One month ago.
☐ Frequency	Every time I have a bowel movement, I see some blood mixed in.
☐ Description (blood before, during, or after defecation)	The blood is mixed in with the brown stool.
☐ Bright red or dark blood	Bright red.
☐ Pain during defecation	No.
☐ Constipation	Well, I have had constipation for a long time, and I keep taking laxatives. At first I got some relief from them, but now they are of no help to me at all.
☐ Frequency of bowel movements	I have had 2 bowel movements a week for the past 6 months.
☐ Diarrhea	I have had diarrhea for the past 2 days.
☐ Urgency	No.
☐ Tenesmus (ineffectual spasms of the rectum accompanied by the desire to empty the bowel)	A little.
☐ Frequency of diarrhea	Three times a day.
☐ Description of the diarrhea	Watery, brown, mixed with blood.
☐ Mucus in stool	No.
☐ Melena	No.
☐ Fever/chills	No.
☐ Abdominal pain	No.
☐ Nausea/vomiting	No.
☐ Diet	I eat a lot of junk food. I don't eat vegetables at all.
☐ Weight changes	I have lost about 10 pounds over the past 6 months.
☐ Appetite changes	My appetite has been the same.
☐ Recent travel	No, but I am thinking of going on a trip with my family next week. Do you think I should stay home?
☐ Contact with people with diarrhea	No.
☐ Exercise	I walk for half an hour every day.

☑ Question	Patient Response
☐ Urinary problems	No.
☐ Current medications	No. I used to take many laxatives, such as bisacodyl, but I stopped all of them when the diarrhea started.
☐ Past medical history (recent antibiotic use)	I had bronchitis 3 weeks ago; it was treated with amoxicillin.
☐ Past surgical history	Hemorrhoids resected 4 years ago.
☐ Family history	My father died at 55 of colon cancer. My mother is alive and healthy.
☐ Occupation	Lawyer.
☐ Alcohol use	No.
☐ Illicit drug use	No.
☐ Tobacco	No.
☐ Sexual activity	With my wife.
☐ Drug allergies	None.

Connecting with the Patient

☐ Examinee recognized the SP's emotions and responded with PEARLS.

Physical Examination

☐ Examinee washed his/her hands.

☐ Examinee asked permission to start the exam.

☐ Examinee used respectful draping.

☐ Examinee did not repeat painful maneuvers.

☑ Exam Component	Maneuver
☐ CV exam	Auscultation
☐ Pulmonary exam	Auscultation
☐ Abdominal exam	Auscultation, palpation, percussion

Closure

☐ Examinee discussed initial diagnostic impressions.

☐ Examinee discussed initial management plans:

　☐ Follow-up tests: Examinee mentioned the need for a rectal exam.

☐ Examinee asked if the SP had any other questions or concerns.

Sample Closure

Mr. Klein, the symptoms you describe may be due to readily treatable problems, such as hemorrhoids, an infection in your colon, or diverticulosis. However, they may also be a sign of more serious disease, such as colorectal cancer. It is crucial that we run some blood tests, a stool exam, and probably a colonoscopy, which involves looking at your colon through a thin tube that contains a camera. I will also need to perform a rectal exam today. Once we make a diagnosis, we should be able to treat your problem. Do you have any questions for me?

Patient Note

History

Physical Examination

Differential Diagnosis

Diagnosis #1

History Finding(s):

Physical Exam Finding(s):

Diagnosis #2

History Finding(s):

Physical Exam Finding(s):

Diagnosis #3

History Finding(s):

Physical Exam Finding(s):

Diagnostic Workup

History

HPI: *55 yo M c/o bright red blood per rectum.*

- *History of constipation 6 months ago, 2 bowel movements a week.*
- *1 month ago noticed blood mixed with stool with each bowel movement.*
- *2 days ago, tenesmus and watery brown diarrhea mixed with blood.*
- *10-lb weight loss in 6 months despite good appetite.*
- *Diet of junk food and no vegetables.*
- *No urgency, mucus in stool, or pain with defecation.*
- *Denies fevers, chills, nausea, vomiting, abdominal pain, recent history of travel, or contact with ill persons.*

ROS: *Negative except as above.*

Allergies: *NKDA.*

Medications: *Used to take many laxatives (bisacodyl), but stopped after the onset of diarrhea 2 days ago.*

PMH: *Bronchitis 3 weeks ago, treated with amoxicillin.*

PSH: *Hemorrhoids resected 4 years ago.*

SH: *No smoking, no EtOH, no illicit drugs. Sexually active with wife only.*

FH: *Father died of colon cancer at age 55.*

Physical Examination

Patient is in no acute distress.

VS: *WNL.*

Chest: *Clear breath sounds bilaterally.*

Heart: *RRR; normal S1/S2; no murmurs, rubs, or gallops.*

Abdomen: *Soft, nondistended, nontender, ⊕ BS, no hepatosplenomegaly.*

Differential Diagnosis

Diagnosis #1: Colorectal cancer	
History Finding(s)	**Physical Exam Finding(s)**
Blood mixed with stool for 1 month	
Family history of colon cancer	
Unintentional weight loss of 10 lbs	

Diagnosis #2: Hemorrhoids	
History Finding(s)	**Physical Exam Finding(s)**
History of hemorrhoids	
Hematochezia	

Patient Note

Diagnosis #3: C difficile *colitis*	
History Finding(s)	**Physical Exam Finding(s)**
Acute diarrhea	
Recent antibiotic exposure	

Diagnostic Workup

Rectal exam, stool for occult blood
Colonoscopy
Stool for C difficile *PCR*
Fecal leukocytes
CBC
Anoscopy
Flexible proctosigmoidoscopy

CASE DISCUSSION

Patient Note Differential Diagnoses

- **Colorectal cancer:** A positive family history coupled with the presence of blood in the stool, a change in bowel habits, and weight loss is consistent with this diagnosis. A rectal exam with stool tested for occult blood should be sent to start the necessary workup.

- **Hemorrhoids:** Recurrent hemorrhoids may explain the patient's hematochezia, but more typical findings in hemorrhoids are fresh blood on the toilet paper or in the toilet bowl.

- **Pseudomembranous (C difficile) colitis:** It is important to ask all patients with acute diarrhea about recent antibiotic exposure, as symptoms of antibiotic-associated colitis may be delayed for up to 6–8 weeks. However, stool rarely contains gross blood. The absence of fever and lower abdominal cramping also makes this diagnosis (and other forms of infectious colitis) less likely.

Additional Differential Diagnoses

- **Diverticulosis:** This is the most common cause of major lower GI bleeding, but it usually presents with larger-volume bleeds occurring in discrete, self-limited episodes.

- **Angiodysplasia:** This is another common cause of lower GI tract bleeding, but as with diverticular disease, it cannot explain the other features of this patient's presentation.

- **Ulcerative colitis:** Although the patient has chronic constipation, the absence of abdominal pain and the recent onset of diarrhea and tenesmus make inflammatory bowel disease a less likely etiology for this patient's month-long hematochezia.

Diagnostic Workup

- **Rectal exam, stool for occult blood:** Useful for detecting masses and hemorrhoids. Always test for occult blood in stool, especially in a patient complaining of visible blood with each bowel movement.

- **Colonoscopy:** A screening colonoscopy should have been offered to the patient at age 45 (10 years before the age at which a first-degree family member was first diagnosed). It should be the initial test performed in patients older than 40 years of age presenting with hematochezia.

- **Stool for C difficile PCR:** A stool C difficile toxin assay has low sensitivity and has been replaced at most institutions with PCR. The C difficile PCR test has a turnaround time of two hours with a sensitivity and specificity higher than 97%.

- **Fecal leukocytes:** Usually present in invasive bacterial infection and in inflammatory bowel disease. Variably present in C difficile colitis.

- **CBC:** To investigate anemia. Leukocytosis could also suggest infection or inflammatory bowel disease.

- **Anoscopy:** Can identify bleeding internal hemorrhoids, rectal ulcers, and traumatic lesions.

- **Flexible proctosigmoidoscopy:** If nondiagnostic, follow up with a barium enema or a colonoscopy.

- **Double-contrast (air contrast) barium enema:** Not as accurate as colonoscopy for the diagnosis of polyps and cancer, and cannot diagnose angiodysplasia. Used primarily when colonoscopy is unavailable or contraindicated.

- **CT—abdomen/pelvis:** Contrast-enhanced exams can detect diverticulosis or masses but generally are not useful in the evaluation of GI bleeding.

CASE 38
DOORWAY INFORMATION

Opening Scenario

Charles Andrews, a 66-year-old male, comes to the clinic complaining of a tremor.

Vital Signs

BP: 135/85 mm Hg

Temp: 98.6°F (37°C)

RR: 16/minute

HR: 70/minute, regular

Examinee Tasks

1. Take a focused history.

2. Perform a focused physical exam (do not perform rectal, genitourinary, or female breast exam).

3. Explain your clinical impression and workup plan to the patient.

4. Write the patient note after leaving the room.

Checklist/SP Sheet

Patient Description

Patient is a 66 yo M.

Notes for the SP

- Exhibit mild muscle rigidity in your wrists and arms—that is, when the examinee tries to move your wrists and arms, stiffen them and move them slowly.
- Lean your back forward slightly and walk in small, shuffling steps.
- Exhibit a resting hand tremor (pill rolling) that disappears with movement.

Challenging Questions to Ask

"Do you think I will get better?"

Sample Examinee Response

"I think your tremor will improve with medication, but I don't know how long the improvement will last. The tremor may be a sign of a larger movement disorder called Parkinson's disease, and we need to do some additional evaluations to explore that possibility."

Examinee Checklist

Building the Doctor-Patient Relationship

Entrance

☐ Examinee knocked on the door before entering.

☐ Examinee introduced self by name.

☐ Examinee identified his/her role or position.

☐ Examinee correctly used patient's name.

☐ Examinee made eye contact with the SP.

Reflective Listening

☐ Examinee asked an open-ended question and actively listened to the response.

☐ Examinee asked the SP to list his/her concerns and listened to the response without interrupting.

☐ Examinee summarized the SP's concerns, often using the SP's own words.

Information Gathering

☐ Examinee elicited data efficiently and accurately.

☑ Question	Patient Response
☐ Chief complaint	I have a tremor in this hand (points to right hand).
☐ Location	Only in the right hand.
☐ Duration	I noticed it about 6 months ago, but lately it seems to be getting worse.
☐ Context	It shakes when I'm just sitting around doing nothing. It usually stops when I hold out the remote control to change the channel.
☐ Alleviating factors	None.
☐ Exacerbating factors	It seems more severe when I am really tired.
☐ Associated symptoms (falls, headaches, TIA symptoms, drooling, changes in voice or handwriting, difficulty with ADLs/IADLs, depression, constipation, rash, etc.)	No, I don't think so. My wife says I've slowed down because I can't keep up with her when we go grocery shopping, but I think that's just because I retired last year.
☐ Prior history of similar symptoms	Well, back in college I occasionally had a hand tremor after pulling an all-nighter and drinking lots of coffee. The tremor was in both hands, but it was worse in the right. It seemed faster than the one I have now.
☐ Caffeine intake	One cup of coffee every morning. I used to drink 3 cups a day, but I've cut back over the past few months.
☐ Alcohol use	None. Both of my parents were alcoholics, so I never touch it.
☐ Past medical history	High cholesterol, treated with diet. Asthma, treated with an albuterol inhaler as needed.
☐ History of head trauma	No.
☐ Family history	My parents died in a car accident in their 40s, and my sister is healthy. I think my father may have had a tremor, but I'm not sure.
☐ Social history	I am married and live with my wife.
☐ Occupation	Retired chemistry professor.
☐ Exercise	No, I'm really not very active anymore.

☑ Question	Patient Response
☐ Tobacco	No.
☐ Illicit drug use	No.
☐ Current medications	Albuterol inhaler as needed. I have not used it in more than a year.
☐ Drug allergies	No.

Connecting with the Patient

☐ Examinee recognized the SP's emotions and responded with PEARLS.

Physical Examination

☐ Examinee washed his/her hands.

☐ Examinee asked permission to start the exam.

☐ Examinee used respectful draping.

☐ Examinee did not repeat painful maneuvers.

☑ Exam Component	Maneuver
☐ CV exam	Auscultation
☐ Pulmonary exam	Auscultation
☐ Neurologic exam	Mental status, cranial nerves, motor exam (including muscle tone), DTRs, cerebellar, gait, sensory exam

Closure

☐ Examinee discussed initial diagnostic impressions.

☐ Examinee discussed initial management plans:

    ☐ Follow-up tests.

    ☐ Possible need to compare an old handwriting sample with a present sample.

☐ Examinee offered support throughout the patient's illness.

☐ Examinee asked if the SP had any other questions or concerns.

Sample Closure

Mr. Andrews, I am sorry to have to tell you this, but on the basis of your history and physical exam, it would appear that you have Parkinson's disease. Your symptoms may improve with medications, but eventually they will return. One indicator of disease progression involves looking closely at your handwriting. Do you think you could bring an old sample of your handwriting with you on your next visit? You should also know that about 25% of the time, patients with your symptoms do not have Parkinson's disease. For this reason, I would like to run a few tests, including some imaging studies of your head and some blood tests. Although we won't have those results before you leave today, I will print out a comprehensive patient pamphlet that will give you resources to help answer your questions as they come up. I want you to know that I will be here to treat you and to help you every step of the way. Do you have any questions for me?

Patient Note

History

Physical Examination

Differential Diagnosis

Diagnosis #1

History Finding(s):   **Physical Exam Finding(s):**

Diagnosis #2

History Finding(s):   **Physical Exam Finding(s):**

Diagnosis #3

History Finding(s):   **Physical Exam Finding(s):**

Diagnostic Workup

Patient Note

History

HPI: *66 yo M c/o right hand tremor for 6 months. It occurs at rest and seems to be getting worse. The tremor is exacerbated by fatigue. There are no alleviating factors (he does not drink alcohol). Reducing his caffeine intake to 1 cup of coffee daily did not seem to help. He denies associated symptoms but does say that his wife complains that he has "slowed down" since retiring last year. Specifically, he seems to be walking more slowly recently (time course unspecified, but within the past year). He had a hand tremor when very fatigued back in college, but it was bilateral and faster than his present tremor.*

ROS: *Negative except as above.*

Allergies: *NKDA.*

Medications: *Albuterol MDI prn (no use in past year).*

PMH: *High cholesterol, treated with diet. Mild asthma.*

SH: *No smoking, no EtOH, no illicit drugs. He is a retired chemistry professor, married and lives with his wife.*

FH: *Father may have had a tremor.*

Physical Examination

Patient is in no acute distress.

VS: *WNL.*

Chest: *Clear breath sounds bilaterally.*

Heart: *RRR; normal S1/S2; no murmurs, rubs, or gallops.*

Neuro: *Mental status: Alert and oriented × 3. Cranial nerves: 2–12 grossly intact. Motor: Right hand resting tremor with "pill-rolling" movement that improves or disappears during purposeful action or posture. Mild muscle rigidity in both wrists and arms, but no frank cogwheeling. Strength 5/5 throughout. DTRs: Symmetric 2+ in all extremities. Cerebellar: ⊖ Romberg, rapid alternating movements and heel-to-shin test normal and symmetric. Gait: Bradykinetic, takes small steps. Walks with back slightly bent forward. Sensation: Intact to soft touch and pinprick.*

Differential Diagnosis

Diagnosis #1: Parkinson's disease	
History Finding(s)	**Physical Exam Finding(s)**
Resting tremor	Low-frequency tremor in upper extremity
	Bradykinetic gait
	Upper extremity rigidity

Diagnosis #2: Essential tremor	
History Finding(s)	**Physical Exam Finding(s)**
Possible family history of tremor	Tremor in distal upper extremity

Diagnosis #3: Physiologic tremor

History Finding(s)	Physical Exam Finding(s)
Resting tremor	Tremor in distal upper extremity

Diagnostic Workup

MRI—brain

CASE DISCUSSION

Patient Note Differential Diagnoses

- **Parkinson's disease (PD):** This is the most common cause of resting tremor (ie, a tremor that is evident with the affected body part supported and completely at rest but improves or subsides with voluntary activity), although some patients with PD also have a postural/action tremor that is indistinguishable from essential tremor (ET, see below). Tremor is usually low frequency (4–6 Hz), begins in one upper extremity, and may later involve the other extremities as well. Leg tremor is more commonly due to PD than to ET. The face, lips, and jaw may be involved, but in contrast to ET, PD does not produce head tremor. Along with the tremor, the patient's bradykinesia and rigidity suggest PD.

- **Essential tremor (ET):** This is the most common neurologic cause of postural tremor (ie, tremor that is apparent when the arms are held outstretched) or action tremor (ie, tremor that increases at the end of goal-directed activity such as finger-to-nose testing). Approximately 50% of cases are familial. Tremor is usually high frequency and often asymmetrically involves the distal upper extremity. The head, voice, chin, trunk, and legs can also be involved. ET is not associated with other neurologic signs and improves following the ingestion of small amounts of alcohol. Differentiation from the classic resting tremor of PD is usually straightforward, as in this case.

- **Physiologic tremor:** This refers to a very low-amplitude, high-frequency (10- to 12-Hz) tremor present in normal individuals. The tremor is often not visible, but when enhanced by medications or other medical conditions, it is the most common cause of postural and action tremors. Conditions that can enhance physiologic tremor include anxiety, excitement, sleep deprivation/fatigue, hypoglycemia, caffeine intake, alcohol withdrawal, thyrotoxicosis, fever, and pheochromocytoma.

Additional Differential Diagnoses

- **Midbrain lesion:** Midbrain injury due to stroke, trauma, or demyelinating disease is a rare cause of a solitary asymmetric resting tremor.

- **Drug-induced tremor:** Many medications can enhance physiologic tremor, notably β-agonists (eg, albuterol), nicotine, theophylline, TCAs, lithium, valproic acid, and corticosteroids. Mercury and arsenic exposure may also contribute to tremor. Neuroleptics and metoclopramide can cause drug-induced parkinsonism, but tremor is often absent in these cases.

- **Psychogenic tremor:** This often manifests with varying frequency and either becomes more irregular or subsides entirely when the patient is asked to perform a complex, repetitive motor task with the contralateral limb.

- **Wilson's disease:** This can cause resting tremor (among other manifestations) but is not considered in patients older than 40 years of age.

- **Hyperthyroidism:** This is associated with fine tremor along with a variety of other classic signs and symptoms.

Diagnostic Workup

- **MRI—brain:** To rule out a structural lesion, particularly in the midbrain or basal ganglia.

- **TSH:** To screen for hyperthyroidism.

- **Heavy metal screen:** To screen for mercury and arsenic toxicity via urine or blood tests.

- **Ceruloplasmin, slit lamp examination for Kayser-Fleischer rings, AST/ALT, CBC, 24-hour urinary copper, liver biopsy:** These tests constitute the screening tests (and diagnostic tests, in the case of liver biopsy) used to evaluate for suspected Wilson's disease. As noted previously, the patient's advanced age precludes consideration of Wilson's disease.

CASE 39
DOORWAY INFORMATION

Opening Scenario

Kristin Grant, a 30-year-old female, comes to the office complaining of weight gain.

Vital Signs

BP: 120/85 mm Hg

Temp: 98.0°F (36.7°C)

RR: 13/minute

HR: 65/minute, regular

BMI: 30

Examinee Tasks

1. Take a focused history.
2. Perform a focused physical exam (do not perform rectal, genitourinary, or female breast exam).
3. Explain your clinical impression and workup plan to the patient.
4. Write the patient note after leaving the room.

Checklist/SP Sheet

Patient Description

Patient is a 30 yo F.

Notes for the SP

None.

Challenging Questions to Ask

"I want to go back to smoking because I have started gaining weight since I quit."

Sample Examinee Response

"I understand that controlling your weight is important to you, but the health risks of smoking far outweigh those associated with weight gain. We also need to determine if something else is contributing to your weight gain and, if so, discuss strategies to deal with it."

Examinee Checklist

Building the Doctor-Patient Relationship

Entrance

☐ Examinee knocked on the door before entering.

☐ Examinee introduced self by name.

☐ Examinee identified his/her role or position.

☐ Examinee correctly used patient's name.

☐ Examinee made eye contact with the SP.

Reflective Listening

☐ Examinee asked an open-ended question and actively listened to the response.

☐ Examinee asked the SP to list his/her concerns and listened to the response without interrupting.

☐ Examinee summarized the SP's concerns, often using the SP's own words.

Information Gathering

☐ Examinee elicited data efficiently and accurately.

☑ Question	Patient Response
☐ Chief complaint	I am gaining weight.
☐ Onset	Three months ago.
☐ Weight gained	I've gained 20 pounds over the last 3 months.
☐ Cold intolerance	Yes.
☐ Skin/hair changes	My hair is falling out more than usual, and I feel that my skin has become dry.
☐ Voice change	No.
☐ Constipation	No.
☐ Appetite changes	I have a good appetite.
☐ Fatigue	No.
☐ Depression	No.
☐ Sleeping problems (falling asleep, staying asleep, early waking, snoring)	No.
☐ Associated symptoms (fever/chills, chest pain, shortness of breath, abdominal pain, diarrhea)	No.
☐ Last menstrual period	One week ago.
☐ Frequency of menstrual periods	I used to get my period every 4 weeks, but recently I've been getting it every 6 weeks or more. The period lasts 7 days.
☐ Start of change in cycle	Six months ago.
☐ Pads/tampons changed a day	It was 2–3 a day, but the blood flow is becoming less, and I use only 1 a day now.
☐ Age at menarche	Age 13.
☐ Pregnancies	I have 1 child; he is 10 years old. I have not had any other pregnancies.
☐ Problems during pregnancy/delivery	No, it was a normal delivery, and my child is healthy.
☐ Miscarriages/abortions	None.

☑ Question	Patient Response
☐ Hirsutism	No.
☐ Current medications	Lithium.
☐ Past medical history	I have bipolar disorder. I was started on lithium 6 months ago; I haven't had any problems since then.
☐ Past surgical history	None.
☐ Family history of obesity	My mother and sister are obese.
☐ Occupation	Housekeeper.
☐ Alcohol use	None.
☐ Illicit drug use	Never.
☐ Tobacco	I quit smoking 3 months ago. I had smoked 2 packs a day for 10 years.
☐ Exercise	No.
☐ Diet	The usual. I haven't changed anything in my diet in more than 10 years. Coffee during the day, chicken, steak, Chinese food. I usually eat out.
☐ Sexual activity	With my husband.
☐ Contraceptives	My husband had a vasectomy 2 years ago.
☐ Drug allergies	No.

Connecting with the Patient

☐ Examinee recognized the SP's emotions and responded with PEARLS.

Physical Examination

☐ Examinee washed his/her hands.

☐ Examinee asked permission to start the exam.

☐ Examinee used respectful draping.

☐ Examinee did not repeat painful maneuvers.

☑ Exam Component	Maneuver
☐ Head exam	Inspected conjunctivae, mouth, and throat
☐ Neck exam	Palpated lymph nodes, thyroid gland
☐ CV exam	Auscultation
☐ Pulmonary exam	Auscultation
☐ Abdominal exam	Auscultation, palpation, percussion
☐ Extremities	Inspected for edema, checked DTRs

Closure

☐ Examinee discussed initial diagnostic impressions.

☐ Examinee discussed initial management plans:

   ☐ Follow-up tests.

   ☐ Lifestyle modification (diet, exercise, relaxation techniques, smoking cessation support).

☐ Examinee asked if the SP had any other questions or concerns.

Sample Closure

Mrs. Grant, most smokers gain an average of 5 pounds when they quit. You have gained 20 pounds over 3 months. This may have resulted from your smoking cessation, but bear in mind that the health risk posed by smoking is far worse than the risk you might incur from excessive weight gain. In addition, there may be other reasons for your weight gain; for example, it may be related to your thyroid gland, or it may be a side effect of the lithium you're taking. I would like to draw some blood to measure your thyroid function and lithium levels. In the meantime, in addition to stopping smoking, you should continue to pursue a healthier lifestyle. Try to decrease the fatty foods you eat and increase the healthy ones, such as fruits and vegetables. Exercising only 30 minutes 3 times a week can also improve your health. Do you have any questions for me?

History

Physical Examination

Patient Note

Differential Diagnosis

Diagnosis #1

History Finding(s):   **Physical Exam Finding(s):**

Diagnosis #2

History Finding(s):   **Physical Exam Finding(s):**

Diagnosis #3

History Finding(s):   **Physical Exam Finding(s):**

Diagnostic Workup

Patient Note

History

HPI: *30 yo F c/o weight gain of 20 lbs over the past 3 months after she stopped smoking. She has a good appetite and reports no change in her diet. For 6 months she has experienced oligomenorrhea and hypomenorrhea, dry skin, and cold intolerance. The patient denies voice change, constipation, hirsutism, depression, fatigue, or sleep problems.*

OB/GYN: *Last menstrual period last week. See HPI for other.*

ROS: *Negative except as above.*

Allergies: *NKDA.*

Medications: *Lithium, started 6 months ago.*

PMH: *Bipolar disorder, diagnosed 6 months ago.*

PSH: *None.*

SH: *2 PPD for 10 years; stopped 3 months ago. No alcohol, no illicit drugs. Sexually active with husband only. Doesn't exercise.*

FH: *Mother and sister are obese.*

Diet: *Consists mainly of lots of coffee during the day, chicken, steak, and Chinese food.*

Physical Examination

Patient is in no acute distress.

VS: *WNL.*

HEENT: *No conjunctival pallor, mouth and pharynx WNL.*

Neck: *No lymphadenopathy, thyroid normal.*

Chest: *Clear breath sounds bilaterally.*

Heart: *RRR; normal S1/S2; no murmurs, rubs, or gallops.*

Abdomen: *Soft, nontender, nondistended, ⊕ BS, no hepatosplenomegaly.*

Extremities: *No edema, normal DTRs in lower extremities bilaterally.*

Differential Diagnosis

Diagnosis #1: Hypothyroidism	
History Finding(s)	**Physical Exam Finding(s)**
Oligo- and hypomenorrhea	
Chronic dry skin	
Chronic cold intolerance	

Diagnosis #2: Smoking cessation	
History Finding(s)	**Physical Exam Finding(s)**
Weight gain following smoking cessation	

Diagnosis #3: Lithium-related weight gain

History Finding(s)	Physical Exam Finding(s)
Ongoing lithium therapy	

Diagnostic Workup

TSH
Serum lithium level
Fasting glucose, cholesterol, triglycerides

CASE DISCUSSION

Patient Note Differential Diagnoses

- **Hypothyroidism:** This patient has classic early symptoms of hypothyroidism, which include weight gain, dry skin, cold intolerance, elevated serum cholesterol, and changes in menstruation patterns. Deepening of the voice, constipation, depression, and fatigue are also symptoms of hypothyroidism. It needs to be ruled out as a cause of her weight gain.

- **Smoking cessation:** Weight gain occurs in most patients following smoking cessation but usually averages only 4.5 lbs (2 kg). However, major weight gain such as that seen in this case may occur. Patients generally report increased appetite and calorie consumption.

- **Lithium-related weight gain:** Weight gain is a common side effect of lithium therapy and may contribute in this case. Other symptoms include cold intolerance, dry skin, confusion, dizziness, headache, lethargy, hair loss, and fatigue.

Additional Differential Diagnoses

- **Familial obesity:** There are strong genetic influences on the development of obesity, but a positive family history does not account for acute weight gain.

- **Pregnancy:** Regardless of the menstrual history given by the patient, pregnancy should be suspected in a woman of childbearing age who has unexplained weight gain.

- **Cushing's syndrome:** This is a rare cause of unexplained weight gain and can usually be diagnosed by physical exam (eg, exam may reveal hypertension, moon facies, plethora, supraclavicular fat pads, truncal obesity with thin limbs, and abdominal striae).

Diagnostic Workup

- **TSH:** To diagnose suspected hypothyroidism.

- **Serum lithium level:** To check if the patient's lithium dosage is appropriate. Lithium has a narrow therapeutic index, and serum levels should be checked every 3–6 months.

- **Fasting glucose, cholesterol, triglycerides:** To screen for medical complications of obesity such as diabetes or hyperlipidemia.

- **Urine hCG:** To rule out pregnancy.

- **Dexamethasone suppression test:** To screen for hypercortisolism. A suppressed morning cortisol following bedtime dexamethasone administration excludes Cushing's syndrome with 98% certainty.

- **24-hour urine free cortisol:** Performed if the dexamethasone suppression test is abnormal. Helps confirm hypercortisolism.

CASE 40
DOORWAY INFORMATION

Opening Scenario

The mother of Theresa Wheaton, a 6-month-old female child, calls the office complaining that her child has diarrhea.

Examinee Tasks

1. Take a focused history.

2. Explain your clinical impression and workup plan to the mother.

3. Write the patient note after leaving the room.

Checklist/SP Sheet

Patient Description

The patient's mother offers the history.

Notes for the SP

Show concern about your child's health, but add that you don't want to come to the office unless you have to because you do not have transportation.

Challenging Questions to Ask

"How sick is my baby?"

Sample Examinee Response

"It is hard for me to give you an accurate answer over the phone. I would like you to bring your baby here so that I can examine her and perhaps run some tests. After that, I should be able to give you a more accurate assessment."

Examinee Checklist

Building the Doctor-Patient Relationship

Entrance

☐ Examinee introduced self by name.

☐ Examinee identified his/her role or position.

☐ Examinee correctly used patient's name and identified caller and relationship of caller to patient.

Reflective Listening

☐ Examinee asked an open-ended question and actively listened to the response.

☐ Examinee asked the SP to list his/her concerns and listened to the response without interrupting.

☐ Examinee summarized the SP's concerns, often using the SP's own words.

Information Gathering

☐ Examinee elicited data efficiently and accurately.

☐ Examinee showed compassion for the SP and her child.

☑ Question	Patient Response
☐ Chief complaint	My baby has diarrhea.
☐ Onset	It started yesterday at 2 P.M.
☐ Progression	It is getting worse.
☐ Frequency of bowel movements	She has about 6 bowel movements per day.
☐ Description of bowel movements	Light brown, watery, large amounts.
☐ Blood in stool	No.
☐ Relationship to oral intake	None.
☐ Previous regular bowel movements	Yes.
☐ Abdominal distention	No.
☐ Appetite changes	She is not as hungry as she used to be.
☐ Activities	Not as playful as she was earlier.
☐ Awake and responsive	She is less responsive and looks drowsy.
☐ Number of wet diapers	None since yesterday.
☐ Dry mouth or sunken soft spot over the head	Yes, her mouth is dry.
☐ Treatment tried	I tried some Tylenol, but it did not help.
☐ Vigorous cry	No, her cry is weak.
☐ Recent URI	No.
☐ Fever	Yes; I took her temperature, and it was 100.5°F.
☐ Breathing fast	No.
☐ Nausea/vomiting	No.
☐ Rash	No.
☐ Shaking (seizures)	No.
☐ Cough, pulling ear, or crying when urine is passed	No.
☐ Day care center	Yes.
☐ Ill contacts in day care center	Not to my knowledge.
☐ Vaccinations	Up to date.
☐ Last checkup	Two weeks ago, and everything was normal.
☐ Birth history	It was an uncomplicated spontaneous vaginal delivery.
☐ Eating habits	Formula with iron; rice cereal at night; occasionally juice.

☑ Question	Patient Response
☐ Current medications	None.
☐ Past medical history	Nothing of note.
☐ Past surgical history	None.
☐ Family history	None.
☐ Drug allergies	None.

Connecting with the Patient

☐ Examinee recognized the SP's emotions and responded with PEARLS.

Physical Examination

None.

Closure

☐ Examinee discussed initial diagnostic impressions.

☐ Examinee discussed initial management plans:

    ☐ Follow-up tests.

☐ Examinee asked if the SP had any other questions or concerns.

Sample Closure

Ms. Wheaton, from the information you have given me, I am concerned that your child may be dehydrated. She hasn't urinated since yesterday, and she is weak and drowsy. It is very hard for me to assess her over the telephone, and I do not want to jeopardize her health in any way. For this reason, I am going to ask you to bring her in for a physical exam and a full assessment, and we will then proceed according to what we find on the exam. I understand that you may have problems with transportation, but we are fortunate to have a social worker here who can help you handle these issues. After we are done on the phone, I will transfer your call to him, and he can help you. Do you have any questions for me?

Patient Note

History

Physical Examination

Patient Note

Differential Diagnosis

Diagnosis #1

History Finding(s):	Physical Exam Finding(s):

Diagnosis #2

History Finding(s):	Physical Exam Finding(s):

Diagnosis #3

History Finding(s):	Physical Exam Finding(s):

Diagnostic Workup

Patient Note

History

HPI: *The source of information is the patient's mother. The mother of a 6-month-old F c/o her child having 1 day of diarrhea, weakness, and drowsiness. The child has had 6 watery brown bowel movements per day. There was no blood in her stool, but she has not urinated since yesterday. She received Tylenol without improvement. The mother reports the child's temperature as 100.5°F and adds that her mouth is dry. The child has no known sick contacts but is in day care. The mother denies any vomiting, lethargy, excessive sleeping, abnormal behavior, or recent URIs. The child had a normal checkup with her pediatrician 2 weeks ago and is up to date on her immunizations. She has a diet of formula with iron and rice cereal at night with occasional juice.*

ROS: *Negative.*

Allergies: *NKDA.*

Medications: *None.*

PMH: *Uncomplicated spontaneous vaginal delivery.*

PSH: *None.*

FH: *Noncontributory.*

Physical Examination

None.

Differential Diagnosis

Diagnosis #1: Viral gastroenteritis	
History Finding(s)	**Physical Exam Finding(s)**
Acute watery diarrhea	
Low-grade fever (100.5°F)	
Day care attendance	

Diagnosis #2: Bacterial diarrhea	
History Finding(s)	**Physical Exam Finding(s)**
Acute diarrhea	
Day care attendance	
Low-grade fever (100.5°F)	

Diagnosis #3: Malabsorption	
History Finding(s)	**Physical Exam Finding(s)**
Watery diarrhea	
Dry mouth	

Diagnostic Workup

Rotavirus enzyme immunoassay/norovirus PCR
Electrolytes
Stool leukocytes, culture, ova and parasitology, and pH

CASE DISCUSSION

Patient Note Differential Diagnoses

- **Viral gastroenteritis:** This is the most common cause of pediatric acute infectious diarrhea. Rotavirus was the most likely cause until the introduction of rotavirus vaccine into the routine infant immunization schedule. Viral gastroenteritis cases are now caused by other viruses (primarily norovirus).

- **Bacterial diarrhea:** The most common types of bacterial diarrhea are *Shigella, Salmonella, Campylobacter jejuni, Aeromonas,* and *Yersinia enterocolitica. E coli* and *Clostridium* species are normal intestinal flora, but pathogenic strains are capable of causing bacterial diarrhea.

- **Malabsorption:** This condition may result from a baby's consumption of juice and may be the culprit in the current patient's case. It is important to counsel parents that juice should not be introduced into the diet of babies in this age group. Some children may have milk intolerance as well. However, milk intolerance would probably not present as acutely as is seen here.

Additional Differential Diagnoses

- **UTI:** Diarrhea in infants may be a nonspecific response to an infection such as UTI or pyelonephritis.

- **Intussusception:** Given the severe nature of this disease, intussusception must be considered in the differential. The classic presentation includes abdominal pain, vomiting, and bloody ("currant jelly") stools. Some 75% of patients with intussusception have only two of these findings. Intussusception is also associated with recent viral illness and low-grade fever.

- **Bacteremia:** Bacteremia/sepsis should be ruled out in any child with high fever, drowsiness, and no urine output.

Diagnostic Workup

- **Rotavirus enzyme immunoassay/norovirus PCR:** Rotavirus can be detected through the rotavirus enzyme immunoassay. Norovirus, previously known as the Norwalk virus, can be detected through PCR amplification. Serum titers for norovirus can be positive within two weeks of initial symptoms.

- **Electrolytes:** Children with diarrhea frequently have metabolic acidosis or other electrolyte abnormalities, such as hyponatremia.

- **Stool leukocytes, culture, ova and parasitology, and pH:** WBCs in the stool would suggest an infectious etiology, and culture may reveal a bacterial pathogen. Microscopy may reveal ova or parasites such as *Giardia,* an infection that is common among day care attendees. Stool pH can distinguish a secretory from an osmotic cause of diarrhea by revealing a pH of > 6 or < 5, respectively.

- **UA:** To assess for pyelonephritis or UTI.

- **AXR:** A plain film abdominal radiograph should pick up characteristics of bowel obstruction in intussusception.

- **Blood cultures:** To rule out bacteremia.

CASE 41
DOORWAY INFORMATION

Opening Scenario

The mother of Adam Davidson, an 8-year-old male child, comes to the office concerned that her son continues to wet the bed.

Examinee Tasks

1. Take a focused history.

2. Explain your clinical impression and workup plan to the mother.

3. Write the patient note after leaving the room.

Checklist/SP Sheet

Patient Description

The patient's mother offers the history; her son is in the waiting room.

Notes for the SP

None.

Challenging Questions to Ask

- "Did I do something wrong to cause this problem?"
- "Is my child going to get better?"

Sample Examinee Response

"There are a few medical problems that can lead to your child's condition, but it's just as likely to be an isolated symptom. Bed-wetting is much more common than most people believe, and there is no reason for you or your child to feel embarrassed or guilty. There are a number of treatment options available for this condition, and after we have run a few tests to rule out any physiologic abnormalities, I will discuss them with you."

Examinee Checklist

Building the Doctor-Patient Relationship

Entrance

☐ Examinee knocked on the door before entering.

☐ Examinee introduced self by name.

☐ Examinee identified his/her role or position.

☐ Examinee correctly used patient's name.

☐ Examinee made eye contact with the SP.

Reflective Listening

☐ Examinee asked an open-ended question and actively listened to the response.

☐ Examinee asked the SP to list his/her concerns and listened to the response without interrupting.

☐ Examinee summarized the SP's concerns, often using the SP's own words.

Information Gathering

☐ Examinee elicited data efficiently and accurately.

☑ Question	Patient Response
☐ Chief complaint	My child wets his bed.
☐ Frequency	Two or three times a week.
☐ Time of day	Only at night.
☐ Onset	I guess he has always had trouble at night. I don't think he has ever gone more than a few nights without an accident.
☐ Have you tried any interventions or drugs in the past?	We ordered one of those nighttime alarms, but everyone in the house could hear it, so we didn't use it for long.
☐ How has the behavior affected the child?	He is ashamed of himself. He avoids overnight trips and sleepovers because of it.
☐ How has the behavior affected you?	It bothers me. I'm afraid he has some underlying disease or abnormality.
☐ Have you ever punished or rewarded him?	I feel irritated sometimes, but I've never punished him. I try to encourage him by rewarding him on dry nights.
☐ Alleviating/exacerbating factors	None that I can think of.
☐ Does the problem increase in times of stress?	I'm not sure, but it probably does.
☐ Late-night eating or drinking	No.
☐ Volume of urine	I don't think it's a large amount, but I'm not sure. The bed is wet all over.
☐ Dysuria	I'm not sure. Sometimes he does complain of pain.
☐ Urinary urgency	No.
☐ Fever	No.
☐ Urine color	Yellow.
☐ Hematuria	No.
☐ Abdominal pain	No.
☐ Constipation	No.
☐ Snoring	No.
☐ Nighttime awakening	No.
☐ Environmental changes related to wetting	No, I can't think of anything. We haven't moved or had any family problems.
☐ Any major stresses?	No, he does well in school and has great friends. I think the only hard thing for him is not being able to attend sleepovers.
☐ Family history of enuresis	Actually, his father had the same trouble as a kid. From my understanding, his father didn't gain full control until he was about 10 years old.

☑ Question	Patient Response
☐ Neurologic history	As far as I know, he has never had any problems of this kind.
☐ Birth history	Normal.
☐ Child weight, height, and language development	He was always on time with his development. He walked early, talked on time, and is reading at a third-grade level.
☐ Current medications	None.
☐ Past medical history	None.
☐ Past surgical history	None.
☐ Drug allergies	No.

Connecting with the Patient

☐ Examinee recognized the SP's emotions and responded with PEARLS.

Physical Examination

None.

Closure

☐ Examinee discussed initial diagnostic impressions.

☐ Examinee discussed initial management plans:

  ☐ Further examination.

  ☐ Follow-up tests.

☐ Examinee asked if the SP had any other questions or concerns.

Sample Closure

Mrs. Davidson, your son's condition is probably an isolated symptom, but I would still like to examine him and run some tests to make sure he does not have an underlying infection or a more serious medical problem. We can then discuss his treatment options. Do you have any questions for me?

Patient Note

History

Physical Examination

Differential Diagnosis

Diagnosis #1

History Finding(s):   **Physical Exam Finding(s):**

Diagnosis #2

History Finding(s):   **Physical Exam Finding(s):**

Diagnosis #3

History Finding(s):   **Physical Exam Finding(s):**

Diagnostic Workup

Patient Note

History

HPI: *The source of the information is the patient's mother. The mother of an 8 yo M c/o her child continuing to wet the bed several times a week. The child has never had a significant period of continence at night. He has no hematuria, fever, or urgency. There is possible dysuria, although the mother is not sure. The mother denies that the child c/o abdominal pain or constipation. The child does not snore or wake up multiple times during the night. There are no exacerbating factors, and there have been no major lifestyle changes or stresses in the family. The problem is causing distress for the child, who has been avoiding sleepovers, as well as for the mother, who is worried about the possibility of an underlying medical condition.*

ROS: *Negative.*
Allergies: *NKDA.*
Medications: *None.*
PMH: *None.*
PSH: *None.*
Birth history: *Normal.*
Developmental history: *Normal.*
FH: *Positive family history of male nocturnal enuresis.*

Physical Examination

None.

Differential Diagnosis

Diagnosis #1: Monosymptomatic primary nocturnal enuresis

History Finding(s)	Physical Exam Finding(s)
Chronic nocturnal enuresis	
Family history of enuresis	

Diagnosis #2: Urinary tract infection

History Finding(s)	Physical Exam Finding(s)
Enuresis	
Possible dysuria	

Diagnosis #3: Secondary enuresis

History Finding(s)	Physical Exam Finding(s)
Nocturnal enuresis	

Diagnostic Workup

Genital exam
UA
Urine culture

CASE DISCUSSION

Patient Note Differential Diagnoses

- **Monosymptomatic primary nocturnal enuresis:** This is a diagnosis of exclusion. This patient's history indicates a primary problem as opposed to a secondary one. The history and physical exam do not provide any related signs or symptoms, suggesting a monosymptomatic pathology. A urine sample must be taken to rule out infection, and old records should be evaluated to ensure that the presentation is not part of a global delay.

- **Urinary tract infection (UTI):** Enuresis may be the only symptom of UTI in children, and screening for UTI should be part of the workup for childhood enuresis. This patient does not have frequency or urgency, but urinary incontinence alone should trigger an evaluation. Additionally, according to the mother, he may have dysuria. A positive UA is presumptive of UTI, and culturing urine can establish a definitive diagnosis and direct treatment.

- **Secondary enuresis:** The patient's mother does not report a major trauma or life or environmental change such as the divorce of parents, a major illness, or abuse that might result in regression to incontinence. This diagnosis is further unlikely because the child has not been continent for any significant period.

Additional Differential Diagnoses

- **Constipation:** Infrequent or hard stools may indicate chronic constipation, which can put pressure on the urinary bladder and decrease its capacity. This may delay continence and look like a primary disorder. Physical examination can reveal impacted stool on the left side.

- **Sleep apnea:** Wetting occurs in all stages of sleep but is associated with particular disorders, such as sleep apnea and narcolepsy. This patient does not present with snoring or upper airway obstruction, and thus there is no indication of apnea that might warrant further evaluation.

- **Functional bladder disorder:** Children with functional disorders void several times a day, hold urine until the last moment, and wet small volumes almost every night, sometimes multiple times a night. This patient has normal voiding patterns during the day and remains continent a majority of nights.

Diagnostic Workup

- **Genital exam:** To evaluate for disorders such as abnormalities of the meatus, epispadias, and phimosis.

- **UA:** To evaluate for a UTI. Clear urine, a negative dipstick, and a negative microscopic examination combined have a negative predictive value between 95% and 98%.

- **Urine culture:** The only 100% specific test for UTI.

- **First-morning urine specific gravity:** To evaluate for insufficient ADH levels as the cause of the patient's nocturnal enuresis. An early-morning urine concentration of < 1.015 may indicate a lack of nighttime and early-morning ADH surges, which may predict a positive response to pharmacologic therapy with DDAVP.

- **U/S—renal:** Should be pursued if bed-wetting continues with multiple treatments, abnormal voiding patterns, or recurrent UTIs confirmed by UA and urine culture.

- **BUN/Cr:** Should be obtained before renal ultrasound to evaluate renal function. To avoid unnecessary blood draws in children, blood for BUN/Cr testing should not be drawn until results from a urine sample are obtained.

CASE 42
DOORWAY INFORMATION

Opening Scenario

The mother of Michaela Weber, an 11-month-old female child, comes to the emergency department after her daughter has a seizure.

Examinee Tasks

1. Take a focused history.

2. Explain your clinical impression and workup plan to the mother.

3. Write the patient note after leaving the room.

Checklist/SP Sheet

Patient Description

The patient's mother offers the history; she is a good historian.

Notes for the SP

Express anxiety about your daughter's condition.

Challenging Questions to Ask

"Is my child going to have permanent brain damage from this?"

Sample Examinee Response

"The most likely explanation for your daughter's seizure is her fever, in which case there should be no permanent damage. There are some causes of seizures that are more serious, though. We will run all the necessary tests to make sure one of those is not the cause."

Examinee Checklist

Building the Doctor-Patient Relationship

Entrance

☐ Examinee knocked on the door before entering.

☐ Examinee introduced self by name.

☐ Examinee identified his/her role or position.

☐ Examinee correctly used patient's name.

☐ Examinee made eye contact with the SP.

Reflective Listening

☐ Examinee asked an open-ended question and actively listened to the response.

☐ Examinee asked the SP to list his/her concerns and listened to the response without interrupting.

☐ Examinee summarized the SP's concerns, often using the SP's own words.

Information Gathering

☐ Examinee elicited data efficiently and accurately.

☑ Question	Patient Response
☐ Chief complaint	My child had a seizure.
☐ Onset	This morning at 11 A.M.
☐ Description of event	We were laying her down for her nap and her body just started shaking.
☐ Duration	It lasted about a minute total.
☐ Postictal symptoms	She seemed sleepy afterward.
☐ Tongue/head trauma	No.
☐ Has this happened before?	No.
☐ Whole-body shaking	Yes.
☐ Family history of seizures	None.
☐ Recent illness	Yes, she has had a temperature and runny nose the past 2 days.
☐ Fevers/chills	Her temperature was 102.9°F last night; she hasn't had any chills.
☐ Rash	No.
☐ Medication for fever	I gave her some Children's Tylenol last night—it helped a little. I didn't take her temperature again, but her forehead still felt hot.
☐ Ear tugging	No.
☐ Nausea/vomiting	No.
☐ Change in bowel habits or in stool color or consistency	No.
☐ Change in urinary habits or in urine smell or color; change in number of wet diapers	Fewer wet diapers than usual.
☐ Appetite changes	She has had Pedialyte and some breast milk but not much else.
☐ Appearance/demeanor (lethargic, irritated, playful, etc.)	She has been more fussy the past couple days, but consolable.
☐ Ill contacts	No.
☐ Day care center	No.
☐ Home environment	She lives with me, my husband, and her 3-year-old brother.
☐ Vaccinations	Up to date.
☐ Last checkup	Two months ago for 9-month checkup.
☐ Birth history	A 38-week vaginal delivery with no complications.
☐ Weight, height, and language development	Normal.

☑ Question	Patient Response
☐ Eating habits	She is breast-fed and eats some table food but hasn't been eating the table food the past couple of days. She takes iron supplements that our pediatrician gave us.
☐ Sleeping habits	She has not slept well the past 3 nights.
☐ Current medications	Just the Tylenol.
☐ Past medical history	None.
☐ Past surgical history	None.
☐ Drug allergies	No.

Connecting with the Patient

☐ Examinee recognized the SP's emotions and responded with PEARLS.

Physical Examination

None.

Closure

☐ Examinee discussed initial diagnostic impressions.

☐ Examinee discussed initial management plans:

   ☐ Follow-up tests.

☐ Examinee asked if the SP had any other questions or concerns.

Sample Closure

Mrs. Weber, it sounds as though your child has indeed had a seizure. The most likely cause is her high fevers; seizures caused by fevers happen in many young children. However, because there are many types of seizures, I would like to examine your child and also do some tests to make sure that the seizures are not being caused by something more serious, like meningitis. Do you have any questions for me?

Patient Note

History
_____
_____
_____
_____
_____
_____
_____
_____
_____
_____
_____
_____
_____
_____
_____
_____
_____

Physical Examination
_____
_____
_____
_____
_____
_____
_____
_____
_____
_____
_____
_____

Patient Note

Differential Diagnosis

Diagnosis #1

History Finding(s):   **Physical Exam Finding(s):**

Diagnosis #2

History Finding(s):   **Physical Exam Finding(s):**

Diagnosis #3

History Finding(s):   **Physical Exam Finding(s):**

Diagnostic Workup

Patient Note

History

HPI: *The source of information is the patient's mother. Patient is an 11-month-old F with a tonic-clonic seizure.*

- *Witnessed this A.M. by parents, lasted approx. 1 minute.*
- *No tongue or body trauma.*
- *Postictal drowsiness noted.*
- *No history of prior seizures.*
- *Patient has had rhinorrhea for past 2 days, fevers to 102.9°F with decreased PO intake, difficulty sleeping, and fewer wet diapers.*
- *No rash, nausea/vomiting, lethargy, or inconsolability.*
- *No sick contacts.*

ROS: *Negative except as above.*
Allergies: *NKDA.*
Medications: *Tylenol.*
PMH/PSH: *None.*
Birth history: *Term uncomplicated vaginal delivery.*
Dietary history: *Breast milk, table foods, and supplemental vitamins.*
Immunization history: *Up to date.*
Developmental history: *Last checkup was 2 months ago and showed normal weight, height, and development.*

Physical Examination

None.

Differential Diagnosis

Diagnosis #1: Simple febrile seizure	
History Finding(s)	**Physical Exam Finding(s)**
Seizure duration < 15 minutes	
No prior history of seizures	
Fever (T_{max} 102.9°F)	

Diagnosis #2: Meningitis	
History Finding(s)	**Physical Exam Finding(s)**
Tonic-clonic seizure	
Fever (T_{max} 102.9°F)	
Decreased appetite	
Decreased urine output	

Diagnosis #3: Hyponatremia	
History Finding(s)	**Physical Exam Finding(s)**
Seizure	

Diagnostic Workup

LP—CSF analysis
CBC
Electrolytes

CASE DISCUSSION

Patient Note Differential Diagnoses

- **Simple febrile seizure:** The most frequent cause of an isolated seizure in a child with a common febrile illness is a febrile seizure. These tend to be familial and may recur with subsequent febrile illnesses but disappear before adulthood. They do not require treatment and do not cause permanent neurologic damage.

- **Meningitis:** In children younger than one year of age, meningitis findings can often be limited to fever and clinical symptoms. The infant might be irritable but is usually easily consolable. Viral meningitis is common in infants and could be likely in this patient considering the baby's poor appetite, high fever, and decreased urine output. A seizure suggests neurologic involvement, and the most important cause to rule out is meningitis.

- **Hyponatremia:** Hyponatremia from various causes can result in pediatric seizures; the classic case occurs when a poor family waters down their infant's formula. There are also congenital causes of hyponatremia, such as congenital adrenal hyperplasia. The occurrence in the setting of fever makes this less likely than the infectious causes.

Additional Differential Diagnoses

- **UTI:** Decreased urine output is not likely secondary to a UTI in this patient. However, given the patient's high fever and gender, a UTI with subsequent pyelonephritis or bacteremia is a possibility.

- **Occult bacteremia:** This child has a fever > 102°F (38.9°C) and no clear source of infection. Bacteremia and sepsis may present in this manner in children younger than one year of age; the incidence is highest in neonates and decreases with age.

Diagnostic Workup

- **LP—CSF analysis:** A fever with seizures may be benign, or it may suggest meningitis. A lumbar puncture is the most definitive test with which to diagnose or rule out meningitis. It allows CSF analysis of cell count and differentials, glucose, protein, Gram stain, culture, viral cultures and PCR, and opening pressure.

- **CBC, electrolytes:** To test for hyponatremia caused by any source. Potassium and glucose levels help in assessing adrenal function. A WBC count > 15,000/μL might be suggestive of occult bacteremia.

- **Blood culture, UA and urine culture:** These tests constitute the sepsis or occult bacteremia workup in children with unexplained high fever. UTI may be occult and must be investigated.

- **CT—head:** Used mainly to rule out brain abscess, encephalitis, or hemorrhage.

- **Electroencephalogram (EEG):** Used to identify epileptiform activity, although a single febrile seizure does not warrant an EEG.

CASE 43
DOORWAY INFORMATION

Opening Scenario

Brian Davis, a 21-year-old male, comes to the office complaining of a sore throat.

Vital Signs

BP: 120/80 mm Hg

Temp: 99.5°F (37.5°C)

RR: 15/minute

HR: 75/minute, regular

Examinee Tasks

1. Take a focused history.
2. Perform a focused physical exam (do not perform rectal, genitourinary, or female breast exam).
3. Explain your clinical impression and workup plan to the patient.
4. Write the patient note after leaving the room.

Checklist/SP Sheet

Patient Description

Patient is a 21 yo M.

Notes for the SP

- Be rude and defensive.
- Make most of your answers a curt "yes" or "no."
- Pretend that you have LUQ tenderness on abdominal palpation.

Challenging Questions to Ask

"Do you think I have AIDS?"

Sample Examinee Response

"What makes you think you might have AIDS? Do you believe that you have been exposed to HIV? It is a possibility, but I will not be able to tell until I have ordered some blood tests."

Examinee Checklist

Building the Doctor-Patient Relationship

Entrance

☐ Examinee knocked on the door before entering.

☐ Examinee introduced self by name.

☐ Examinee identified his/her role or position.

☐ Examinee correctly used patient's name.

☐ Examinee made eye contact with the SP.

Reflective Listening

☐ Examinee asked an open-ended question and actively listened to the response.

☐ Examinee asked the SP to list his/her concerns and listened to the response without interrupting.

☐ Examinee summarized the SP's concerns, often using the SP's own words.

Information Gathering

☐ Examinee elicited data efficiently and accurately.

☑ Question	Patient Response
☐ Chief complaint	Sore throat.
☐ Onset	Two weeks ago.
☐ Runny nose	No.
☐ Fever/chills	Mild fever over the past 2 weeks, but I didn't take my temperature. No chills.
☐ Night sweats	No.
☐ Cough	No.
☐ Swollen glands and lymph nodes	Yes, in my neck (if asked); a little painful (if asked).
☐ Rash before or after onset of symptoms	No.
☐ Jaundice	No.
☐ Chest pain	No.
☐ Shortness of breath	No.
☐ Abdominal pain	I've had some discomfort here (points to the LUQ) constantly since yesterday.
☐ Radiation	No.
☐ Severity on a scale	4/10.
☐ Relationship of food to pain	No.
☐ Alleviating/exacerbating factors	None.
☐ Nausea/vomiting	No.
☐ Change in bowel habits	No.
☐ Change in urinary habits	No.
☐ Headache	No.
☐ Fatigue	I have been feeling tired for the past 2 weeks.
☐ Ill contacts	My ex-girlfriend had the same thing 2 months ago. I don't know what happened to her because we broke up around that time.
☐ Weight changes	Yes, I feel that I am losing weight, but I don't know how much.

✓ Question	Patient Response
☐ Appetite changes	I don't feel like eating anything at all.
☐ Current medications	Tylenol.
☐ Past medical history	I had gonorrhea 4 months ago. I took some antibiotics.
☐ Past surgical history	None.
☐ Family history	My father and mother are alive and in good health.
☐ Occupation	Last year in college.
☐ Alcohol use	Yes, on the weekends.
☐ Illicit drug use	No.
☐ Tobacco	Yes, I smoke a pack a day. I started when I was 15 years old.
☐ Sexual activity	I have a new girlfriend.
☐ Use of condoms	Yes.
☐ Active with men, women, or both	Men and women.
☐ Number of sexual partners during the past year	Two.
☐ History of STDs	I told you, I had gonorrhea 4 months ago, and I was cured after a course of antibiotics.
☐ Drug allergies	No.

Connecting with the Patient

☐ Examinee recognized the SP's emotions and responded with PEARLS.

Physical Examination

☐ Examinee washed his/her hands.

☐ Examinee asked permission to start the exam.

☐ Examinee used respectful draping.

☐ Examinee did not repeat painful maneuvers.

✓ Exam Component	Maneuver
☐ Head and neck exam	Examined nose, mouth, throat, lymph nodes; checked for sinus tenderness
☐ CV exam	Auscultation
☐ Pulmonary exam	Auscultation
☐ Abdominal exam	Auscultation, palpation, percussion
☐ Skin/lymph node exam	Inspected for rashes, lesions, lymphadenopathy

Closure

☐ Examinee discussed initial diagnostic impressions.

☐ Examinee discussed initial management plans:

    ☐ Follow-up tests (including consent for HIV testing).

    ☐ Safe sex practices.

    ☐ Help with smoking cessation.

    ☐ Recommendation to avoid contact sports because of the possible increased risk of traumatic splenic rupture.

☐ Examinee asked if the SP had any other questions or concerns.

Sample Closure

Mr. Davis, it is likely that you have acquired the same infection your girlfriend had. This may be no more than a transient viral infection, or it may represent a more serious illness such as HIV. We will need to run a few tests to help us make the diagnosis. I recommend that we obtain an HIV test, and we will also need to obtain a throat swab and an ultrasound of your abdomen. In the meantime, I strongly recommend using condoms to avoid an unwanted pregnancy and to prevent STDs. Since infectious mononucleosis is one of the diseases that might account for your symptoms, I also recommend that you avoid contact sports for at least 3 weeks because of the possible risk of traumatic rupture of your spleen, which could be fatal. Also, since cigarette smoking is associated with a variety of diseases, I advise you to quit smoking; we have many ways to help you if you are interested. Do you have any questions for me?

Patient Note

History

Physical Examination

Differential Diagnosis

Diagnosis #1

History Finding(s):   Physical Exam Finding(s):

Diagnosis #2

History Finding(s):   Physical Exam Finding(s):

Diagnosis #3

History Finding(s):   Physical Exam Finding(s):

Diagnostic Workup

Patient Note

History

HPI: *21 yo M c/o sore throat for the past 2 weeks. Two weeks ago he had a mild fever and fatigue, but he denies any chills, runny nose, cough, night sweats, shortness of breath, or wheezing. The patient also notes LUQ abdominal pain since yesterday. The pain is 4/10 and constant with no radiation, no relation to food, and no alleviating or exacerbating factors. He has poor appetite and subjective weight loss. His ex-girlfriend had the same symptoms 2 months ago.*

ROS: *Negative except as above.*

Allergies: *NKDA.*

Medications: *Tylenol.*

PMH: *Gonorrhea 4 months ago, treated with antibiotics.*

PSH: *None.*

SH: *1 PPD since age 15; drinks heavily on weekends. Multiple female and male partners; uses condoms.*

FH: *Noncontributory.*

Physical Examination

Patient is in no acute distress.

VS: *WNL.*

HEENT: *Nose, mouth, and pharynx WNL.*

Neck: *Supple, bilateral cervical lymphadenopathy.*

Chest: *Clear breath sounds bilaterally.*

Heart: *RRR; normal S1/S2; no murmurs, rubs, or gallops.*

Abdomen: *Soft, nondistended, ⊕ BS, no hepatosplenomegaly, mild LUQ tenderness on palpation.*

Skin: *No rash.*

Differential Diagnosis

Diagnosis #1: Infectious mononucleosis	
History Finding(s):	**Physical Exam Finding(s):**
Sore throat for 2 weeks	LUQ tenderness
LUQ pain	Lymphadenopathy
Recent history of ill contact	

Diagnosis #2: Acute HIV infection	
History Finding(s):	**Physical Exam Finding(s):**
Sore throat for 2 weeks	
Two sexual partners over past year, active with men and women	
Treated for gonorrhea 4 months ago	

Diagnosis #3: Streptococcal pharyngitis

History Finding(s):	Physical Exam Finding(s):
Sore throat for 2 weeks	Lymphadenopathy
Low-grade fever	
History of cigarette smoking	

Diagnostic Workup

CBC with peripheral smear
Monospot test
Anti-EBV antibodies
HIV antibody and viral load
Throat culture

CASE DISCUSSION

Patient Note Differential Diagnoses

- **Infectious mononucleosis:** The differential diagnosis for "sore throat" includes many pathogens. This patient's LUQ pain suggests splenomegaly, which could limit the differential (for a unifying diagnosis) to an infectious mononucleosis caused by EBV or, less commonly, by CMV infection. The physical exam is notoriously insensitive for detecting splenomegaly and may be misleading, as in this case. This patient also presents with cervical lymphadenopathy, a typical feature of infectious mononucleosis. However, he does not exhibit exudative pharyngitis, another feature with which infectious mononucleosis is commonly associated.

- **Acute HIV infection:** Acute HIV infection can be associated with fever, lymphadenopathy, sore throat, and a generalized maculopapular rash. This stage of disease typically occurs within one month of exposure to the virus and can last up to several weeks. Symptoms eventually resolve on their own.

- **Group A streptococcal pharyngitis:** Clinical features in patients with sore throat that predict group A streptococcal pharyngitis include tonsillar exudates, tender anterior cervical lymphadenopathy, a history of fever (temperature > 100.4°F/38°C), and absence of cough. "Strep throat" must be recognized and treated to prevent acute rheumatic fever.

Additional Differential Diagnoses

- **CMV infection:** CMV can mimic infectious mononucleosis or acute HIV infection. Patients can present with mild flulike symptoms, including fever, lymphadenopathy, and fatigue. However, patients may also be asymptomatic, requiring a high index of suspicion for clinical testing.

- **Other infectious etiologies:** Other infections that can present with nonspecific symptoms include *Neisseria gonorrhoeae*, *Mycoplasma* (although lower respiratory symptoms usually predominate), rubella, and *Chlamydia trachomatis*.

Diagnostic Workup

- **CBC:** Findings are nonspecific, but leukocytosis may be seen in bacterial infection, and a lymphocytosis may be seen in viral infection.

- **Peripheral smear:** Can reveal atypical lymphocytes in infectious mononucleosis.

- **Monospot test (heterophil agglutination test):** Usually becomes positive in EBV-associated mononucleosis within four weeks of onset of illness.

- **Anti-EBV antibodies:** Antibodies to various EBV antigens can be detected, such as IgM antibody to viral capsid antigen (VCA) and to nuclear antigen (EBNA). There is also a PCR to detect EBV in serum.

- **HIV antibody and viral load:** Check antibody via ELISA and Western blot to exclude preexisting HIV infection, and check viral load to document acute infection.

- **Throat culture:** The gold standard for diagnosing bacterial pharyngitis.

- **Rapid streptococcal antigen:** Has high negative predictive value (ie, it can accurately confirm the absence of group A streptococcal pharyngitis).

- **CMV antibody titers/CMV PCR:** To check for CMV infection.

Opening Scenario

Jay Keller, a 49-year-old male, comes to the ED complaining of passing out a few hours earlier.

Vital Signs

BP: 135/85 mm Hg

Temp: 98.0°F (36.7°C)

RR: 16/minute

HR: 76/minute, regular

Examinee Tasks

1. Take a focused history.

2. Perform a focused physical exam (do not perform rectal, genitourinary, or female breast exam).

3. Explain your clinical impression and workup plan to the patient.

4. Write the patient note after leaving the room.

Checklist/SP Sheet

Patient Description

Patient is a 49 yo M, married with 3 children.

Notes for the SP

None.

Challenging Questions to Ask

"Do you think I have a brain tumor?"

Sample Examinee Response

"I think it's unlikely. To make absolutely sure, however, we will do a CT scan, which is a special imaging study of the brain. That will help us see the structure of the brain and rule out any bleeding or tumor."

Examinee Checklist

Building the Doctor-Patient Relationship

Entrance

☐ Examinee knocked on the door before entering.

☐ Examinee introduced self by name.

☐ Examinee identified his/her role or position.

☐ Examinee correctly used patient's name.

☐ Examinee made eye contact with the SP.

Reflective Listening

☐ Examinee asked an open-ended question and actively listened to the response.

☐ Examinee asked the SP to list his/her concerns and listened to the response without interrupting.

☐ Examinee summarized the SP's concerns, often using the SP's own words.

Information Gathering

☐ Examinee elicited data efficiently and accurately.

☑ Question	Patient Response
☐ Chief complaint	I passed out.
☐ Describe what happened	This morning I was taking the groceries to the car with my wife when I suddenly fell down and blacked out.
☐ Loss of consciousness before, during, or after the fall	I think I lost consciousness and then fell down on the ground.
☐ Duration of loss of consciousness	My wife told me that I did not respond to her for several minutes.
☐ Palpitations before the fall	Yes, just before I fell down, my heart started racing.
☐ Sensing something unusual before losing consciousness (sounds, lights, smells, etc.)	No.
☐ Spinning/lightheadedness	I felt lightheaded right before the fall.
☐ Shaking (seizure)	Yes, my wife told me that my arms and legs started shaking after I fell down.
☐ Duration of shaking	She said around 30 seconds.
☐ Bit tongue	No.
☐ Lost control of the bladder	No.
☐ Weakness/numbness	No.
☐ Speech difficulties	No.
☐ Confusion after regaining consciousness	No.
☐ Headaches	No.
☐ Chest pain, shortness of breath	No.
☐ Abdominal pain, nausea/vomiting, diarrhea/constipation	No.
☐ Head trauma	No.
☐ Similar falls, lightheadedness, or passing out before	No.
☐ Gait abnormality	No.
☐ Weight changes	No.

☑ Question	Patient Response
☐ Appetite changes	No.
☐ Current medications	Hydrochlorothiazide, captopril, aspirin, atenolol.
☐ Past medical history	High blood pressure for the past 15 years; heart attack 1 year ago.
☐ Past surgical history	Appendectomy.
☐ Family history	My father died from a heart attack at age 55, and my mother died in good health.
☐ Occupation	Clerk in a video store.
☐ Alcohol use	Yes, I drink 3–4 beers a week.
☐ CAGE questions	No (to all 4).
☐ Illicit drug use	No.
☐ Tobacco	No, I stopped a year ago. I had smoked a pack a day for the previous 25 years.
☐ Sexual activity	Yes, with my wife.
☐ Drug allergies	No.

Connecting with the Patient

☐ Examinee recognized the SP's emotions and responded with PEARLS.

Physical Examination

☐ Examinee washed his/her hands.

☐ Examinee asked permission to start the exam.

☐ Examinee used respectful draping.

☐ Examinee did not repeat painful maneuvers.

☑ Exam Component	Maneuver
☐ Head and neck exam	Inspection (head, mouth), carotid auscultation and palpation, thyroid exam
☐ CV exam	Palpation, auscultation, orthostatic vital signs
☐ Pulmonary exam	Auscultation
☐ Extremities	Palpated peripheral pulses
☐ Neurologic exam	Mental status, cranial nerves (including funduscopic exam), motor exam, DTRs, cerebellar, Romberg test, gait, sensory exam

Closure

☐ Examinee discussed initial diagnostic impressions.

☐ Examinee discussed initial management plans:

   ☐ Follow-up tests.

☐ Examinee asked if the SP had any other questions or concerns.

Sample Closure

Mr. Keller, I need to run some tests to determine the reason you passed out this morning, so I am going to get a CT scan of your head to look for bleeding or masses, and I will then order some blood tests to look for infections or electrolyte abnormalities. You mentioned that your heart was racing just before you passed out, so I will also ask you to wear a heart monitor for 24 hours. Doing so is just like having a constant ECG, and it will allow us to detect any abnormal heartbeats you might have. We will start with these tests and then go from there. Do you have any questions for me?

Patient Note

History

_____
_____
_____
_____
_____
_____
_____
_____
_____
_____
_____
_____
_____
_____
_____
_____
_____
_____
_____

Physical Examination

_____
_____
_____
_____
_____
_____
_____
_____
_____
_____
_____
_____
_____
_____
_____

Patient Note

Differential Diagnosis

Diagnosis #1

History Finding(s):   *Physical Exam Finding(s):*

Diagnosis #2

History Finding(s):   *Physical Exam Finding(s):*

Diagnosis #3

History Finding(s):   *Physical Exam Finding(s):*

Diagnostic Workup

History

HPI: *49 yo M c/o 1 episode of syncope that occurred a few hours ago. He was taking the groceries to the car with his wife when he suddenly felt lightheaded, had palpitations, lost consciousness, and fell down. He was unconscious for several minutes. His wife recalls that his arms and legs started shaking for 30 seconds after he fell down. He denies subsequent confusion, weakness or numbness, speech difficulties, tongue biting, or incontinence.*

ROS: *Negative except as above.*
Allergies: *NKDA.*
Medications: *HCTZ, captopril, aspirin, atenolol.*
PMH: *Hypertension for the past 15 years; MI 1 year ago.*
PSH: *Appendectomy.*
SH: *1 PPD for 25 years; quit smoking 1 year ago. Drinks 3–4 beers/week, CAGE 0/4, no illicit drugs.*
FH: *Father died from an MI at age 55.*

Physical Examination

Patient is in no acute distress.

VS: *WNL, no orthostatic changes.*
HEENT: *NC/AT, PERRLA, no funduscopic abnormalities, no tongue trauma.*
Neck: *Supple, no carotid bruits, 2+ carotid pulses with good upstroke bilaterally, thyroid normal.*
Chest: *Clear breath sounds bilaterally.*
Heart: *Apical impulse not displaced; RRR; normal S1/S2; no murmurs, rubs, or gallops.*
Extremities: *Symmetric 2+ brachial, radial, and dorsalis pedis pulses bilaterally.*
Neuro: *Cranial nerves: 2–12 grossly intact. Motor: Strength 5/5 throughout. Sensation: Intact to pinprick and soft touch bilaterally. DTRs: Symmetric 2+ in upper and lower extremities, ⊖ Babinski bilaterally. Cerebellar: Romberg, finger to nose normal. Gait: Normal.*

Differential Diagnosis

Diagnosis #1: Convulsive syncope	
History Finding(s):	**Physical Exam Finding(s):**
Loss of consciousness lasting several minutes	
Arms and legs shaking for 30 seconds	
No subsequent confusion or weakness	

Patient Note

Diagnosis #2: Cardiac arrhythmia

History Finding(s):	Physical Exam Finding(s):
Loss of consciousness preceded by palpitations and lightheadedness	
Taking a β-blocker (atenolol)	
No subsequent confusion or weakness	
History of MI	

Diagnosis #3: Seizure

History Finding(s):	Physical Exam Finding(s):
Loss of consciousness lasting several minutes	
Arms and legs shaking for 30 seconds	
Sudden onset	

Diagnostic Workup

CBC
Electrolytes
ECG and Holter or event monitor
CT—head or MRI—brain
EEG

CASE DISCUSSION

Patient Note Differential Diagnoses

- **Convulsive syncope:** Seizure-like activity often occurs after syncope and is due to global cerebral hypoperfusion. There is no EEG correlate, and a seizure workup is not required.

- **Cardiac arrhythmia:** Cardiac syncope typically occurs without warning, although a history of palpitations may indicate the presence of an underlying arrhythmia. This patient's history of MI increases his risk of developing ventricular tachycardia, and β-blocker therapy may contribute to bradyarrhythmia.

- **Seizure:** Seizures usually occur unpredictably in a manner unrelated to posture or exertion. They may stem from a variety of causes, including metabolic factors, trauma, vascular factors, and brain tumors. Tonic-clonic seizures are often accompanied by tongue biting, incontinence, and prolonged confusion or drowsiness postictally.

Additional Differential Diagnoses

- **Vasovagal syncope:** This often occurs in the setting of emotional stress or pain and may be due to excessive vagal tone with resulting hypotension. Syncope is often heralded by nausea, sweating, tachycardia, pallor, and feeling "faint." This is also the mechanism of syncope in postmicturition syncope.

- **Drug-induced orthostatic hypotension:** The patient's antihypertensive medications increase his risk for orthostatic hypotension and syncope. However, lightheadedness and syncope in this condition are usually postural (ie, they occur when getting up from a lying or seated position), and this patient's orthostatic vital signs were normal.

- **Aortic stenosis:** This and other mechanical causes (eg, hypertrophic obstructive cardiomyopathy, atrial myxoma) are commonly exertional or postexertional and occur without warning. The lack of a murmur and other physical findings makes this unlikely in this case.

Diagnostic Workup

- **CBC, electrolytes:** To rule out anemia, evidence of hyperviscosity, or electrolyte imbalance that could lead to arrhythmia or other causes of syncope.

- **ECG and Holter or event monitor:** To evaluate possible arrhythmia.

- **CT—head:** The test of choice to exclude intracranial hemorrhage. Also rules out tumor, trauma, prior stroke, or abscess.

- **MRI—brain:** Provides better anatomic detail than CT. Indicated when focal neurologic signs and symptoms are present. MRA is helpful when vertebrobasilar insufficiency is suspected (ie, when syncope is accompanied by other brain stem signs).

- **EEG:** To evaluate suspected seizure activity.

- **Echocardiography:** To rule out mechanical causes of syncope (eg, severe aortic stenosis, atrial myxoma, severe LVH with small residual cavity size, and hypertrophic obstructive cardiomyopathy).

- **CXR:** To rule out lung mass, cardiomyopathy, or other pathology.

- **Prolactin:** Often elevated within 30–60 minutes of a generalized seizure (it is useless after that time interval). Must be compared to baseline prolactin levels.

Top-Rated Review Resources

HOW TO USE THE DATABASE

This section is a database of recommended clinical science review books, sample examination books, and commercial review courses marketed to medical students studying for the USMLE Step 2 CS. For each book, we list the **Title** of the book, the **First Author** (or editor), the **Current Publisher**, the **Copyright Year**, the **Edition**, the **Number of Pages**, the **ISBN Code**, the **Approximate List Price**, and the **Format** of the book. Most entries also include **Summary Comments** that describe their style and utility for studying. Finally, each book receives a **Rating.**

The rating scale is composed of six letter grades that reflect the detailed student evaluations. Each book receives one of the following ratings:

A+	Excellent for boards review.
A	
A–	Very good for boards review; choose among the group.
B+	
B	Good, but use only after exhausting better sources.
B–	

The **Rating** is meant to reflect the overall usefulness of the book in preparing for the USMLE Step 2 CS examination. This is based on a number of factors, including the following:

- The cost of the book
- The readability of the text
- The appropriateness and accuracy of the book
- The quality and number of sample questions
- The quality of written answers to sample questions
- The quality and appropriateness of the illustrations (eg, graphs, diagrams, photographs)
- The length of the text (longer is not necessarily better)
- The quality and number of other books available in the same discipline
- The importance of the discipline on the USMLE Step 2 CS examination

Please note that **the rating does not reflect the quality of the book for purposes other than reviewing for the USMLE Step 2 CS exam.** Many books with low ratings are well written and informative but are not ideal for board preparation. We have also avoided listing or commenting on the wide variety of general textbooks available in the clinical sciences.

Evaluations are based on the cumulative results of formal and informal surveys of hundreds of medical students from medical schools across the country. The summary comments and overall ratings represent a consensus opinion, but there may have been a large range of opinions or limited student feedback on any particular book.

Please note that the data listed are subject to change because:

- Publishers' prices change frequently.
- Individual bookstores often charge an additional markup.
- New editions come out frequently, and the quality of updating varies.
- The same book may be reissued through another publisher.

We actively encourage medical students and faculty to submit their opinions and ratings of the clinical science review books listed here so that we may update our database (see "How to Contribute," p. xvii). In addition, we ask that publishers and authors submit review copies of clinical science review books, including new editions and books not included in our database, for evaluation. We also solicit reviews of new books or suggestions for alternate modes of study that may be useful in preparing for the examination, such as flash cards, computer-based tutorials, commercial review courses, and Internet Web sites.

Disclaimer/Conflict of Interest Statement

None of the material in this book, including the ratings, reflects the opinion or influence of the publisher. All errors and omissions will gladly be corrected if brought to the attention of the authors through the publisher.

A

USMLE Step 2 CS Core Cases
$40.00   Review

BROTTMAN

Kaplan, 2013, 408 pages, 3rd edition, ISBN 9781609788896

A review book of case-by-case presentations.

Pros: Features an introductory section on appropriate phraseology for the exam and how best to interact with patients. Also includes 43 cases that cover a variety of specialties. This edition also offers information and tips regarding note writing.

Cons: Some reviewers felt that cases were too simple and lacking in detailed differential diagnoses.

Summary: A great review book with a variety of clinical cases and updated information about note writing.

B+

USMLE Step 2 Clinical Skills Triage
$39.95   Review

SCHWECHTEN

Oxford University Press, 2010, 268 pages, 1st edition, ISBN 9780195398236

An organized case-by-case presentation of patient encounters.

Pros: Offers 40 cases that simulate actual examination scenarios covering the most common complaints and diagnoses, including telephone encounters and difficult conversations. Information is organized linearly into "Symptoms," "Diagnosis," and "Treatment" sections and is then summarized by "Take Home Points." Cases are written with sample dialogue that simulates appropriate doctor-patient communication. Includes integrated tables and figures plus 100 full-color images that help clarify and organize information.

Cons: Some readers may find that cases are not sufficiently detailed. The format of the practice cases does not facilitate practice with a partner. Content has not been updated to reflect recent changes to the exam and patient note format.

Summary: A succinct but thorough review of the most common clinical conditions.

B

NMS Review for the USMLE Clinical Skills Exam
$44.95   Review

ARIAS

Lippincott Williams & Wilkins, 2007, 296 pages, 2nd edition, ISBN 9780781766937

A sleek review book presented in a non-workbook format.

Pros: Provides extensive coverage of physical exam techniques and signs/symptoms, and includes a wealth of basic science information. Chapters devoted to the physical exam and note writing cover OB/GYN, neurology, psychology, pediatrics, and trauma medicine. Also features 91 review cases covering internal medicine and family practice, surgery and orthopedics, OB/GYN, the nervous system, pediatric and phone medicine, and trauma medicine.

Cons: Some of the material may not be sufficiently high yield for the Step 2 CS exam. Cases are compressed into a one-page format with a written patient note, a differential diagnosis, a diagnostic workup plan, and a short paragraph on clinical correlation. Some readers may find that the information provided is too general and lacking in specific details about what is needed for the exam. Content has not been updated to reflect recent changes to the exam and patient note format.

Summary: A good book for both Step 2 CS and Step 2 CK preparation that provides a large number of concise cases. However, the text does not provide a step-by-step approach to the patient exam or patient note.

B Core Concepts for USMLE Step 2 CS: A Focused and Goal-Oriented Approach

$44.95 Review

SHARMA

CreateSpace, 2010, 380 pages, 1st edition, ISBN 9781453608043

A thorough text that reviews core clinical concepts in the context of the Step 2 CS exam.

Pros: Features 61 common clinical cases described in detail. Incorporates solid clinical skills for evaluating a patient in preparation for the Step 2 CS exam. The text thoroughly explains the expectations of standardized patients and examiners so that test takers are better prepared, which is especially useful for IMGs. Also includes specific exam elements such as ethical dilemmas, counseling, and phone interviews.

Cons: If you are not used to the integrated format of the content, you may not find this text appropriate. Some found the suggested interview questions and the differential diagnoses inadequate. The format of the practice cases makes it challenging to practice with a partner. Content has not been updated to reflect recent changes to the exam and patient note format.

Summary: A clear and thorough concept-oriented review book that is useful for all Step 2 CS test takers.

B The Ultimate Guide and Review for the USMLE Step 2 Clinical Skills Exam

$39.95 Review

SWARTZ

Elsevier, 2006, 402 pages, 1st edition, ISBN 9781416037279

A large workbook-style review text.

Pros: Easy to read and printed in a large point size. Includes a detailed chapter outlining the basics of the exam. Approximately 20 pages are devoted to communication skills, and an additional 10 pages are devoted to a guide to U.S. culture. A standardized patient grading checklist is included with each case.

Cons: Because the workbook format takes up a significant amount of space, only 30 review cases are provided. Content has not been updated to reflect recent changes to the exam and patient note format.

Summary: May be best suited to examinees who seek practice documenting checklists and patient notes. The lengthy sections on communication skills and U.S. culture make it more suitable for IMGs. Those who seek a quick review might be better served by a more concise text.

B⁻

CS Checklists: Portable Review for the USMLE Step 2 CS
ROONEY

$34.95   Review

McGraw-Hill, 2007, 348 pages, 2nd edition, ISBN 9780071488235

A pocket-sized text presented in workbook format.

Pros: Provides detailed descriptions of the components of a complete health history, physical exam, and patient note write-up, presented in bullet-point format. Also features 55 cases organized by chief complaint along with a brief paragraph on history. A patient history checklist, a physical exam checklist, and physical exam findings are provided as well. One-page "answers" listed at the end of the book include a differential diagnosis, an appropriate workup, and a brief paragraph on clinical correlation. Also features a case index with diagnoses and corresponding page numbers.

Cons: Offers limited general information on the physical exam and on how to perform and interpret exam findings, and the formatting may be somewhat confusing. The management discussion includes referrals, which are not required on the actual Step 2 CS exam. Content has not been updated to reflect recent changes to the exam and patient note format.

Summary: A concise text that contains all the information needed for Step 2 CS review. Cases are streamlined to allow for practice without taking up copious amounts of space. However, the content may not be as accurate or detailed as other, more thorough sources. Overall, a high-yield book that may require additional texts if more in-depth information is needed on the physical exam.

USEFUL WEB SITES

The following is a collection of online resources and Web sites that may also help you prepare for the Step 2 CS exam:

http://www.usmleworld.com
http://www.kaptest.com/Medical-Licensing/Step2cs.html
http://usmlecsprep.com

ACRONYMS AND ABBREVIATIONS

Abbreviation	Meaning
AAMC	Association of American Medical Colleges
ABG	arterial blood gas
ACE	angiotensin-converting enzyme
ADH	antidiuretic hormone
ADHD	attention-deficit hyperactivity disorder
ADLs	activities of daily living
AFB	acid-fast bacillus
AIDS	acquired immunodeficiency syndrome
ALT	alanine aminotransferase
ANA	antinuclear antibody
ANCA	antineutrophil cytoplasmic antibody
AP	anteroposterior
AST	aspartate aminotransferase
AXR	abdominal x-ray
BNP	B-type natriuretic peptide
BP	blood pressure
BPH	benign prostatic hypertrophy
BPPV	benign paroxysmal positional vertigo
BS	bowel sounds
BUN	blood urea nitrogen
CBC	complete blood count
CC	chief complaint
CCP	cyclic citrullinated peptide
CD	cluster of differentiation
CEA	carcinoembryonic antigen
CHF	congestive heart failure
CIS	Communication/Interpersonal Skills [CS score]
CK	Clinical Knowledge [exam]
CMV	cytomegalovirus
CNS	central nervous system
c/o	complains of
COPD	chronic obstructive pulmonary disease
CPK	creatine phosphokinase

Abbreviation	Meaning
CPK-MB	creatine phosphokinase, MB fraction
Cr	creatinine
CRP	C-reactive protein
CS	Clinical Skills [exam]
CSA	Clinical Skills Assessment
CSEC	Clinical Skills Evaluation Collaboration [testing center]
CSF	cerebrospinal fluid
CT	computed tomography
CTA	computed tomography angiogram
CV	cardiovascular
CVA	costovertebral angle
CXR	chest x-ray
D&C	dilatation and curettage
DDAVP	1-deamino (8-D-arginine) vasopressin
DEXA	dual-energy x-ray absorptiometry
DFA	direct fluorescent antibody [test]
DHEAS	dehydroepiandrosterone sulfate
DI	diabetes insipidus
DIC	disseminated intravascular coagulation
DM	diabetes mellitus
DNA	deoxyribonucleic acid
DSD	dementia syndrome of depression
dsDNA	double-stranded deoxyribonucleic acid
DSM	*Diagnostic and Statistical Manual* [of Mental Disorders]
DTR	deep tendon reflex
DVT	deep venous thrombosis
EBNA	Epstein-Barr nuclear antigen
EBV	Epstein-Barr virus
ECFMG	Educational Commission for Foreign Medical Graduates
ECG	electrocardiogram
ED	emergency department, erectile dysfunction

Abbreviation	Meaning
EEG	electroencephalogram
ELISA	enzyme-linked immunosorbent assay
EMG	electromyogram
ENT	ear, nose, and throat
EOMI	extraocular movements intact
ERCP	endoscopic retrograde cholangiopancreatography
ESR	erythrocyte sedimentation rate
ET	essential tremor
EtOH	ethyl alcohol
FAST	focused assessment with sonography for trauma [scan]
FH	family history
FSH	follicle-stimulating hormone
FSMB	Federation of State Medical Boards
FT_3	free triiodothyronine
FT_4	free thyroxine
G6PD	glucose-6-phosphate dehydrogenase
GERD	gastroesophageal reflux disease
GH	growth hormone
GI	gastrointestinal
HbA_{1c}	hemoglobin A_{1c}
HBsAg	hepatitis B surface antigen
HBV	hepatitis B virus
hCG	human chorionic gonadotropin
HCTZ	hydrochlorothiazide
HEENT	head, eyes, ears, nose, and throat
5-HIAA	5-hydroxyindoleacetic acid
HIDA	hepatobiliary iminodiacetic acid [scan]
HIV	human immunodeficiency virus
HPI	history of present illness
HPV	human papillomavirus
HR	heart rate
HRT	hormone replacement therapy
HSV	herpes simplex virus
IADLs	instrumental activities of daily living
ICE	Integrated Clinical Encounter [CS score]
Ig	immunoglobulin
IMED	International Medical Education Directory
IMG	international medical graduate
IV	intravenous
IVP	intravenous pyelography
IWA	Interactive Web Application
JVD	jugular venous distention
KOH	potassium hydroxide
KUB	kidney, ureter, bladder [imaging]
LAD	lymphadenopathy

Abbreviation	Meaning
LDH	lactate dehydrogenase
LH	luteinizing hormone
LLQ	left lower quadrant
LMP	last menstrual period
LOC	loss of consciousness
LP	lumbar puncture
LUQ	left upper quadrant
LVH	left ventricular hypertrophy
MCP	metacarpophalangeal [joint]
MDD	major depressive disorder
MDI	metered-dose inhaler
MDMA	methylenedioxymethamphetamine ("Ecstasy")
MI	myocardial infarction
MRA	magnetic resonance angiography
MRCP	magnetic resonance cholangiopancreatography
MRI	magnetic resonance imaging
MTP	metatarsophalangeal [joint]
MVA	motor vehicle accident
MVS	mitral valve stenosis
NBME	National Board of Medical Examiners
NC/AT	normocephalic/atraumatic
NKDA	no known drug allergies
NRMP	National Residency Matching Program
NSAID	nonsteroidal anti-inflammatory drug
N/V	nausea or vomiting
OASIS	Online Applicant Status and Information System
OCP	oral contraceptive pill
OSA	obstructive sleep apnea
OTC	over the counter
PA	posteroanterior
PCOS	polycystic ovary syndrome
PCP	phencyclidine ("angel dust")
PCR	polymerase chain reaction
PD	Parkinson's disease
PERRLA	pupils equal, round, and reactive to light and accommodation
PFT	pulmonary function test
PID	pelvic inflammatory disease
PMH	past medical history
PMI	point of maximal impulse
PN	patient note
PPD	pack per day; purified protein derivative [tuberculin skin test]
prn	pro re nata [as needed]
PSA	prostate-specific antigen
PSH	past surgical history

Abbreviation	Meaning
PT	prothrombin time
PTSD	posttraumatic stress disorder
PTT	partial thromboplastin time
RA	rheumatoid arthritis
RBC	red blood cell
RF	rheumatoid factor
RLQ	right lower quadrant
ROS	review of systems
RPR	rapid plasma reagin
RR	respiratory rate
RRR	regular rate and rhythm
RUQ	right upper quadrant
SEP	Spoken English Proficiency [CS score]
SH	social history
SIADH	syndrome of inappropriate [secretion of] antidiuretic hormone
SLE	systemic lupus erythematosus
SOB	shortness of breath
SP	standardized patient
SPECT	single-photon emission computed tomography
STD	sexually transmitted disease
T_3	triiodothyronine
T_4	thyroxine
TB	tuberculosis

Abbreviation	Meaning
TCA	tricyclic antidepressant
TEE	transesophageal echocardiography
TIA	transient ischemic attack
TIBC	total iron-binding capacity
TM	tympanic membrane
TMJ	temporomandibular joint
TOEFL	Test of English as a Foreign Language
TSE	test of spoken English
TSH	thyroid-stimulating hormone
TTE	transthoracic echocardiography
UA	urinalysis
URI	upper respiratory infection
U/S	ultrasound
USMLE	United States Medical Licensing Examination
UTD	up to date [vaccinations]
UTI	urinary tract infection
VCA	viral capsid antigen
VDRL	Venereal Disease Research Laboratory
V/Q	ventilation-perfusion [scan]
VS	vital signs
WBC	white blood cell
WNL	within normal limits
XR	x-ray
yo	year old

► **NOTES**

INDEX

sleep complaints
    anxiety and, 405
    depression and, 443
    fatigue, 98–99
    insomnia, 100–101, 397–406
    key history/physical exam, 98–
        99
    narcolepsy, 462
    nightmares, 443
    night sweats, 100
    obstructive sleep apnea (OSA),
        405
    tremor and, 488
small bowel cancer
    abdominal pain and, 114
    diarrhea and, 118
smoking
    asking patient about, 51
    bronchitis and, 469, 471
    challenging questions on, 71, 76
    counseling patients on, 77, 466,
        493, 526
    dysphagia and, 110
    erectile dysfunction and, 122
    hearing loss and, 295
    hematuria and, 119
    laryngeal cancer and, 240, 242
    laryngitis and, 241, 242
    low back pain and, 132
    lung cancer and, 376
    pancreatic cancer and, 385
    pneumonia and, 376
    tremor and, 488
    weight gain after quitting, 493,
        496, 498
Snellen eye chart, 57
snoring
    fatigue and, 98
    insomnia and, 100
social history, asking patient
        about, 51
social phobia, 108
somatoform disorder, 135
sore throat
    key history/physical exam, 101–
        102
    practice case for, 523–531

special patients, 65–67
spherocytosis, 303
sphincter of Oddi, in jaundice, 329
spinal fracture, 249
spinal stenosis, 132
spinal x-ray, 168
splenic infarct, 114
splenic rupture
    abdominal pain and, 114
    motor vehicle accident and, 178
splenomegaly
    mononucleosis and, 531
    sore throat and, 101
Spoken English Proficiency (SEP)
        score, 6
spontaneous abortion. See
        also pregnancy
    abdominal pain and, 116, 424
    challenging questions on, 76
    vaginal bleeding and, 125
sprained ankle, 358
SPs. See standardized patients (SPs)
Spurling's sign, 245, 248
sputum, examining, 46, 315
standardized patients (SPs), 4, 40.
        See also patients
    scoring done by, 5
    simulations of physical exam
        findings, 61–63
stomach cancer. See gastric cancer
stool
    bloody, 119, 472–480
    currant jelly appearance, 506
    greasy, 385, 386, 387, 403
strangulated hernia, 136
strength, joint, 60
streptococcal pharyngitis, 530, 531
streptococcal tonsillitis.
        See tonsillitis
stress fracture, 130, 357, 358
stress incontinence, 122
stridor, 414
stroke
    challenging questions on, 75
    dementia and, 433, 434
    numbness/weakness and, 96, 97,
        98

subarachnoid hemorrhage, 88
subdural hematoma
    confusion/memory loss and, 91,
        434
    numbness/weakness and, 97
substance use
    asking patient about, 51
    chest pain and, 148, 150
    in children, 138
    constipation and, 116
    depression and, 92
    erectile dysfunction and, 122
    fatigue and, 98
    hallucinations and, 460
    hypotension and, 96
    insomnia and, 100, 405
    joint/limb pain and, 128
    loss of consciousness and, 95
    low back pain and, 132
    nongonococcal septic arthritis
        and, 348
    palpitations and, 108
    PCP intoxication, 460, 462
    psychosis and, 93, 461, 462
    tremor and, 488
    weight change and, 108, 109
suicidal ideation, 92, 443, 444
summary technique, 11, 45
superficial venous thrombosis, 131
support, in patient
        communication, 44
surgery
    challenging questions on, 72,
        77
    patient fears of, 69
swallowing. See dysphagia
symmetric arthritis, 348
syncope. See consciousness, loss of
syphilis
    Ménière's disease and, 295, 339
    sore throat and, 102
syringomyelia, 97
systemic lupus erythematosus (SLE)
    diagnostic criteria, 348
    joint/limb pain and, 129, 131,
        347, 348
systemic sclerosis, 110

ABOUT THE AUTHORS

Tao Le, MD, MHS

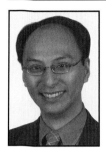

Tao developed a passion for medical education as a medical student. He currently edits more than 15 titles in the *First Aid* series. In addition, he is the founder and editor of the *USMLE-Rx* test bank and online video series as well as a cofounder of the *Underground Clinical Vignettes* series. As a medical student, he was editor-in-chief of the University of California, San Francisco (UCSF) *Synapse*, a university newspaper with a weekly circulation of 9000. Tao earned his medical degree from UCSF in 1996 and completed his residency training in internal medicine at Yale University and fellowship training at Johns Hopkins University. He subsequently went on to cofound Medsn, a medical education technology venture, and served as its chief medical officer. He is currently conducting research in asthma education at the University of Louisville.

Vikas Bhushan, MD

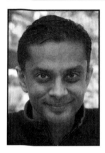

Vikas is a writer, editor, entrepreneur, and teleradiologist on sabbatical. In 1990 he conceived and authored the original *First Aid for the USMLE Step 1*. His entrepreneurial endeavors include a student-focused medical publishing enterprise (S2S), an e-learning company (medschool.com/Medsn), and an ER teleradiology practice (24/7 Radiology). Firmly anchored to the West Coast, Vikas completed a bachelor's degree at the University of California, Berkeley; an MD with thesis at UCSF; and a diagnostic radiology residency at the University of California, Los Angeles. His eclectic interests include technology, information design, photography, South Asian diasporic culture, and avoiding a day job. Always finding the long shortcut, Vikas is an adventurer, a knowledge seeker, and an occasional innovator. He enjoys novice status as a kiteboarder and single father and strives to raise his children as global citizens.

Mae Sheikh-Ali, MD

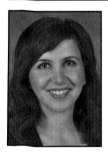

Mae is currently an associate professor of medicine and an associate program director for the Endocrinology Fellowship Program at the University of Florida College of Medicine, Jacksonville. She earned her medical degree from Damascus University School of Medicine in Syria. She completed her residency training in internal medicine at Drexel University College of Medicine in Philadelphia and endocrinology fellowship training at Mayo Clinic College of Medicine, Jacksonville, Florida. She is an editor and contributing author of several editions of *First Aid for the USMLE Step 2 CS* and the *Underground Clinical Vignettes* series. Mae is passionate about medical education and is taking an active role in teaching and empowering medical students, residents, fellows, and patients. She is currently pursuing an academic career in endocrinology with a focus on vitamin D, obesity, and diabetes research projects.

Kachiu Cecilia Lee, MD, MPH

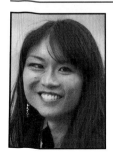

Kachiu received her medical degree and master's degree in public health from Northwestern University and then served as chief resident in her dermatology residency at Brown University. After completing her residency, she will begin fellowship training in laser surgery at Massachusetts General Hospital's Wellman Center for Photomedicine (Harvard Medical School). Kachiu intends to pursue an academic career with a research emphasis on epidemiology, health services, and medical education. As the first physician in her family, she hopes to play a critical role in helping medical students and residents fulfill their career aspirations. She has contributed to several projects in the *First Aid* series, including the *USMLE-Rx* test bank, *First Aid for the USMLE Step 1*, and *First Aid for the USMLE Step 2 CS*. In her leisure time, she enjoys photography, playing piano, and exploring New England with her husband and daughter.

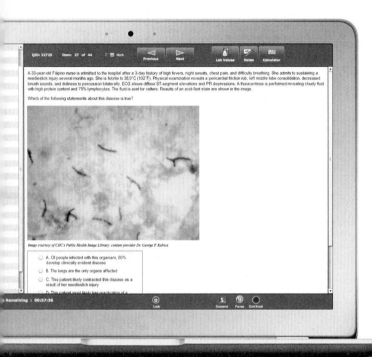
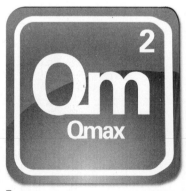